THINKING ABOUT THINKING

This book examines cognition with a broad and comprehensive approach. Drawing upon the work of many researchers, McDowell applies current scientific thinking to enhance the understanding of psychotherapy and other contemporary topics, including economics and health care. Through the use of practical examples, his analysis is accessible to a wide range of readers. In particular, clinicians, physicians, and mental health professionals will learn more about the thought processes through which they and their patients assess information.

Philip E. McDowell, LCSW, has a private practice in Lowville, New York. He earned a Lifetime Achievement Award from the New York State Office of Mental Health in 2002.

THINKING ABOUT THINKING

Cognition, Science, and Psychotherapy

Philip E. McDowell

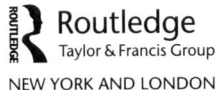
NEW YORK AND LONDON

First published 2015
by Routledge
711 Third Avenue, New York, NY 10017

and by Routledge
27 Church Road, Hove, East Sussex BN3 2FA

Routledge is an imprint of the Taylor & Francis Group, an informa business

© 2015 Taylor & Francis

The right of Philip E. McDowell to be identified as author of this work has been asserted by him in accordance with sections 77 and 78 of the Copyright, Designs and Patents Act 1988.

All rights reserved. No part of this book may be reprinted or reproduced or utilised in any form or by any electronic, mechanical, or other means, now known or hereafter invented, including photocopying and recording, or in any information storage or retrieval system, without permission in writing from the publishers.

Trademark notice: Product or corporate names may be trademarks or registered trademarks, and are used only for identification and explanation without intent to infringe.

Library of Congress Cataloging-in-Publication Data
McDowell, Philip E., author.
  Thinking about thinking : cognition, science, and psychotherapy / Philip E. McDowell.
    p. ; cm.
  Includes bibliographical references and index.
  I. Title.
[DNLM: 1. Mental Processes—physiology. 2. Brain—physiology. 3. Cognition. 4. Psychotherapy. WL 337]
  QP360.5
  612.8′233—dc23
  2014030932

ISBN: 978-1-138-82396-9 (hbk)
ISBN: 978-1-138-82397-6 (pbk)
ISBN: 978-1-315-74175-8 (ebk)

Typeset in Bembo
by Apex CoVantage, LLC

Printed and bound in the United States of America by Publishers Graphics, LLC on sustainably sourced paper.

After great inference, I came to the conclusion that I hadn't the foggiest idea what cognition was.
—Richard Powers
Galatea 2.2

It's disorienting to grasp that the world itself is neutral and that all the familiarity and unfamiliarity I feel is being carried around in my head.
—Verlyn Klinkenborg
New York Times
June 3, 2009

We humans can tolerate suffering but we cannot tolerate meaninglessness.
—Archbishop Desmond Tutu

Sensation tells us a thing is.
Thinking tells us what it is this thing is.
Feeling tells us what this thing is to us.
—Carl Gustav Jung

Figures 1.1, 1.3, 2.2 and 2.6: Katherine McDowell Patterson

Figures 4.5, 4.6 and 4.7: from *On the Origin of the Human Mind* by Dr. Andrey Vyshedskiy. Published by MobileReference. Copyrights MobileReference and Dr. Andrey Vyshedskiy

Figure 4.1: adapted from *How the Mind Works*, Steven Pinker, Penguin Press, 1997, page 87.

Figures 4.2 and 4.3: adapted from *How the Mind Works*, Steven Pinker, Penguin Press, 1997, page 103.

CONTENTS

List of Illustrations	*viii*
Introduction	*ix*

1	Thinking about Psychology	1
2	Thinking about the Brain	42
3	Thinking about Emotions	68
4	Thinking about Thinking	90
5	Thinking about Our Selves	141
6	Thinking about Science and Contemporary Issues	174
7	Re-Thinking Psychotherapy	221

Bibliography	*245*
Index	*255*

ILLUSTRATIONS

1.1	Human Eye	22
1.2	Ponzo Illusion	23
1.3	Human Ear	24
2.1	Gross Brain Organization	45
2.2	Neuron	47
2.3	Brain Lobes	49
2.4	Brodmann's Areas	50
2.5	Association Areas	50
2.6	Synapse	58
4.1	Knowledge Representation of "Cat"	95
4.2	Computer Model of "Cat" and "Squirrel"	97
4.3	Neural Model of "Cat" and "Squirrel"	98
4.4	Visual Illusion/Ambiguity	99
4.5	Triangular Representation of a Neuronal Ensemble	116
4.6	Pyramid Model of a Neuronal Ensemble	117
4.7	Polyhedron Model of a Neuronal Ensemble	117
5.1	Drawing by Adult Survivor of Childhood Abuse: Initial Presentation	158
5.2	Drawing by Adult Survivor of Childhood Abuse: Early in Therapy	159
5.3	Drawing by Adult Survivor of Childhood Abuse: After Therapeutic Rapport Is Established	159
6.1	Utility and Prospect Theories Psychological Model	180

INTRODUCTION

I have been a practicing psychotherapist for over 40 years. The essence of psychotherapy—the art and science of using (primarily) verbal communication, which is one expression of cognition, to address problems of thinking, feeling, and behaving—is *thinking about thinking*.

I received my graduate training in psychotherapy at the University of Michigan in the 1960s. The knowledge and skills I acquired were labeled *social casework*. The practice of psychotherapy was limited to psychiatrists and a small group of others who had undergone training at a recognized psychoanalytic institute in keeping with the teachings of Sigmund Freud and his followers. Since then, there has been a proliferation of research in the psychological and neurological sciences, due in part to new technologies and increased funding. The resulting findings have profound implications for the practice of psychotherapy, yet I am struck by the apparently immense gap between research and practice. This book is my modest attempt to bridge that gap.

This book is not designed to be a complete exploration of the subject. My intended audience includes psychotherapists; students of neuroscience, philosophy, psychology, and psychotherapy; and general readers who desire a better grasp of how we try to understand ourselves and the environments in which we function. I have provided references in the manner accepted by scientific publications, as well as recommendations for further reading, in the bibliography. I also recommend that anyone interested in the latest thinking about psychology and neuroscience become a subscriber to *Scientific American Mind* magazine.

An early scientific principle entitled Occam's razor suggests that given alternative explanations we should choose the simplest until the more complex provides more compelling evidence—a historical rendition of the modern acronym KISS: Keep It Simple, Stupid. This parsimony is congruent with my Scottish heritage, so

I have tried to apply it to the consideration of an obviously complex subject. In doing so, I also have had to contend with Einstein's razor: "Everything should be made as simple as possible, but no simpler." Here the great scientist warns that oversimplification can lead to false conclusions. I hope that I have had some success in conveying the depth and richness of cognition without rendering it unrecognizable to my intended audience.

Research findings should lead to hypothesis formulation, testing, and replication. Reports in the popular press do not always make clear the degree to which findings have been supported by rigorous application of the scientific method, resulting in what has been referred to as "brain porn." Neuroscientific explanations, even irrelevant ones, can imbue an argument with unwarranted credibility. I have tried to avoid this pitfall by citing esteemed science thinkers and researchers, while selectively referencing a few popular science writers, including Malcolm Gladwell, Sarah Begley, and Wray Herbert.

The clinical vignettes are altered to protect the identities of the patients. Some have a kind of fairy tale quality to them due to my distilling a vast amount of clinical data to illustrate the utility of a specific intervention. All are anecdotal and do not represent scientific evidence of the effectiveness of a particular intervention. Any resemblance to actual persons or patients is coincidental.

Ultimately, this book about thinking is about *my* thinking. It is *my* interpretation of the scientific data, combined with my professional and personal life experiences. I owe a great debt to the thousands of patients who over the years have trusted me with their most intimate thoughts and feelings. Many colleagues have enriched my understanding of how we think, especially those during my 29 years as director of the Lewis County (New York) Community Mental Health Center.

Thanks to Ruth Spina for her thoughtful review of the first draft of this book and for her helpful comments on matters scientific. Joanne Freeman has been a delight to work with as an editor, smoothing my text so that even I could understand what I was trying to say. George Zimmar of Taylor and Francis has encouraged and challenged me and deserves special gratitude for taking a chance on this first-time author.

Finally, my beloved wife, Martie, and daughters, April and Kate, have been a constant source of support and inspiration, shaping the way I think in the most positive way.

1
THINKING ABOUT PSYCHOLOGY

In the beginning of heaven and earth
There were no words,
Words came out of the womb of matter
And whether a man dispassionately
Sees to the core of life
Or passionately sees the surface
The core and the surface
Are essentially the same,
Words making them seem different
Only to express appearance.
If names be needed, wonder names them both:
From wonder into wonder
Existence opens.
—Tao Te Ching
(translated by Witter Bynner)

As the blade of a sword cannot cut itself,
As a fingertip cannot touch itself,
So a thought cannot see itself.
—Robert Allen,
A Thousand Paths to Zen

Featuring works made from the 1960s to today, "Telling Secrets" centers on the participatory role of the viewer in contemporary art and the strategies that artists use to encourage multiple interpretations of their work. Prior to the twentieth century, most art aimed to tell familiar stories or reflect everyday life and accepted social mores. Twentieth century art movements such as abstraction, performance and conceptual have fostered

> *a more interpretive role for the viewer. Contemporary artists relish the fact that the "meaning" of works of art is not fixed but rather shaped by each viewer.*
> National Museum of Women in the Arts, "Telling Secrets: Codes, Captions and Conundrums in Contemporary Art," October 9, 2009 to January 10, 2010

Prepare yourself for a wild ride. This opening sentence provides a clue to my mental state as I sit at the keyboard to begin my book. At one level, I am conveying what I expect you to experience, but I am also acutely aware that I am directing the sentiment at myself. I've made a decision to try to examine and express one of the most elusive human experiences. Because I am doing this through writing, I have but one medium through which to communicate my thinking: language. Written language, to be precise.

Much language is basically metaphorical. It compares an object or concept to similar or different objects or concepts to create understanding. In *I Is an Other*, James Geary (2011) cites linguistic research that suggests people use a metaphor every 10 to 25 words; most of the other words are a means to connect the metaphors. Thus, what Stephen Pinker refers to as "pedestrian poetry" (1997, p. 358) is not some frill but rather represents the essence of how we express our thinking linguistically. Because our thinking is imprecise, so are our metaphors. As we increase our awareness of thinking, we begin to recognize patterns, as well as similarities and differences among patterns. Creativity involves discovering new patterns and blending old ones to find new meaning.

Language is a means by which we express our thinking. What might thinking be like for a person without language? This question has been explored intellectually by philosophers, in more practical terms by Anne Sullivan in her work with the blind and deaf Helen Keller, and more recently by Susan Schaller in *A Man Without Words* (2012).

In English, we use different types of metaphors to represent different topics. In *Metaphors We Live By*, George Lakoff and Mark Johnson (2003) cite the following examples.

Ideas are represented by food metaphors: Some ideas are half-baked, we devour an interesting book and digest new facts, and we regurgitate our knowledge on tests.

Money is expressed through liquid metaphors. The title of stockbroker is derived from the French *brocheur*, which refers to the tavern worker who taps the keg to get the beer flowing. Thus, we drain our funds, skim off the top, sponge off others, and dip into savings.

The behavior of the stock market is represented by two kinds of metaphors, depending on the direction it is heading. A rising market is represented as a

> living creature, climbing and soaring with intent. A falling market is expressed through inanimate terms, as it tumbles, falls, and slides downward.
>
> Relationships are described using the language of health. Some marriages are thought of as sick, others as healthy.

We experience the world as analog via our senses. Both light and sound are transmitted to our eyes and ears as continuous and variable waves. People interpret these phenomena and express their interpretation digitally through language. An analogy is the transmission of information via a telephone line, which is analog, to the receiving unit, which transforms it into a digital format, which is then experienced as a voice. Metaphor is a digital means of interpreting an analog. Thus, I create the comparison with a wild ride and suggest you should be ready for the unexpected. Since you have chosen to read this book/take the ride, you likely have some expectation that there will be challenges ahead. So, through six simple words, 27 symbols we label as letters, placed in a specific order on a page, I have expressed an expectation of a subjective experience. Each reader, in turn, will interpret those symbols, and indeed, all that follow, in a somewhat different way.

Meaning is created not only by words, but also by manipulating visual symbols and representations. We process these non-narratives somewhat differently than words, adding another dimension to communication. Accordingly, I have included various illustrations and tables to supplement the narrative. Hopefully, they will assist the reader in sharing my interpretations.

Differences of interpretation are what distinguish each of us as human beings and constitute the focus of this book. Why do some people like opera while others find it boring? Why does one person find Sarah Palin a source of hope and inspiration while others think her inexperienced and inarticulate? Why do people who experience the same traumatic event process and remember it very differently? Why do siblings report vastly different memories of their childhoods, even identical twins who experienced the same events at the same time through very similar genetic makeups?

> Stanislas Dehaene (2009) is interested in understanding how the human brain adapted to the challenge of reading. In *Reading in the Brain*, he notes that the same brain areas are activated in reading, no matter the language or culture. Further, all the writing systems worldwide use the same basic shapes. Research on the brains of monkeys identifies neurons that preferentially respond to certain naturally occurring shapes that are comparable to those basic shapes. Dehaene hypothesizes that the left hemisphere of the brain "recycles" these shapes into a code for languages.
>
> In *Harnessed: How Language and Music Mimicked Nature and Transformed Ape to Man*, Mark Changizi (2011) postulates that not only does written

> language emanate from the shapes our ancestors saw in nature, but that the spoken word is the result of our auditory systems adapting to process the sounds of nature most efficiently. His evidence: The most common sounds found in nature that are essential to our survival (the patter of footsteps, the hiss of predators) occur in all human languages more often and consistently than would be expected by chance. Thus, language and music evolved from the sound waves we process best. Both Dehaene and Changizi are creating hypotheses from their observation of associations that lead to the identification of patterns.

As we think about thinking, we will observe thinking and try to create an understanding of thinking through interpretations of what we observe. Thus, thinking is both the tool and object of study. Is that possible? Or a hopeless conundrum? Most scientists will warn us at this point about the *observer effect*, which posits that the act of observing changes the observed. This theory can be applied to sociological or psychological inquiry, in which the act of observation creates a rather clear intervening variable. For example, introducing an outside observer to a group or culture affects the ways in which the subjects perceive, think, feel, and behave. Asking people what they think (for example, by using opinion polls) can influence the way they think in multiple ways, through the wording of the question, the context and timing of the inquiry, the choices presented. Many of us have received "polls" from an elected representative seeking our participation in public policy issues by posing a question such as, "Do you (1) support increased funding for our military? or (2) want our country taken over by commie/pinko terrorists?" Or "(1) Do you favor funding food stamps? or (2) Should hungry people suffer the consequences of their moral turpitude?" Reducing complexity to binary choice influences responses.

Study in the physical sciences faces a similar problem of the measurement itself affecting its outcome. In quantum mechanics, which is the study of the behavior of subatomic particles, the act of measuring the path of an electron fundamentally changes experimental outcomes.

Then there is the problem of defining what we are examining. What is thinking? Most of us can agree on the physically observable: It is an eight-letter word. A thought itself has no physical qualities; it is the product of a complex interaction among material entities within the brain, the body, and the environment. Here I invoke philosopher Ludwig Wittgenstein's notion of *private language*. The meaning of a word cannot be precisely located: It is relative to the observer. Human language is wondrously complicated, but like quantum mechanics, it is ultimately imprecise and observer dependent.

Words also have different meanings in different contexts. So, too, for the words "think" and "thinking." For example, "I think Joe is a jerk" is an expression of *emotions* that result from my mental processing of the sensory stimuli from the being named Joe. "I think the Cubs will win the World Series" expresses an eternal hope but an irrational conclusion. The thought that 8 + 8 = 16 is factual, devoid of emotion. "I think, therefore I am" is a different sort of computation. A dream is a visual, auditory, and verbal expression of thought. A song running through my head, whether expressed out loud in the shower or experienced silently when I am in public, is an expression of thinking. When a patient in therapy describes "feeling smothered" by the actions of a partner, I think by virtue of my training and experience that she might be connecting her perceptions with a similar, perhaps traumatic, prior life experience. All are thoughts involving different parts of the brain.

Language is one means to express our thinking. Steven Pinker, Johnston Professor of Psychology at Harvard, conceptualizes language as a discrete combinatorial system (1997). Written language starts with *mentalese*, the electrochemical activity among neurons, which connect to phenomes (basically letters in English) that connect to morphemes (the smallest meaningful bits, or syllables), that build into words, then phrases and sentences. Spoken language is based on the same combinatorial principles but is expressed by the speaker through the conversion of encoded discrete symbols (digital) into sound waves (analog), then converted from analog to digital by the listener into meaning.

> Written and spoken language is the primary tool in psychotherapy. However, there are other means of expressing our thinking and feeling that are the basis for other forms of psychological healing. Visual art is an effective means of expression for children who have not developed the requisite language and for adults whose expressive language may be impaired by physical or psychological limitations. Similarly, dance and other movement therapies provide added routes of expression, while yoga combines physical and mental activities that can change the way we experience our environment. Even aromas have been touted by some as having therapeutic benefits.
>
> Highly effective teachers enhance learning by utilizing multiple modes of presentation that can be processed by multiple sensory systems. In a similar way, highly effective psychotherapists create synergy by combining verbal, visual, and motor interventions.

Noam Chomsky (1983), professor emeritus in the Department of Linguistics and Philosophy, Massachusetts Institute of Technology, asserts two fundamental characteristics of language. While there are a finite (but ever growing) number of words in any language, there are an unlimited number of sentences. There is plenty of room for new ideas. Thus, Chomsky says that language cannot be a limited recipe of responses. Rather, the brain must have some program or mechanism to build new combinations in meaningful ways. Strings of random words have meaning only by chance. The brain has the ability to place different kinds of words in an order and context that produces meaning.

The second characteristic of language is derived from observation of young children as they acquire language. Grandson Brian Philip sees a small, red rubber ball roll by as his doting PopPop says "ball." He doesn't learn that "ball" refers to a rolling motion, or rubber, or red. He quickly grasps the word as referring to the object. Numerous studies of infant perception and language acquisition have led many researchers to interpret their observations as confirming an innate, intuitive, and universal human capacity to make meaning and create language. Pinker refers to this as the language instinct.

The complexity of language has become more evident as researchers have tried to program robots to comprehend and express it. To do so requires a comprehensive understanding of all the rules that govern word meaning and use. As such programs are developed, researchers are becoming increasingly aware that they do not have such an understanding. One simple example is the role of context in finding the meaning of a homonym, one of a group of words that share the same spelling and pronunciation but have different meanings. In 1987, psycholinguists Cyma van Petten and Marta Kutas wrote a paper describing lexical priming, the rapid process by which people can discern the meaning of a homonym from other words used in context. Take the word "bank." "Phil cashed his check at the bank" has meaning because of the proximity and context of "cashed" and "check" (the latter also a homonym). "Phil drove the golf ball into the bank of the stream," a not uncommon happening, connotes a different meaning for "bank" by coupling it with "stream" (yet another homonym). The amount of programming code required to discern different meanings of the same words would be astronomical. Humans must have some means other than symbol computation to process the sight and/or sound of these short strings of letters and discover the intended meaning.

Understanding how the brain works is often intuited from findings about abnormal brains. Schizophrenia is a devastating psychiatric disorder characterized by gross deviance from normal interpretations of stimuli. For example, a person with schizophrenia might interpret Jerry Seinfeld's voice on TV as that of God speaking to him. Neuroscientists have found that persons categorized as having symptoms of schizophrenia are unable to distinguish between the contextually appropriate and inappropriate meaning of a homonym. They also have an impaired ability to distinguish their own actions from those of others, a possible explanation for auditory hallucinations (interpreting internal voices as coming from someone else).

Words define discrete entities, but the world around us is not so constructed. Think about color. Scientists tell us that the phenomenon we call color consists of a continuous dimension of wavelengths. Our sensory systems are unable to detect wavelengths as such. Visible electromagnetic wavelengths are in the 400–700 nanometer range. We are unable to perceive 650 nm, 570 nm, 510 nm, or 475 nm as such. Rather, we are able to construct instruments that can measure wavelengths. Discrete colors (red, yellow, green, and blue) are the labels/interpretations we attach to our perception of specific wavelengths (more accurately, small ranges of wavelengths) to make meaning of the visual stimulation we process. The same is true of sound. In music, Western culture converts analog sound waves to digital notes, just as we interpret spoken language. The sound of "cat" and "sat" are acoustically similar, but we don't create a meaning in between them. Speech sounds are processed discontinuously, or digitally.

Steven Pinker (1997) concludes that human language has a unique design that is distinct from those of other creatures. It is *infinite*, with no limit to the number and combination of words and sentences. It is *digital*, built on discrete elements, not a continuum. And it is *compositional*, deriving its meaning from the principles governing the arrangement of its components.

Languages have evolved as a means to express interpretations of the world around us, which we experience through our senses. At the same time, the particular language we speak can influence the way we experience reality by shaping and limiting the nature of the thoughts we can express. Language is encoded and processed digitally to create meaning from an analog world. Meaning, in turn, is derived by comparing and contrasting objective stuff or subjective concepts to something else.

Language is a *process*. An analogy is based on the analysis of similarities. The only thing that can be completely similar is the exact same thing. German mathematician and philosopher Gotttfried Leibniz (1646–1716) referred to this as the "indiscernibility of identicals." So analogous analysis must also be cognizant of differences in order to effectively create meaning. The processes I choose to compare with thinking are the scientific method, on the one hand, and psychotherapy, on the other.

At first blush, these two processes seem to be very different. Scientific method is structured: make observations, form a hypothesis, test the hypothesis, come to a reasoned conclusion. It is open to scrutiny, subject to objective measurement, and replicable. Psychotherapy is largely unstructured, conducted in private, and rarely directly observed. It involves subtle, complex objective and subjective dynamics between two or more people, and outcomes may or may not be measurable. This distinction between the objective and measurable, and the subjective and indiscernible, is the basis of Descartes's body-mind dilemma, referred to as *dualism*. In this context, the mind is not the brain, an identifiable physical object. Rather, the mind comprises the unique subjective experiences of thinking and emotion.

Recent studies suggest that the body has a significant influence on those outcomes we label mental. For example, the physical qualities of temperature and texture can affect our social perceptions and behaviors. The distinction between mind and body is linguistic. They are not identical, but one is a manifestation of the other. Advances in research using new technologies are breaking down the distinctions between what we experience subjectively as thinking and what can be physically observed within the brain that creates the experience. Scientists are beginning to observe the physical underpinnings of the experience of thinking.

J is a 34-year-old married father of three with no prior history of psychiatric symptoms requiring treatment. He was referred by his primary care physician after appearing in the emergency room with classic panic attack symptoms: hyperventilation, heart arrhythmia, chest pain, and fear of dying. No physical basis could be found for his symptoms.

J denied any significant current stressors: His marriage was stable, his finances were secure, his family had not undergone any changes, his job was rewarding. When I tried to obtain a history of his childhood and youth, however, he was unable to remember anything prior to age eight. His parents were deceased, he had no siblings, and his wife met him in college and had no knowledge of his younger years.

The role of a therapist is to help the patient make meaning of his symptoms or problems so that the patient can make changes that he chooses. When the initial presentation does not provide a clear path to meaning, the therapist can begin to experience failure anxiety. This discomfort can then motivate the therapist to push harder, to begin to make meaning out of insufficient information. In J's case, there might be a temptation to push him to fill his memory gaps. In extreme cases, a therapist might unwittingly play a role in creating false memories.

Over a two-month period, J reported a slow diminution in the frequency and intensity of the panic episodes. After five sessions, we chose to discontinue further psychotherapy, with the understanding that he could return at any time. He has not done so. But one of a therapist's most important mandates was achieved: Do no harm.

One hypothesis might be that J had experienced "body memory" of a repressed childhood trauma, possibly triggered by some stimulus of which he had no awareness. He was clearly not ready to pursue the course of meaning-making, though. Perhaps he never will be. To push a patient to go where he is not ready to go runs the risk of re-traumatization.

The mind-body connection seems evident, yet it is poorly understood. Helping a patient construct a coherent, meaningful understanding of sudden, acute symptoms of anxiety is not always possible, or necessary.

Another basis for comparison is purpose. Both the scientific method and psychotherapy involve an overall strategy to achieve a goal. The goal of the scientific method is to discern meaning in the world around us by using logical processes to evaluate measurable phenomena. From an evolutionary perspective, the purpose of psychotherapy is to *think about thinking* in order to enhance and enrich survival.

In addition, understanding of both the scientific method and psychotherapy can be attained through consideration of their properties. Steven Pinker, Christof Koch, Vilayanur Ramachandran, Daniel Kahneman, Andrey Vyshedskiy, and other experts in psychology and neuroscience referenced in this book reflect the scientific analysis of the properties of thinking, from fuzzy stereotypes to rule-based generalization and computation. Both the professional literature I cite and my own anecdotal experiences consider the application of our understandings of cognition to psychotherapy.

All three levels of analysis challenge our thinking. Welcome to the wild ride.

A Starting Place: Classical, Intuitive Psychology

We need to start our journey somewhere, and since I am the self-appointed tour guide in charge of the itinerary, our starting point will be psychology—specifically, cognitive-behavioral psychology.

In the 1960s, the debate in the psychotherapy field was between classical Freudian psychoanalysis, complete with unconscious processes and conflicts between instincts and the superego, and Skinnerian behavioral psychology, which focused on objective behavior and denied unconscious processes and emotions. As a graduate student at the time, I was more impressed by the emotional level of the disagreements and the egos of the combatants than the intellectual rigor of the debate. When I entered the office of Stuart Finch, MD, esteemed director of the University of Michigan Children's Psychiatric Hospital, I was struck by the portrait of Sigmund Freud hanging above his desk, which I likened to a picture of the Pope behind the desk of a bishop. I don't doubt that somewhere a committed behaviorist had a similar picture of B. F. Skinner decorating his or her office.

> Russian psychologist Ivan Pavlov demonstrated *classical conditioning* over a hundred years ago by training dogs to salivate by pairing food with an auditory stimulus, a ringing bell. In a similar pairing of stimuli, his students were able to train the immune systems of animals to respond to nonpathogenic stimuli. More recently, Manfred Schedlowski and Gustavo Pacheco-Lopez (2010) at the University of Duisberg-Essen demonstrated the potential to train the immunosuppressive response in humans. In a double-blind study, he had one group of subjects drink an odd-tasting concoction containing an immunosuppressant for three days; the other group drank the concoction with placebo. In subsequent trials that included only placebo for up to 11 days, the experimental group showed elevated levels of immunosuppressants in their blood, while the controls did not.

The fields of neuroscience, psychology, and psychotherapy have evolved significantly since that time. Extensive research has broadened greatly our knowledge of these fields, including our understanding of thinking. Cognitive-behavioral psychology has transcended the rigid dogma of behaviorism by incorporating newer findings from the study of perception and emotions. It has become the most researched school of psychotherapy and is now considered by many practitioners to be the most effective type of verbal therapy.

Psychology is the study of how living creatures process stimuli from outside themselves and from within their own bodies in order to behave in ways that will enhance their survival. Let us examine this definition. "Psychology" is a label/word created to try to encompass a variety of phenomena, most of which are subjective and thus not readily accessible to direct observation and measurement. "Study" is a label/word that connotes a desire to understand via further examination. "Living creatures" is one of those labels that is usually self-evident in its daily use (your dog versus a rock) but that confounds the brightest in its ethical applications (think abortion or euthanasia). "Process" is a word derived from the Latin *pro* (forward) and *cedere* (to go), which expresses an abstract via a concrete, easily understood image. "Stimuli" is the plural of the Latin verb for "goad" or "incite." "Outside ourselves or from within our own bodies" references our consciousness, our interpretation of ourselves as distinct from that which we deem to not be part of ourselves. Some people think this ability distinguishes us from other living creatures, but there is no way to objectively measure that assertion. Buddhist thinking, on the other hand, minimizes the distinction between self and non-self, asserting that it contributes to human suffering. "Behave" is a label that attempts to distinguish the observable from the subjective human experience.

Finally, there is "survival." In and of itself, this word is generally understood and emotionally neutral. However, when the context within which it is used is the origin and change over time (evolution) of that which we call life itself, it becomes the center of a highly emotional debate, one that could be the subject of another (lengthy) book that examines how we think. As for me, I am more interested in understanding how such differences in thinking develop and become divisive than in staking out a particular position. For the purposes of this book, let's say that survival is a fairly obvious goal of most living creatures, regardless of the philosophical or religious context within which it is considered. When humans behave in ways that threaten their survival (attempt suicide, live unhealthy lifestyles), we label it abnormal or pathological, although in limited situations we reframe life-threatening behavior as heroic (when in combat or saving another life).

The emotions that arise in defense of the supposed intellectual, social, and political implications of Darwin's theories of evolution and natural selection detract from a clear understanding of two fundamental concepts that are often confused. *Evolution* refers to changes in species over time and was recognized as a concept long before Darwin, although it was explained earlier by different mechanisms. Darwin's theory posited for the first time that *natural selection* was the cause of evolution. Natural selection joined two different, independent ideas. One, Pinker notes, is that a trait has a function that enhances reproduction. The second is that the organism's ancestors reproduced better than their competitors did. Any good scientific theory makes strong predictions that may later be proven false. Natural selection would be disproved if someone were to discover a trait that enhanced reproduction but that didn't appear at the end of a lineage of organisms that could have used it to help in their reproduction. No such discovery has yet been made, however.

Tim Harford (2011a), a journalist for the *Financial Times* and author of such books as *Adapt: Why Success Always Starts with Failure* and *The Undercover Economist*, notes that all complex systems are the product of trial and error, variation and selection. These processes apply equally to the evolution of species, organizations, and societies. Indeed, scientific thinking itself can be conceptualized as an evolutionary process in which ideas mutate unexpectedly into new theories that compete with others until the most useful persist and proceed to compete with yet other evolving theories in a never-ending process. The notion that this process will lead to an end, an ultimate truth, is likely a product of conceptualizations born of navigating our daily lives (more in chapter 6).

Classical psychology can be divided into four areas of study: perception, cognition (including memory, learning, thinking, and intelligence), emotion (including motivation and decision making), and behavior. Of these, only perception corresponds to readily identifiable areas of physiological functioning. The study of psychology began before there was a comprehensive understanding of the brain. In contrast, the study of neuroscience is organized around topics associated with neural functioning, such as fear, rage, sex, and language. Thus, there is a seeming disconnect when the two sciences try to collaborate. Each has a body of knowledge that has grown from very different perspectives. Classical psychology evolved out of philosophy and is based on the intuition that there are two distinct human psychological experiences: thinking and emotion. However, this binary distinction between subjective experiences is arbitrary. It might just as well have been between mathematical and interpersonal psychology, contemplative and action-oriented psychology, or sexual and other-than-sexual psychology.

The principles and concepts on which any discipline is based create a framework for study and furthering understanding, but also have the side effect of constraining the very inquiry they support. This illustrates the concept of *path dependence*: Choices are made as concepts develop. Newer concepts build on the original ones until a whole body of knowledge is created. The original concepts survive even after they outlive their usefulness. This reflects a tension between stability and chaos. Both are required for survival.

One example of path dependence is the impact of the internal combustion engine on modern history. The engine was designed and constructed based on the technology and resources available in the 1800s. As its applications increased, so did the demand for petroleum products to fuel it. After some 150 years, the ever-increasing demand has been a major driver of world economic and political thinking and behaving.

An example at the systems level is how we pass on knowledge to our youth through a system of education. Historically, adults taught children within the context of the home or tribe. Teaching in groups led to the establishment of a physical location. Schools with one room were consolidated as populations increased and over time developed into massive institutional bureaucracies with heavy capital investments, structured hierarchies of academic expectation, homogenized instruction that largely disregarded individual learning styles and interests, and competing vested interests not always aligned with optimum academic achievement. The current efforts at educational reform are severely hampered by their dependence on decisions regarding changes to the existing investments in our concepts and institutions. Reforms in health care, mental health care, and services to the developmentally disabled are similarly constrained.

We might be able to imagine a better way to meet the educational needs of our society. To do so would require eliminating some concepts and their applications. One small example might be the notion that all children enter kindergarten at age five, or that all children spend a majority of their school hours sitting at a desk, processing (or not) auditory and visual stimuli. There is ample evidence that these practices are not responsive to the educational readiness and needs of all students, yet we persist in engaging them, even in the face of better alternatives.

In an analogous way, *eliminativism* refers to a belief that the common conceptions of the mind, including such notions as sensation, experience, thinking, and feeling, are filled with problems that limit our ability to understand. Specifically, the concepts within folk (intuitive) psychology defy reduction to natural science, to a materialistic basis; thus, our ability to create meaning of our own cognition is constrained by our older, outdated concepts of the mind.

Recognizing these constraints, we need to understand the basic tools that constitute effective thinking. The raw material, or *input*, for thinking is sensory stimulation. We experience the world through our senses, our perceptions, although perception is incomplete, inconsistent, and fallible.

We process the input using four interrelated tools (Hall, 2005), all of which, like perception, are fallible. First is *memory*, which is essential for any higher order thinking. Memory is stored in neural networks and activated by electrical and chemical processes throughout the body, not just in the brain. It is highly fallible and inconsistent. We can repeatedly remember basic mathematical facts, such as $2 + 2 = 4$, $9 \times 6 = 54$, but the act of remembering more complex experiences alters the neural networks in small, and sometimes not-so-small, ways. We recall social interaction at a party or the details of an accident or crime differently at different times and under changing circumstances. We never remember these complex events in exactly the same way. Memory is a fundamental but unreliable aspect of cognition. The inaccuracy of memory in the healthy brain is magnified in people impaired by dementia. As long as they can remember at least some words, they can express some of their sensory experience. As they are robbed of more and more memory, though, they sometimes can't even identify a loved one and may lose even their most basic vocabulary. In the final stage of dementia, thinking as expressed through language ceases.

A second tool in processing sensory stimuli is *association*. We link one memory to another, and new sensory experiences to old ones. These associations are based on some type of similarity, such as similar form or similar temporal experience, and are often multiple. For example, when I try to recall a name, I can often identify the number of letters in it, the first letter, and its nationality before I can retrieve the full name. Presumably the name is stored in a neural network that has multiple connections to other networks.

This notion of *distributed internal representations* of our experiences also likely applies to motor functions. Chapter 4 notes the evolutionary advantages of such distribution, as opposed to a simple, localized encoding strategy: the ability to represent similar items by overlapping but non-identical patterns, the ability to generalize, and the ability to compensate when neural connections degrade by trauma, disease, or aging.

> While dining with friends, I observed the phenomenon of a group employing their individual distributed encoding processes in an interactive way. During a discussion of favorite movies, we would try to remember a title or the name of an actor by searching for and verbalizing our associations, which would trigger further associations within the group. The synergistic power of our interactive distributed encoding led us (eventually) to identify all our favorites. When such naturalistic attempts at discovery fail, we can turn to a computer-based search engine to help us make these connections.

Our initial impression of a person is based on associations with memories of similar people we have met. We may not be conscious of the sensory stimuli to which we make associations. It might be a subtle cue: body language, facial features, hairdo, details of dress, vocabulary, or intonations of speech. David Eagleman (2011) cites a study that illustrates the unconscious nature of significant associations: Men rate women whose eyes are dilated as more attractive but have no awareness of the basis for their decision. Such associations may be weak and malleable, subject to change as more sensory input about that person is processed. Alternatively, such an association may be strong, so that we avoid or ignore further sensory input that might challenge it.

Associations can be triggered by disparate sensory stimuli. A smell can be paired with memories of a location, a meal, or a lover. Hearing phrases can trigger memories of songs in which those phrases appear. The sight of a vintage car can stimulate memories of youthful adventures. The feel of a new pair of shoes can conjure up memories of going to the Buster Brown Shoe Store as a child. The smell of the sea air can be tied to memories of a romantic vacation.

Building on the creation of associations is the third and more complex tool of thinking, *pattern discernment*. Here we create meaning by identifying similarities among different sensory inputs and their associated memories. This tool is the basis for creating categories, for labeling phenomena, and for language itself. Categories of physical objects are generally taught to us. Based on certain similarities, we identify certain four-legged creatures as dogs and others as cats, even though some very small dogs might appear more similar to cats than to the largest canines. Other patterns have more personal meaning, as noted by Wittgenstein. Thus, I discern a pattern of behaviors and characteristics in another person and label that person a friend, while someone else does not. In the political arena, people discern very different patterns from the same governmental policies or public figures. Think taxes, health care, gun regulation, abortion, or President Obama. Each of us screens out, discounts, or reinterprets those stimuli that do not conform with our preexisting hypothesis, model, or belief—a phenomenon called *confirmation bias*. We can always find evidence to support our thoughts and beliefs. This differs from scientific thinking, which seeks evidence to refute a hypothesis.

The brain's ability to discern patterns is an immense cognitive strength but also underlies a flaw. In our constant effort to make meaning, we create internal patterns (realities) that do not exist externally. *Pareidolia* refers to our inclination to create patterns to make meaning of the stimuli. Visual pareidolia creates patterns out of random visual stimuli. Look at a cloud and you might see the shapes of animals, faces, or religious figures. A devout Catholic woman once showed me a snapshot of clouds, taken from the window of an airplane, that looked to her like Jesus. I was unable to create that pattern despite her considerable effort to show me. Some projective psychological tests such as the Rorschach ask the subject to identify patterns from inkblots, from which the psychologist interprets meaning about the subject's cognitive and emotional functioning. I can discern multiple animal figures when I look at the fieldstone walls in my cellar, which is over 200 years old.

Our survival as social creatures relies heavily on facial recognition, which occurs within the visual cortex. One result is our preference to discern the pattern of a human face from vague visual stimuli. Another is the ability to infer emotion from minimal visual inputs. The latter seems to include a cultural component. People in Eastern cultures tend to focus on the eyes to interpret emotions, while Westerners intuit from the mouth. Persons with some psychiatric and/or developmental disorders avoid eye contact, thereby limiting facial cues that contribute to more effective interpersonal skills.

As we acquire language up to age four, our brains rely on a limited number of *phonemes*, the discrete components of speech that we learn to create understanding of language. Auditory pareidolia is the interpretation of meaningful language from random sounds. Examples include interpreting the stimuli created by the breeze blowing through trees as a word or hearing supposedly hidden messages when music is played backward. In both cases, suggestibility can play a major role. You are more likely to "hear" a message when told what to listen for.

We rely on pattern discernment to make sense of our environment, but these patterns can lead us astray. Skinner (1948) noted that when presented with food at regular intervals pigeons would create behavioral rituals to pair with the stimulus. He concluded that the birds "believed" their behavior could generate the food. Further, he compared such pattern generation to human superstitions, such as rituals like rain dances and certain religious practices. In science, a common error is to use a pattern as confirmation of an understanding rather than as the basis for hypothesis generation and testing. Patterns are a starting point for creating understanding, not the truth itself.

Another evolved interpretive tendency is to assign *agency* to discerned patterns. Our ancestors' chances for survival were enhanced by interpreting the rustling in the leaves as a predator rather than as a random gust of wind. This survival benefit comes at a cost—the interpretation of agency where none exists. An extreme form of this hyperactive agency detection is conspiracy theory, the assumption of agency behind a discerned pattern. Such illusions can be emotionally compelling. Much of our political experience is grounded in highly emotional beliefs distilled from the selective processing of visual and auditory stimuli via pattern recognition and agency assignment. We are driven to believe we know far more than is possible.

A fourth tool of thinking is *reason*. Going beyond association and pattern discernment, reason moves from one idea to another via logical inference. Like association and pattern discernment, reason is subject to multiple flaws. At the same time, reason, used correctly, can overcome the flaws and limitations of our basic neurology.

Induction is the process of deriving general principles from particular instances and offers probable, but not certain, support for a conclusion. I observe that all the swans I have ever seen, in person or in pictures, are white. I conclude that all swans are white. Indeed, most are, except for the rare black ones. *Deduction* is the process of inferring particular conclusions, which are irrefutable, from general truths. Example: All men are mortal. I am a man. Therefore, I am mortal.

Dialectic is the process of finding basic principles through probing assumptions via a question-and-answer format. Socrates used this process to debunk false opinions. Plato, Hegel, and Marx utilized similar processes to advance their unique paradigms.

Analogies involve a process that finds comparisons between otherwise disparate entities. This process underlies taxonomies, or systems of classification. The similarities among dogs and cats earn them admission to the category of mammals. Their differences place them in separate categories of canines and felines.

Abstraction is the process of generalizing by distilling information to retain only what is relevant to a specific purpose. Take the word "ball." It is generally associated with a geometric shape, a circle, and can refer to balls used for such disparate purposes as playing golf, providing bearings for moving wheels, and containing large quantities of beer. However, the use of the word "ball" is not consistent, varying with the intended purpose. Thus, a football is not round yet qualifies when included among a group of objects used in sports; a hockey puck does not despite its roundness. Psychology includes many abstract concepts whose use varies with the intent of the user. Imprecision in the use of abstractions creates considerable cognitive confusion and emotional distress. Psychology is not alone in this regard: think philosophy, economics, politics, physics, virtually every area of human inquiry.

Reason is distinct from *rationalization*. The former starts with premises and moves forward to conclusions via logical processes. Rationalization starts with a conclusion, then seeks evidence to support it. One example is creationism, which starts with a literal interpretation of scripture, then works backward to explain it through the notion of intelligent design. This requires ignoring massive amounts of scientific data in order to avoid *cognitive dissonance*.

We will use these tools of thinking to examine our thinking about psychology, the brain, and thought itself.

Perception and Our Senses

"Perception" is a word that describes the processing of stimuli by specialized sense organs. The study of perception focuses on the interface between the external sources of stimuli and the areas of the brain where they are processed to create motor activity and meaning. These are not necessarily separate phenomenon; our somatic responses to stimuli contribute to the meaning we create.

Humans have five fundamental senses (visual, auditory, olfactory, tactile, and gustatory) and five associated organs (eye, ear, nose, skin, and taste buds in the mouth and throat) that receive and organize the different types of stimuli. Stimuli interact with the sense organs by way of different media: sound via waves, sight via light, and smelling, touching, and tasting via direct contact of the stimuli with the sensor. The stimuli cause a biochemical and electric reaction that is transmitted by the nerves to the brain. Everyone's sensory processes, from receptors to the transmission of information to the brain, are different. In addition, we process stimuli from within our own bodies through the *somatosensory system*. Included in this system is the *proprioceptive*, which gives us information about our body's movements and positions, and the *vestibular*, which assists balance.

The study of perception includes the ways in which our sensory systems fail us, be it through illusions that expose sensory system shortcomings, via brain lesions or hallucinations, or through sensory processing that seems to underlie emotional/behavioral difficulties. For example, in the past, we assumed that childhood psychiatric disorders were the result of environmental stimuli. There is increasing evidence that the processing of those stimuli, as much or more than the stimuli themselves, underlies maladaptive behavior. For example, the cluster of behaviors labeled attention deficit hyperactivity disorder (ADHD) seems to correlate with impairment of sensory processing within the frontal cortex, resulting in reduced ability to curb expressions of impulses. A child with auditory processing difficulties might have difficulty functioning in environments with multiple sources of auditory stimulation, such as school hallways, gym class, or the school bus. In the future, the assessment of sensory integration will become an increasingly important part of a comprehensive understanding of a person's psychological functioning. Interventions to build on sensory strengths and remediate deficits will become more common.

Psychotic disorders among adults also can be conceptualized as due to sensory processing malfunctions, as illustrated by the following vignette.

A boy experienced significant disruption in his formative years. His mother, diagnosed as suffering from bipolar disorder, had psychotic episodes that included physically abusing the boy, including attempts to stab him with a kitchen knife. In addition, the boy was sexually abused by a peer and sexually assaulted in college. He received periodic psychotherapy for depression in his adolescent and collegiate years. He was sustained during those turbulent times by a support system of peers and caring adults. After attending graduate school, he accepted professional employment in an area geographically removed from his support system.

As the stress of his employment increased, he began to think that he saw and heard evidence that his co-workers and others were mocking him and trying to undermine his career. Sadly, as his thoughts of persecution increased in frequency and intensity, they became self-fulfilling. His concentration was impaired, his job performance declined, and he was let go. He was diagnosed with severe depression with psychotic features and underwent a series of inpatient admissions while undergoing outpatient psychotherapy and pharmacotherapy.

He eventually did achieve a sustained state of relative stability, free of gross paranoid ideation. However, he needed to remain isolated from situations that exposed him to multiple auditory stimuli. When in public settings, he experienced multiple human voices and described an inability to concentrate on any one conversation. The voice of the person sharing his table in a restaurant became blended into the general din. He could only pick up a few words from one conversation, and then a few more from the many others around him. He was unable to make coherent meaning from the cacophony of auditory stimuli he was trying to process. His anxiety would increase, compounding the difficulties. The out-of-control interpretation mimicked that of his previous trauma.

By creating an alternative understanding of his difficulties, he was able to implement strategies to limit his sensory inputs and explore additional meanings of those inputs.

Everyone processes each of the senses somewhat differently. In some cases, individuals have exceptional abilities. Master painters likely see subtleties of color, texture, and spatial relations to which most of us are oblivious. Accomplished musicians seem more attuned to tone and rhythm. Professional wine tasters are certainly more sensitive to the subtleties of vintage wines than most of us. On the opposite end of the spectrum of sensory processing are those inputs that do not get organized into a functional response, labeled as *sensory processing disorders*. They can cause mild to severe problems. One might over- or under-respond to light, sound, touch, taste, or smell or to multiple sensory stimuli.

Q, a seven-year-old boy, was referred by his pediatrician after a behavior checklist completed by the parents was suggestive of oppositional defiant disorder, characterized by poor temper control, arguing with adults, defiance of requests or rules, intentional annoying and blaming of others, irritability, anger, and vindictive behavior. Historically, this complex of symptoms has been interpreted as the result of poor parenting.

Q's parents reported a normal developmental history. No psychological trauma, social stressors, or parenting abnormalities were identified. His preschool years were stable in a consistent environment. When Q entered kindergarten, however, he exhibited separation anxiety in the form of temper tantrums and panic when his mother would leave him. He became aggressive when peers came up behind him or touched him unexpectedly and would withdraw to the back of the classroom, vigilant of the actions of others. His behavior was especially disorganized in the hallway, the lunchroom, and the bus. He exhibited a limited tolerance of sensory inputs, especially visual, auditory, and tactile.

An evaluation by an occupational therapist revealed a variance of more than two standard deviations from the norms on multi-sensory processing. Q was experiencing sensory overload in any environment that included unfamiliar or unexpected inputs, causing him high levels of anxiety and defensiveness. He was the victim of a sensory processing disorder, not bad parenting. Indeed, it was the sensitivity of the parents, their intuition that

> their son couldn't cope with more than small doses of sensory stimulation, that led to the early diagnosis and subsequent interventions.
>
> Successful remediation for Q involved regular occupational therapy, individual and small-group special education services, and classroom modifications by which sensory exposure could be increased gradually as his tolerance improved. Psychotherapy involved helping both Q and his parents think in constructive terms about his condition and about ways to compensate by taking advantage of his strengths: intelligence, creativity, curiosity, and a motivation to succeed.
>
> The behaviors Q first exhibited in his early kindergarten days could be interpreted by themselves as early indications of a budding psychopath. Gathering more pertinent information revealed a very different interpretation, one with clear choices for a more positive outcome. Clearly, a diagnosis is only as good as the information that the diagnostician has available to process.

Our sensory organs are inundated with far more sensory stimuli than the brain can process. It has been estimated that we process only 2% to 5% of all the input available. In *The Doors of Perception*, Aldous Huxley (2004) called this function a "reducing valve." As a result of these structural and filtering differences, everyone experiences the world differently. For example, a couple recently shared with me their experience of attending a Buffalo Bills home game. They sat together, surrounded by the identical sensory stimuli. The man remembered the excessive drinking of the surrounding spectators and their constant use of the f-word, yet the woman recalled only one man swearing and otherwise reported it as an exciting experience. The man focused on the crowd, while the woman stated, "I was watching the game." Same stimuli but markedly different sensory processing and recall. When counseling couples, I emphasize the different ways in which each experiences the world, including each other. A relationship is functional and satisfying to the extent that both members can interpret their differences as acceptable and interesting rather than as a threat or source of contention.

> The considerable variability in the sensory functioning of humans raises obvious philosophical questions: Is it possible to describe an objective reality? Are there indisputable facts, or just individual interpretations? Is the notion that "everything is interpretation" an interpretation itself?

Moreover, different creatures rely on different senses as their primary way of processing the world. Dogs, like Maxine the family beagle, rely on smell as the primary means of experiencing their environment. That is not to say that olfactory perception is unimportant to humans. We are capable of identifying between five and ten thousand different smells. Indeed, olfactory stimuli are a critical part of the human sexual response, even though we are not as conscious of it as we are of the impact of visual and tactile stimuli. For us, smell operates on a more subliminal level. For example, it's said you will sell your house more quickly, and at a higher price, if you have bread baking in the oven when the prospective buyers tour.

In addition to their refined olfactory sensitivity, our household cats depend on the tactile sensations received through their numerous lengthy and nerve-receptor-rich whiskers. In the fields around our house, the cats' main prey are moles, voles, and mice. These rodents have an eye on each side of their head that is capable of moving independently, with no overlapping field of vision. Their survival depends on their ability to constantly scan above for birds of prey. To perceive straight ahead, they move their whiskers repeatedly at different angles, from which they create a three-dimensional image in their brain.

Among humans, taste is a source of great sensual pleasure to those endowed with multiple gustatory receptors and fortunate enough to enjoy access to a variety of food sources. Unlike some other creatures, however, we cannot rely on taste alone to protect us from harmful food intake. We do interpret the smell and taste of rotten food or feces as noxious, and thus avoid consuming them. On the other hand, we lack the olfactory and gustatory abilities to distinguish a poisonous mushroom from one that is edible. Other creatures possess such discriminative powers. Humans have to rely on visual processing combined with the higher level cognitive functions of reading and remembering to make such distinctions (or, like me, you can buy your mushrooms at the local grocery store and trust that they know the difference).

> In attempting to define the distinction between *normal/healthy* and *abnormal/pathological* in our modern, science-driven culture, mental health professionals often invoke the concept of *functional impairment*. A condition is worthy of intervention/treatment if it limits the ability of people to do what they need to do to fulfill their social or occupational roles. Such a paradigm is culturally defined. The personality characteristics of the men who were successful in settling the American West (highly energetic, restless, and primed to make quick decisions) do not serve young males well in a typical present-day classroom.
>
> Some researchers have tied a genetic variant, DRD4-7R, to personality traits of curiosity and restlessness. Others have suggested an association between gene haplotypes and attention deficit hyperactivity disorder (Grady et al., 2005), although this finding has not been consistently replicated (Castellanos et al., 1998) The challenges of scientific research represent the complexities of making meaning using objective, rule-driven procedures. Such challenges will be considered further as our journey continues.

In our day-to-day interpersonal lives, we humans rely largely on visual and auditory stimuli in our attempts to make sense of ourselves and our surroundings. Therefore, I will devote more attention to these two sensory processes.

Seeing the Light

The role of the eye is to gather light, then to convert it into electrical activity that can be sent to the brain for processing (interpretation). In the simplest creatures, the eye does nothing more than register the presence or absence of light. More complex creatures, such as flies, have eyes with compound lenses. Humans, like all animals with a skull and a backbone, have eyes like little cameras, the purpose of which is to focus light rays on a sheet of neurons called the *retina* (see Figure 1.1). The *cornea* and *lens* refract the light rays so they are focused on the retina while the *pupil* controls the amount of light, allowing in more under low light conditions and restricting light in bright conditions. Because the cells that make up the retina are classified as neurons, the retina is considered to be part of the *central nervous system*. Here the distinction between the concepts of perception and interpretation becomes blurred.

The retina contains two types of sensitive light-gathering neurons, *rods* and *cones*. The importance of vision to humans is underscored by the fact that rods and cones represent 70% of all the sensory cells in our bodies. When the molecules of these cells absorb light, they break into two parts: one a derivative of Vitamin A, the other the protein *opsin*, a specialized molecule that can convey information from the outside to the inside of a cell. The opsin initiates a process that sends an electrical impulse to the brain via the *optic disc*, made up of *retinal ganglion cells* (RGCs) that leave the eye and begin the *optic nerve*. Opsins can be traced back to certain molecules in bacteria and are thought to play a role in vision in such apparently diverse creatures as insects, clams, and humans.

However, the eye does not transmit a complete picture of the world to the brain. As we will consider in chapter 5, the brain has the remarkable capacity to create a complete, subjective visual experience from incomplete visual stimuli. The RGCs are the only neurons that project outside the eye via the optic nerve to the brain. Some RGCs transmit data about form and color. Others send information about movement. Most of the sensory input to the eye is never sent to the brain, because there are far fewer RGCs (about 1 million) than there are rods (120 million) and cones (6 million) gathering data. RGCs respond to changing stimulation in the retina by increasing or decreasing their rates of firing, sending some one million bits of information per second. The brain recreates these electrical bits into the subjective experience we think of as vision. The blue in my sweater is my brain's subjective interpretation of the electrical impulses from the RGCs, combined with the label "blue" stored in my memory.

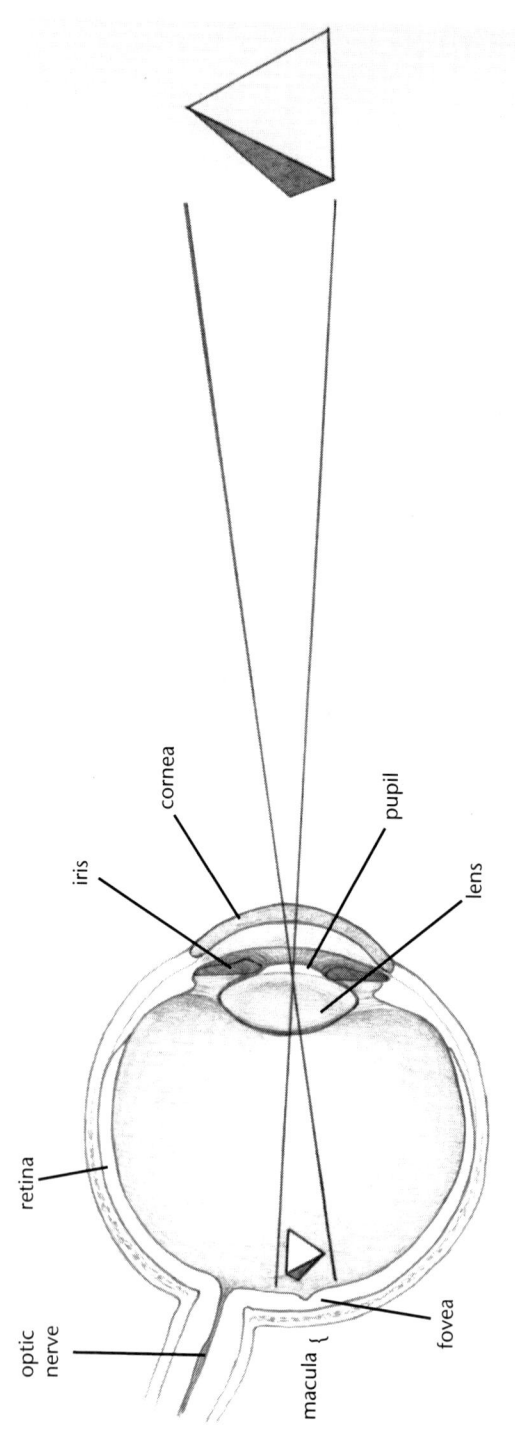

FIGURE 1.1 Human Eye

The perceptual illusion refers to our belief that our perceptions are accurate and direct, that our brain reproduces sensory stimuli truthfully and consistently. The reality is that each sensory system analyzes, deconstructs, then reconstructs stimuli based on its own built-in structures and protocols, including those encoded by prior experience. Thus, the brain does not passively record the environmental stimuli; it actively constructs it. To quote neuroscientist Vernon Mountcastle, "Sensation is an abstraction, not a replication, of the real world" (Kandel, 2006).

Illusions begin with sources of visual stimulation that confuse or challenge our perceptual processes. A common example is the Ponzo illusion (Figure 1.2). The converging railroad ties confound our perception, and we interpret the upper horizontal bar as being farther away, and therefore larger, than the lower horizontal bar. Functional magnetic resonance imaging (fMRI) studies by Geraint Rees (Schwarzkopf & Rees, 2013) at University College London reveal that the magnitude of the perceived size differences were correlated with the size of the viewer's primary visual cortex (V1) at the back of the head: The smaller the V1, the bigger the perception of the size difference.

Perception of distance is affected by somatic experiences. Studies show that subjects judge a water bottle to be closer if they are thirsty, a hill to be higher if they are tired, an out-of-reach object closer if they are told they can use a conductor's baton to reach it. Thus, that thing we call perception is not just the product of sense organs interacting with the brain. A multitude of bodily sensations, via the somatosensory system, influence our perceptions of the world around us.

People who have been blind and subsequently have their sight restored cannot initially make meaning of the visual stimuli. They experience a chaos of color, shape, and motion. Vision is learned. For a child, such learning is part of the developmental process. For an adult with restored vision, learning to see is a different process.

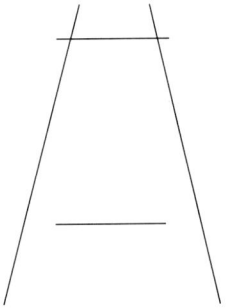

FIGURE 1.2 Ponzo Illusion

How We Hear

In addition to vision, our interpretations of our social functioning rely largely on hearing. The ear collects sound waves from the air and processes them into electrical bits that are then transmitted to the brain, where they are further processed into what we experience subjectively as sound. There is no sound around us, but there are lots of sound waves. Our ears are capable of processing those waves within a range of frequencies. The question "If a tree falls in the forest, and no one is there to hear it, does it make a sound?" is not the deep philosophical puzzle we might have thought in our youth. It is a simple matter of language, word definition, and thinking. The answer, of course, is that the falling tree doesn't make a sound. It makes sound waves. The brain creates sound from the waves it receives and processes.

The ear is usually conceptualized as having three parts (Figure 1.3). The flap of cartilage and skin that we commonly refer to as the ear is technically referred to as the *pinna* and is found only in mammals. The pinna funnels sound waves into the ear canal, at the end of which is the eardrum, separating the outer and middle ear. Sound waves cause the eardrum to vibrate. These vibrations are sent across the middle ear cavity by a series of three tiny bones, which focus the energy of the vibration in the dense fluid within the inner ear. Only mammals have these three bones. Amphibians and reptiles have one, while fish have none. Paleontologist Neil Shubin (2008) describes the fascinating evolution from one

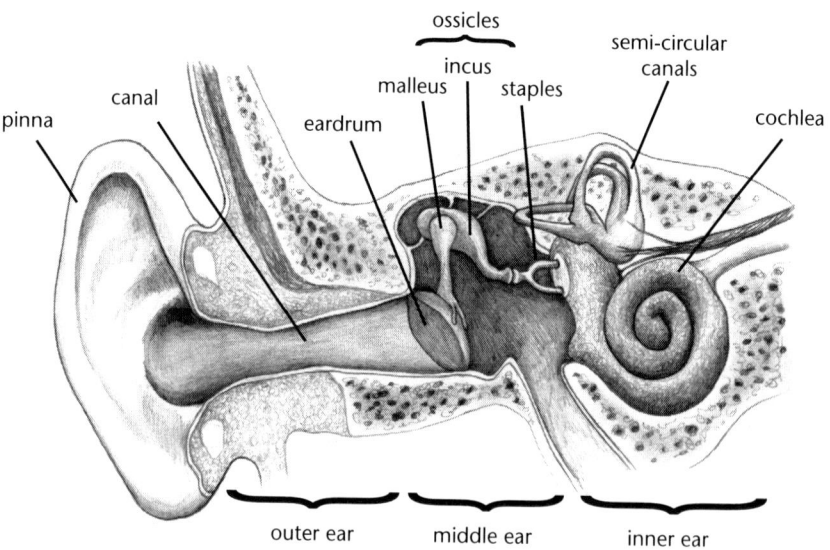

FIGURE 1.3 Human Ear

to three bones (the two additional bones were jaw bones in our ancient ancestors) in *Your Inner Fish*.

The inner ear contains the *cochlea*, a coiled membrane with multiple chambers filled with gel. The *organs of Corti* contain the receptors for the vibrations, which are transmitted as pressure waves along the basilar membrane of the organ of Corti. The membrane vibrations excite hair-like projections that are similar to the photoreceptors in the retina. The movement of these hairs stimulates electrical impulses to the brain. It also sends electrical impulses to the brain that are interpreted as position and acceleration of the head: hence, the inner ear's role in balance, as well as sound. The auditory nerve connects to a number of areas of the brain, described further in chapter 2.

Humans have the capacity to distinguish a number of qualities in the sound waves it processes. Loudness is measured in decibels, pitch in hertz. Different sounds of the same loudness and pitch can be distinguished by their timbre, or harmonic quality. The latter accounts for our ability to identify different instruments playing the same note at the same loudness.

Moreover, we can discern the location and movement of sound waves with a high degree of accuracy. In the woods, we can identify the location of a moving deer from the sound waves emitted by crunching leaves and moving branches, confirming it visually. (The deer more likely first locates us olfactorily, then seeks visual and auditory confirmation.) We have more difficulty seeking visual confirmation of the location of a jet plane because sound and light travel at different speeds, thereby representing different locations in time.

Other human auditory capacities are less well understood, including the ability to distinguish patterns of speech that allow us to identify people on the telephone and a parent's ability to hear the sound of a crying infant amid the chaotic sounds of an action movie on the television. This latter capacity illustrates the importance of separating valued sound from background noise. A hearing aid must do more than increase decibel levels. It must also help the person filter out unwanted sounds and focus on those that are desired. Changing one variable of sound perception can cause unintended consequences in others, illustrating the non-linear nature of the system.

Hearing, like seeing, is a highly personal, subjective, and dynamic experience. Like taste, auditory and visual stimuli will be processed differently at different stages of our lives. As a child, I interpreted the taste of pickles and olives as unpleasant; as an adult I find they stimulate my reward center. When I was a teen, loud, harsh "music" stimulated emotions of excitement associated with sexual stimulation. As an adult, I prefer softer vocal and orchestral stimuli that promote feelings of relaxation and contentment. The muted hues seem more pleasant now compared to the brighter, bolder colors I was drawn to years ago. The stimuli haven't changed, but the subjective experience has.

> A mother once complained to me that her child's teacher had misinterpreted the child's difficulties in the classroom as an attention deficit. The mother explained that her child paid *too much* attention. He took in everything: the movement of other students, the sounds from outside the classroom, the smells from the cafeteria. He just didn't pay attention to the limited amount of stimuli that the teacher preferred. This observation applies not only to attention deficit disorders. The autism spectrum disorders (ASDs) have been defined historically in terms of social and communication impairments. Now a greater than normal capacity for perception has been identified (Herbert, 2010a). In research involving solving complex problems while confronted with irrelevant stimuli, ASD subjects were more capable than normal subjects at successfully completing a task (such as sorting objects by color, shape, and size) while processing data (such as the day's stock market results) irrelevant to the primary task. However, people with increased perceptual capacity pay a price in social settings.

We assume that the external world consists only of things that we can perceive, yet there is ample evidence that this is not so. We know that the human ear and brain can process sound waves within a limited range. Dogs can hear within a spectrum that includes sound waves beyond our range. The human eye can only process objects of a certain size, although technological advances of magnification have greatly expanded that range, thereby changing fundamental concepts of both microscopic and cosmic happenings. It is conceivable that there are some types of visual stimuli that our eyes cannot detect, given that we process only 10 trillionths of the light spectrum. The same is true of the other sensory systems. Indeed, there is likely a whole array of sensations we do not have the capacity to process because they are not essential to our survival. While a few people may have sensory processing abilities beyond the "normal" because of genetic mutation and adaptation, such abilities will become common only when survival so dictates. If climate change results in the elimination of our traditional food supplies and an explosion of both toxic and nutritionally beneficial mushrooms, surviving humans will necessarily develop the sensory capacity to discern the difference.

Integrating Sensory Input

Classifying a sensory experience that originates in the eye as separate from another that starts in the ear is helpful in creating understanding of each but can limit understanding of their mutuality. Early conceptualizations suggested that the brain processed each in discrete areas. That notion has been abandoned based on new understandings. First it was discovered that blind babies acquired some aspects of speech more slowly than their sighted counterparts, suggesting that visual perception of the mouth was important to speech development.

Next came the McGurk effect (McGurk & MacDonald 1976): Subjects watching a video clip of someone repeatedly and silently mouthing "ga" while listening to the same person saying "ba" will report hearing "da." Integrating the visual "ga" with the auditory "ba" creates a new interpretation, "da." Current neuroimaging techniques reveal that auditory perception of a familiar voice stimulates activity within a face recognition area of the brain, the fusiform gyrus. Indeed, it is now believed that the sensory processing areas of the brain are, in fact, multisensory, able to compensate when one sensory stimulus is impaired. For example, when a person is blindfolded for as little as an hour and a half, her visual cortex begins to respond to tactile stimuli.

We think of each sense as a discrete experiencing of our environments, yet the brain does not process them discretely. Rather, our brains create meaning via multiple combinations of sensory perceptions. In rare cases, individuals experience a single sensory modality in multiple ways, a condition referred to as *synesthesia*. In *Born on a Blue Day*, Daniel Tammet (2006) describes his unusual ability to see numbers as shapes, colors, textures, and motion and relates how he utilizes this perceptual abnormality to achieve prodigious feats of memory.

> Despite a diagnosis of autism, Temple Grandin (1976) has achieved fame and success. She found peace as a teenager by being surrounded by farm animals. After receiving a doctoral degree in animal science from the University of Illinois at Urbana-Champaign in 1989, she transformed those experiences into new insights into the more effective handling of both farm animals and persons labeled on the autistic spectrum. Using environmental modification, she discovered ways to soothe anxiety in both animals and autistic persons. She explains her unusual insights by stating, "I don't think like other people. I think in pictures, and I connect them." Abnormal perception and thinking are one route to creativity.

Interpreting Sensory Data

The brain is inundated with sensory data in the form of electrical activity. In fact, the amount of sensory data coming into the brain is far more than can be processed completely. An important function of the brain is to screen and prioritize competing data as it enters. This is akin to the spam filter on your computer. Your brain is constantly receiving tactile data on the interaction between your body and the surfaces it is touching. The brain filters out most of this data unless there is a reason to act on it: If your muscles are getting tight, you will change your position, or if your skin signals discomfort from coolness you will shift the comforter or turn up the thermostat.

The same filtering phenomenon occurs with all the senses. Your brain receives auditory stimuli from the clock ticking or the traffic outside but doesn't interpret it without cause. Olfactory data is filtered unless a sensation interpreted as appealing or dangerous or offensive is received, such as the pot you left unattended on the stove giving off burnt particles that come in contact with the sensory receptors in your nose. Like every step in the sensory process, there is a range of individual experiences. At the extremes are those with limited ability to filter sensory stimuli, such as those with ADHD and those with highly developed filtering abilities, which manifest as heightened powers of concentration.

It is estimated that the average brain filters out at least 95% of incoming sensory data. The task for the brain is to *make meaning* of the rest, to *interpret* chemical and electrical stimuli in a manner that increases the likelihood of survival. It does so in two ways: through emotions (more in chapter 3) and by organizing the various sensory stimuli that seem to go together and assign words to them. Thus, a lot of what we think of as thinking is in words.

Think of as thinking? Remember, we are using thinking to examine thinking. We have created a word, an abstraction, to represent the subjective experience of making meaning of our sensory input. Thinking is more than that, of course. We store sensory experiences in a related process we call memory. We combine past and present sensory experiences and refer to it as learning. We think about ourselves and label it consciousness. Because thinking is a subjective experience, thinking about thinking is a subjective interpretation of a subjective experience.

For example, I look out my window and interpret the visual stimuli to include bark, twigs, and branches. I have learned to associate these labels with these particular stimuli. In addition, I label the chemical and electrical input from the rods and cones in the back of my eye, sent to the brain via the optic nerve, as brown, one of the limited colors I can interpret in the color-deprived landscape of a northern New York winter. Finally, I label the whole of this part of my visual input as a tree.

Thinking is not done exclusively with words. In each hemisphere of the brain, we are able to think visually. In one, usually the right, we have the capacity to visually synthesize, which can be a powerful tool in psychotherapy. It can be easier to alter a visual thought than one locked in language. For example, a patient may have memories of a negative experience associated with a specific person, place, or time. These thoughts may elicit emotions and behavior that prevent the person from completing a task or fulfilling an obligation. In some cases of specific phobias, there is no identifiable experience or association connected with the intense anxiety. No amount of talking, of thinking analytically, seems to weaken the association. However, when the person is in a relaxed emotional state (perhaps, but not necessarily, hypnosis or meditation), the therapist may introduce visual images in which he describes multiple sensory experiences and suggests to the patient alternative mental representations of the stimulus (directly perceived or stored in memory).

> T is a successful professional with no history of psychological difficulty. He has had a lifelong fear of flying that never interfered with his life since he could find alternative means of travel. However, circumstances now require him to fly across the country on short notice. After a history reveals no significant trauma or other anxiety symptoms that limit his functioning, I offer the option of hypnosis. T is skeptical but desperate. I effect induction and employ deepening techniques, then suggest that he visualize himself in a comfortable outdoor environment by the ocean because this is one of his special relaxing places. I suggest multiple, pleasing sensory images: a blue sky, warm sun, gently cooling breeze touching his skin, the rhythmic sound of breaking waves, the smell of the salty sea air. Note I suggest that T integrate four sensory modes in his imagination: visual (blue sky), tactile (warmth and cooling of his skin), auditory (rhythmic wave action), and olfactory (salty sea air). My anecdotal experience is that integrating multiple sensory stimuli has a synergistic effect. I then suggest that while remaining in this comfortable ocean ambience, he picture himself sitting equally comfortably on an airplane (a visualization within a visualization) on the runway as he begins to experience the precursors of panic: mild tension in his chest, slightly increased breathing. Finally, I suggest that he experience a slow shrinking of his mild anxiety until it is concentrated solely under the fingernail of his right pinky. Upon awakening, he seems mildly confused but otherwise unaffected. He calls a week later to report a successful round-trip flight, free of anxiety symptoms. Since then, he has reported a number of successful flights, even many years later.
>
> This vignette is an example of the potential power of sensory integration to change behavior. One possible interpretation of the success of this intervention is that T has created new associations between the sensory experience of an airplane and a positive emotional state. His thinking has changed.

With the evolution of psychology has come refined concepts and ideas and new understandings. The language that develops to express these understandings has meaning limited to the nature of the knowledge at the time the language was created. New knowledge also creates new uses for old language. Aristotle's understanding of thinking has some commonality with modern neuroscientific concepts but is far from the same.

One subspecialty within the field of psychology involves the study of thinking. I will use the term *cognition* to refer to the phenomenon of thinking, which includes such topics as learning, memory, and intelligence. *Metacognition* refers to thinking about thinking.

Another area of study in psychology is emotion, or *affective states*. There is continuing debate in the field about the exact distinction between thought and emotion and the roles each play in processing stimuli to produce behavior. Plato believed that rational thought distinguished humans from other animals. This distinction between thought and emotion persisted through Freudian psychology, with the concepts of id (emotional instincts) and ego (the thinking self). As psychologists have struggled to understand where thinking ends and emotions begin, they have used a construct of linear processes to frame the question in terms of which comes first. For example, cognitive-behavioral theory posits that thinking comes first and shapes the emotion:

$$\text{Perception} \longrightarrow \text{Thinking} \longrightarrow \text{Emotion} \longrightarrow \text{Behavior}$$

The therapeutic strength of this conceptualization does not necessarily lie in its scientific validity but in its practical utility. From a therapeutic perspective, it is probably not important whether we conceptualize thinking or emotion as preceding the other. Distinguishing between thinking and feeling as separate entities has long historical roots, and psychology research has been heavily influenced by this conceptualization. Knowledge builds on previous knowledge, but at some point concepts can become barriers to understanding. Someday, neuroscience may have to move away from the emotion/thinking dichotomy in order to better understand the workings of the brain.

Western intellectual history includes this dichotomy between rational thinking and emotions. Some philosophers have concluded that morality is the product of rational thought, the antithesis of emotional behavior. Neuroscience, however, has challenged this historical dualism. Jeanette Norden of Vanderbilt University thinks that feelings, the mental representations of emotions, are necessary for rational behavior. She cites a case, referenced in chapter 3 of her book *Understanding the Brain* (2007) and included by Antonio Damasio in *Descartes' Error* (1994), in which a patient lost the ability to experience emotions post-surgically and as a result suffered "paralysis by analysis."

Norden defines rational thinking as the weighing of options. In common parlance, "rational" usually refers to intellectual conclusions that subscribe to some predefined standard, usually that of the person making the judgment. In science, "rational" refers to a process, not an outcome. Rational thinking in different people can lead to different conclusions, depending on the stimuli that are processed, the capacities of the perceptual system, the neural pathways developed in previous processing of similar stimuli (memory, including emotions), and a myriad of other factors that influence current brain processing (the neurological equivalents of mood, alertness, hormonal influences, etc.). Indeed, rational thinking in the same person leads to different conclusions at different times. Our opinion of the family dog might depend on whether we have just perceived him/her making a mess on the new carpet or snuggling against us when we are feeling lonely. Likewise, our rational decision regarding who will receive our

Thinking about Psychology 31

vote in an election can change frequently over the course of a long campaign. Our personal "truth," which consists of basic constructs labeled beliefs, is also subject to these same psychological processes.

The interpretation of stimuli, then, involves both of those subjective experiences that we separate into thought and feeling. The very differentiation is a construct that psychologists and philosophers have developed to create meaning/understanding of how we interpret stimuli. A more helpful model combines thought and emotion into an interactive process called *interpretation:*

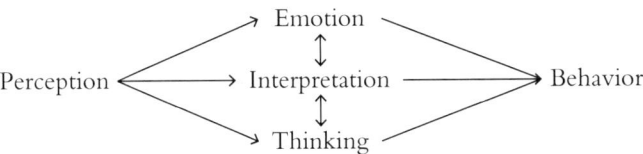

Our cognitions and emotions affect each other.

> K is a veteran of four combat deployments with the 10th Mountain Division, where he served in the infantry. He had been diagnosed with severe posttraumatic stress disorder and, when he first referred himself to me, demonstrated severe anxiety, isolation, and distortions of perception and interpretation. He calls me his "brain mechanic" and has made significant progress in separating his combat experiences from his civilian life in upstate New York. When he learned about the publication of this book, he was eager to offer the following vignette, which he entitled "Perception Is Not Reality" in hopes that non-combatants can begin to appreciate the psychological impact of combat stress:
>
> "Abu Grabe, Iraq. 2004. Above Route Michigan near the intersection of Route Red Devil, there was a crater large enough to swallow an Abrams tank, and on some dark nights with no light from the moon the crater did, in fact, swallow a tank. AQI (Al-Qaeda Iraq) liked to place improvised explosive devices (IEDs) in craters from already detonated IEDs. Using these craters was faster for them and camouflaged them from our units.
>
> "My section's task was to overwatch the large crater along Route Michigan to allow freedom of movement for coalition forces. One day my section was called off our overwatch to investigate some small arms fire coming from the nearby neighborhood. Once we arrived, we cordoned off the area that the small arms fire came from. Then my squad started clearing the houses, looking for the AQI gunners. After an hour of searching, our section was released.
>
> "Upon returning to our overwatch site, we dismounted to clear the area before moving the trucks in. I was on the point and noticed that while we were gone AQI shot mortars exactly where our observation point was

> located. In my head/mind, I can see clearly as if it was yesterday hundreds of unexploded mortar rounds point back to the point of origin. I can see them all around my section, and a few of the mortar rounds were run over by the tires of the trucks. I can still see the 'Oh, shit' look on my driver's face. Although I remember this and it seems as real as this pen I'm writing with, I know there might have been only two, maybe three unexploded mortar rounds. Even though I know the truth, I can't fully accept that as reality. I can't accept that the danger was less than what my mind is perceiving as reality. I get frustrated trying to accept the 'real' reality."

Thinking Scientifically

Psychology is the science of human perception, thinking, feeling, and behaving. Defining the term "science" is easy at one level. Such concepts as objective, logical, and analytical come to mind. When I asked a friend the difference between scientific and unscientific thinking, she replied, "Science is right." Such dichotomous thinking (black/white, right/wrong) is both simplistic and a disservice to the complexity of the subject. For one thing, science often has been proven wrong. Indeed, it is this very ability to prove itself wrong that distinguishes science from other forms of thinking.

One characteristic of science is the nature of the things it examines and the kinds of questions it pursues. Science deals with questions that lend themselves to measurement. Examples of questions that can be pursued by scientific inquiry include: How is the boiling point of water affected by the addition of a specific amount of a certain soluble substance? Is there a correlation between physicians' displays of empathy and better health outcomes in patients with the common cold?

Questions that do not lend themselves to scientific scrutiny include: Do humans have a soul? Does God exist? Empathy is a subjective experience that people can generally agree upon, while "soul" and "God" refer to beliefs for which there is no widespread agreement about either their existence or their nature.

The scientific queries contain terms that can be *operationalized*, or converted into measurable terms. Scientists can agree that boiling point is an observable change in state that can be affixed to a numerical equivalent on a thermometer. The amount and nature of a substance that can be absorbed by water can be clearly defined. The term "empathy" may be a bit more slippery. Here, though, science can break down a subjective experience into observable components. A group of diverse people might be queried as to what they observe that leads them to interpret the physician as being empathetic. A consensus, or significant majority, might agree that they feel empathy when the doctor takes at least five minutes with them, maintains eye contact, examines their throat and ears, and asks at least three questions about their symptoms. An empathy rating could then be constructed, measuring each element on a five-point scale, adding them together for a total empathy score. The definition of a common cold might be subject to consensus by practitioners, and the health outcome can be measured by the severity and duration of symptoms. The extent to which the objective measurement is both accurate and appropriate is referred to as *validity*. (A 2009 study by Rakel et al. found that the duration of a common cold was one day shorter when the physician was viewed as empathetic. Science can demonstrate a relationship, or correlation, between physician empathy and a specific health outcome. Whether empathy is the *cause* of the outcome is less clear.)

An *abstraction* is a concept derived from the essential, selected characteristics of related phenomenon. The study of psychology is replete with abstract concepts: intelligence, empathy, personality, emotions, even cognition itself, to name a few. In order to study psychology in a scientific manner, these abstractions are operationalized via various tests, inventories, and checklists. The resulting data can lead to better understanding, but can also create an illusion, *reification*, whereby the abstraction is confused with objective reality.

Science is not necessarily a superior or "right" way of thinking. It is concerned with a certain kind of inquiry, subject to certain rules. A commonly created duality is that between science and religion. Highly emotional arguments are presented to rationalize the superiority of one over the other, as if it is an either/or dichotomy. Such conflict can arise from language: Each explores questions of *why*. This binary distinction dissolves, however, when the focus of each is made clearer. Physicist V. V. Raman notes that in his native Tamil language, there is a distinction between *why* as causative and *why* as an investigation of purpose. (Tippett, 2010) Science is concerned with causation, *how* phenomena happen. Religion explores questions of purpose, including lack thereof. Conflict arises when each field violates the boundaries of its legitimate field of inquiry.

The science of psychology is concerned with the interpretation of sensory inputs. Some early philosophers of science, such as John Locke (1632–1704) and the *logical positivists*, asserted that sensory experience was the ultimate source of concepts and knowledge. Much of the language and many of the concepts of modern science derived from sensory experience originated with the logical positivists.

Karl Popper (1963) tried to define the line between science and pseudo- and non-science and concluded that the line is *not* that science is supported by observation. He was very much influenced by the three major intellectual challenges of the era: Einstein's theory of relativity, Marx's theory of history, and Freud's theory of psychology, all of which were thought to be scientific. But Popper concluded otherwise. Marx and Freud were pseudo-scientists, he decided, because observation found confirming evidence for their theories everywhere. Further,

Marx and Freud could interpret seemingly negative evidence as confirmation of their theories. Thus, Popper thought that the two criteria for scientific inquiry, the power to explain and confirmation by multiple observations, could lead to invalid conclusions.

But how could Popper say that Einstein's theory, based largely on thought experiments involving hypothetical speeding trains and moving passengers, qualified as real science? General relativity included an unlikely prediction: Light is bent by the gravitational field of the sun. Thus, Einstein provided the criteria by which his theory could be proven false. In fact, subsequent research by Arthur Addington confirmed Einstein's prediction. Popper thought that Marx and Freud expressed important ideas, just as I think *soul* and *God* are important ideas. However, they do not meet a necessary condition of science, the ability to be proven wrong. Instead, they require faith. That said, the ability to falsify its claim, as with Einstein's theory of relativity, is not a sufficient condition to reject a scientific theory. Scientists did not reject all of Newtonian physics when it failed to correctly predict the orbit of Uranus. Rather, they developed an additional theory to explain the discrepancy, the existence of an as-yet-undiscovered planet—Neptune.

As the school of thinking labeled "logical positivism" evolved, it posited two kinds of meaningful statements. One was *analytical*, or literally true by its very meaning, requiring no empirical evidence. "Psychologists study the mind" is such a statement. More important, the concepts of *cause* and *effect* represent *a priori* knowledge. Their relationship is necessary by their meaning via *deductive logic*. To illustrate the distinction between deductive and inductive thinking:

Deduction: working from the general to the specific
Example: theory to hypotheses to observation to confirmation
Theory: Gravity works equally on all objects, free of all intervening variables.
Hypothesis: A rock and a feather will fall at equal acceleration and velocity in a vacuum.
Observation: A rock and feather are dropped from equal heights within a vacuum tube.
Confirmation: The measurements of acceleration and velocity are equal.

Induction: working from specific observation to generalizations and theories
Observation: Certain diseases seem to occur in clusters.
Pattern: People in environments with poor water sanitation seem to contract certain illnesses more frequently and with greater severity.
Tentative hypothesis: An unobserved cause of illness is related to the poor sanitation.
Theory: Germs cause certain illnesses via contagion.

Logical positivism also identified a second type of meaningful statement—a *synthetic statement*, or a claim requiring verification. On further examination, however, this requirement becomes problematic. Some statements by their very nature are unverifiable. We accept that water boils when it reaches a temperature of 100° C, but it cannot be verified that "All water boils at 100° C" because we could never test all water. Further, physicists theorize that heat increases the *probability* that water molecules will speed up, eventually transforming from a liquid to a gas. The introduction of such probability theory into science in the twentieth century introduced another level of complexity to scientific thought. It is not unscientific to assert that someday someone could put his teakettle on a hot burner and it will freeze! If that example is not enough, logical positivism's requirement for verification also rules out statements about all kinds of unobservable phenomenon. (Think quarks and dark matter.)

Thus, the criteria for distinguishing science from pseudo- or non-science are far from clear. Science at once requires both sensory experience and the capacity to go beyond it. Meaning comes from those parts of a theory that can be tested by observation and from our mind's capacity for creating *deductive* relationships among the theory's parts.

> The proper practice of science requires both the application of appropriate measurement procedures and the use of control groups, where possible. However, there are many complex phenomena that cannot be directly studied with control groups. In studying phenomena such as global warming, there needs to be open sharing of all relevant findings. The apparent withholding of certain data by some climate researchers in order to strengthen their theories is a violation of scientific processes and casts a pall over an entire field of inquiry. Research findings on climate change have far-reaching consequences economically and politically. Therefore, climate scientists can face strong incentives to hoard or manipulate findings. Good science requires dispassion, which is not an innate human characteristic.

The modern scientific method was born of the thinking of Francis Bacon (1561–1626), Rene Descartes (1596–1650), and Sir Isaac Newton (1643–1727), who emphasized deductive reasoning to find a theory from the data. John Stuart Mill (1806–1873) devised methods to reach a causal hypothesis from direct observation. His method of agreement would infer a connection between observed phenomena and observed outcomes. For example, one might observe that many people who smoke cigarettes are later diagnosed with lung cancer. The method of agreement would infer a cause-and-effect relationship and assume that cigarette smoking always causes lung cancer. However, further observation reveals that not all people who smoke develop lung cancer and that lung cancer is diagnosed in people who have never smoked. This example shows that any phenomenon that is not *always* present when the outcome occurs is not necessary for that outcome. Rather than a consistent cause and effect, what the research actually reveals is a correlation between the two phenomena.

Mill's method of difference would look at this case differently. Here, all cases of the outcome (lung cancer) would be compared to all the conceivable circumstances (including smoking, exposure to other contaminants, a family history of lung cancer, infectious agents, presence of other cancer-like processes), and if only one circumstance is shared in all cases, it would be inferred to be the cause. In this case, the method shows that one circumstance (smoking) is not sufficient to cause the outcome (lung cancer). Mill's joint method of agreement and difference combines the two methods in hopes of establishing necessary and sufficient conditions for an outcome. This requires very strong data that is not usually available in most complex cases of causality.

> When one billiard ball strikes a second, the first can reasonably be deemed to have *caused* the second to move. Yet another way to conceptualize cause in this case is with the concept of *force*. While the first billiard ball was the *material cause* of moving the second, a law of physics (for every action, there is an equal and opposite reaction) asserts a phenomenological explanation.

Approximately 400 BC, Aristotle conceived of the *doctrine of four causes*. As explained by Daniel Robinson (1989), using the example of a silver bowl, a *material cause* is the substance that constitutes it, in this case silver. The *formal cause* is its shape, or form, which conforms with an abstract idea. The physical process of hammering and molding the silver is the *efficient* cause. Finally, the reason that a thing is done, in this case to create a beautiful object, is the *final cause*.

Using a computational framework, Thomas Griffiths and Joseph Tenenbaum (2005) make a distinction between the strength of a causative agent and what they refer to as "causal structure." The causal structure determines whether an effect results from the cause, while the strength of a causative agent is concerned with measuring the degree of the effect. Each requires a different statistical approach. Causal structure is measured by statistical hypothesis testing, strength by measures of effect size. Griffiths and Tenenbaum propose a Bayesian statistical approach to causal induction that combines two components: structure learning and parameter estimation.

> Thomas Bayes, 1702–1776, was a Presbyterian minister and mathematician who developed a theory of probability, later expanded by Frenchman Pierre Simon Laplace and others, that was fundamentally different from the most commonly used, *frequency theory*. The latter is based on multiple observations of phenomena that are averaged and charted and, in the case of

random variables, distributed in a bell curve. The probability of an outcome can be calculated based on the distribution of these observations. *Bayes' rule* as developed by Laplace involved a *new way of thinking*. Instead of predicting effects from cause, Bayes wondered about the inverse: how to infer the cause from the (observed) effect. Both Bayes and Laplace expressed the idea in words, not as an equation: The probability of a cause, given an event, is proportional to the probability of the event, given its cause. This notion was later refined by mathematical applications and the expansion of computational speed and capacity, resulting in the ability to weigh the relative contributions of multi-variant causation. These refined applications of *inverse probability* have been used in such diverse endeavors as breaking the Nazi enigma code during World War II, locating ships and airplanes lost at sea, and creating a new understanding of the role of cigarette smoking in lung cancer (McGrayne, 2011).

Let's take a break from the theoretical and look at how cause-and-effect analysis is applied by scientifically trained professionals in everyday life. The outcome to be examined is death. There are all sorts of somatic phenomena that correlate with death: The heart stops beating, the brain's electrical activity slows and ceases, the lungs stop absorbing oxygen and emitting carbon dioxide, and the liver ceases to cleanse the blood of toxins. Science tries to go beyond physical observation to explanation. To understand this less-than-upbeat aspect of scientific inquiry, I just had to stroll across the driveway to interview my longtime neighbor and 50-year county coroner veteran, John Hermann, MD. John (now deceased) explained that a standard death certificate lists a proximate cause—the physiological mechanism of death (which rarely stands alone)—followed by contributing causes listed as "due to." Using deductive thinking, the coroner develops a theory and hypotheses about causation, makes observations through examination of the corpse, uses related medical documentation and information gathered from other sources, and either confirms or negates his theory/hypothesis.

A simple case involving a heart attack would list as the proximate cause coronary occlusion due to coronary arteriosclerosis, or cardiac arrest due to generalized arteriosclerosis. A sudden death by a gunshot wound might list the proximate cause as hypovolemic shock (massive loss of blood) due to the laceration of the aorta due to a gunshot wound. A death after 10 days in intensive care following a gunshot wound could result in a death certificate with a proximate cause of multi-organ failure due to irreversible shock due to a lacerated aorta due to a gunshot wound.

The coroner breaks down the concept of cause into the immediate proximate cause (physiologic mechanism of death) and the contributing causes, which can emanate from other somatic sources (fatigue, intoxication) and from factors outside the body (road conditions, chronic cigarette smoking).

A challenge in science is to determine the degree of evidence necessary to logically confirm a theory. Jeffrey Kasser (2001) at North Carolina State University cites the example of copper conducting electricity. The statement that "All copper conducts electricity" goes beyond any possible observation, since it is not possible to test every bit of copper everywhere. David Hume (1711–1776) argued that no number of observations of the sun rising would support a conclusion that the sun will rise tomorrow. However, millennia of observation do establish a pattern, thought of as a *law*, that predicts the next sunrise. Thinking is the process of making meaning from our sensory stimulation, or observation. The more and varied the observations, the more comprehensive and accurate the interpretation. Some ancient societies interpreted the rising sun as a phenomenon controlled by a specific god. Discoveries in astronomy and advances in mathematics produced a very different interpretation of the same observed phenomenon. In a different vein, Karl Popper focused on falsification, not confirmation. In his view, the best that science can offer is that a hypothesis or theory can withstand strenuous efforts to prove it false, thereby resulting in corroboration. Observation from the beginning of recorded human history corroborates the theory that the sun will rise tomorrow. It is an induction inherent in the notion of rationality.

Science and Rationality

Science is a method of inquiry based on rational thought. Rationality and intelligence are not the same. In his book *What Intelligence Tests Miss: The Psychology of Rational Thought*, Keith Stanovich (2009) coins the term *dysrationalia*, the inability to think and behave rationally despite adequate intelligence. He argues that we face increasingly complex problems (read global warming, cancer, terrorism, hunger) that require increasingly more accurate, rational responses. Instead, we waste resources and impair effectiveness through irrational risk assessment, medical treatments, and unnecessary projects. Stanovich points out two causes of dysrationalia: faulty processing and faulty content.

A processing problem arises from choosing the wrong cognitive mechanism. Some of these mechanisms involve great computational power, allowing us to solve many problems slowly, but with great accuracy. These approaches require greater concentration and impair our ability to perform other cognitive tests. Other mechanisms are quick and require little concentration. Most brains prefer the fast, low-effort approach, sometimes at the expense of accuracy. Stanovich considers the following example, based on the work of computer scientist Hector Levesque, of the University of Toronto.

> *Example #1:* Sam is looking at Karen, while Karen is looking at Dave. Sam is married, Dave is not. Is a married person looking at an unmarried person?
>
> A) Yes   B) No   C) Cannot be determined

The vast majority of respondents choose C. Their quick, low-computational approach focuses on Sam and Dave, whose marital status is given. Since Karen's is not, this approach concludes that we cannot determine Karen's marital status, so we can't answer the question. Rational thinking makes clear that Karen's marital status is irrelevant. If she is married, the answer is Yes because she is looking at Dave. If she is unmarried, the answer is Yes because Sam is looking at her. If choice C were eliminated and instruction given that a correct response is still possible, more subjects would be forced to think in a disjunctive ("either/or") manner.

As noted in Stanovich (2009), Nobel Prize–winning psychologist Daniel Kahneman and his colleague Shane Frederick present another challenge to our computational styles.

Example #2: A cup of coffee and a roll cost $1.10 in total. The coffee costs $1 more than the roll. How much does the roll cost?

Many highly intelligent students at prestigious colleges gave the wrong answer of 10 cents. If the roll costs 10 cents, then the coffee costs $1.10 ($1 more) for a total of $1.20. A 5 cent roll yields the correct total.

A variation on the shortcut processing problem is the bias toward ourselves, further elaborated in chapter 5. Stanovich (2009) and his colleague Richard West presented American subjects with two scenarios involving a car that was eight times more likely than a typical family car to kill occupants of another car in a crash. When the car was identified as German, about three-quarters of American responders said it should be banned in the United States. When the vehicle was said to be a Ford Explorer, the percentage saying it should be banned on American streets fell significantly. Political and moral judgments typically involve a self-bias that leads to dysrationalia.

Stanovich also notes that the second source of dysrationalia is in content problems and involves the lack of specific knowledge about rules, data, procedures, strategies, probability, logic, and scientific inference. He presents the following:

Example #3: Imagine that the XYZ syndrome is a serious condition that affects one person in 1,000. Imagine also that the test to diagnose the disease always indicates correctly when a person actually has the XYZ virus. Finally, suppose that this test occasionally misidentifies a healthy individual as having XYZ. The false-positive result of 5% means that the test wrongly indicates that the XYZ virus is present in 5% of the cases where the person does not have the virus. A person chosen at random tests positive for XYZ syndrome. Based on the test result alone, what is the probability, expressed as a percentage, that the individual actually has *XYZ*?

Another health research example from Stanovich further illustrates the danger of dysrationalia:

Example #4: Using 250 subjects, the results of a test of the efficacy of a medical intervention are as follows:

	# Patients Improved	# Patients/No Improvement
Treatment	200	75
No treatment	50	15

Question: Was the treatment/intervention effective?

In chapter 6 we will examine more closely how our health-care system, among others, is often driven by dysrationalia, whether deliberately or by error. Save your answers to examples 3 and 4 until then.

A final example of the gap between intelligence and rational thinking is illustrated in the testing of hypotheses.

Example #5: Four cards are displayed: A   K   8   5

Each card has a letter on one side and a number on the other. Two are letter up, two are number up. The hypothesis to be tested: For these four cards, if one has a vowel on one side, it has an even number on the other. Which card or cards must be turned to test the hypothesis?

For this question, 90% of subjects get it wrong. Most people get the first step, turning over the A. The problem arises with the next step. About half pick the 8 to go with the A, but a consonant on the back of 8 neither confirms nor disproves the hypothesis. The problem does not mention consonants. We are only testing if vowels have even numbers. To prove or disprove, we need not confirm the rule, but only falsify it. Remember Popper's demarcation between science and non-science? Pick the 5 card. A vowel on the back would disprove the hypothesis. In *Incognito*, David Eagleman (2011) theorizes that this common logical error is evidence that human psychology has evolved to solve social, not rational, problems.

Stanovich (2009) argues that people labeled intelligent, as commonly conceived and measured by IQ tests, are only slightly more likely to use disjunctive thinking when situations do not clearly demand it. Most of us apply irrational reasoning to complex (and not-so-complex) challenges. In addition, Stanovich thinks that intelligence does not encompass all cognitive skills. This should be obvious from extreme examples, like the idiot savant Raymond (Dustin Hoffman) in *Rain Man*, who could calculate dates and playing cards but lacked basic social/interpersonal judgment. Yet we continue to use cognitive economy when labeling our interpretations of the competency of others. Why? Because from an evolutionary perspective, this economy has supported our survival. Survival on the savannah required quick responses utilizing our primitive brains. The evolution of more complex problem-solving capacities is a relatively recent occurrence.

A final thought about science and thinking. Science is based on a deterministic model and seeks to discover causes and correlations. In a deterministic paradigm, there is no probability *if all conditions are known*. The more scientific knowledge expands, the more variables are discovered that influence events, rendering them more and more complex. Such complexity is possible to describe only statistically. When we lack enough information to create a statistical model, we think of events as *random*.

How has the ride been so far? Each reader will be processing these pages differently. Words and phrases will have different meanings to different readers, whose minds will wander at different places, filtering out different visual stimuli. Each reader will have to contend with varied sensory stimuli that might be competing for attention (traffic, noisy neighbors, fighting children, even the unusual quiet of a peaceful evening in the country). When you consider all the variables that go into our interpretations of identical stimuli, it is remarkable that we are able to agree on much of anything on our shared journeys. Often we find the differences in our interpretations of the same experience more exciting than the experiences themselves. Think about a good discussion of a book, a movie, or a trip to a new venue. I hope that one thing most of us can agree on up to this point in our journey is that thinking is part of the subjective experience of processing and interpreting sensory stimuli.

In the next chapter, we will examine how thinking about the brain has evolved over time. Later, we will look at models of cognition that challenge the classical psychology conception of the brain as a central planner. Growing out of findings in artificial intelligence, computation, and representation, these models erase the distinctions between perception, cognition, and behavior.

2
THINKING ABOUT THE BRAIN

The mind is just the brain doing its job.

—Simon LeVay

I recall a science fiction movie, *The Fantastic Voyage*, from my childhood. A person was shrunk to a minute size; placed inside a tiny, clear container; and injected into the bloodstream of another person. What followed was a fantastical visual tour of the inside of a human body. I cannot begin to recreate such an experience via words on paper, but I hope to convey a tiny bit of the wonderment as our trip explores the brain itself.

Early civilizations had very limited knowledge of how the human body worked. There were no X-rays or MRIs to examine the internal workings of a living body, no microscopes to study tissue at the cellular level, no laboratory capacity to understand the chemistry of the blood. Our ability to think is limited by the quality and amount of the stimuli we receive and process. One physical finding that was apparent to early students of anatomy was that there was a steady thumping sensation within their own chests and in the chests of everyone they examined. Dissection of the deceased led to the conclusion that the thumping sensation must originate in a fist-sized mass of muscles that was labeled the heart. This evolved to mean "the vital center of one's being, emotions and sensibilities" (*American Heritage Dictionary*), reflecting the early belief that the heart was the center of thinking, of the "soul." The early Egyptians extracted the brains of their deceased pharaohs and discarded them, retaining the heart for mummification. Aristotle (384–322 BC) thought the only function of the brain was to cool the passions of the heart, the center of perception and thinking. Until the Renaissance, the thinking of Galen (c. 130–200 AD) prevailed: The soul, or mind, consisted of spirits emanating from the heart; the brain rendered nobility to the spirits.

Based on observations from crude dissections, Leonardo da Vinci (1452–1519) concluded that perception and thinking did, indeed, rest in the head—more specifically, in the hollow areas of the brain now called ventricles, rather than in the cellular substance. The notion that the mind and the body are distinct entities was advanced by René Descartes (1596–1650). The labels "mind" and "soul" were used to distinguish humans from other animals. Animals might have brains, but they lacked the capacity to make moral judgments for the body. Descartes concluded that this unique human capacity resided in the pineal gland, a somewhat curious conclusion since animals also possess pineal glands. Seventeenth-century English anatomist Thomas Willis and artist Christopher Wren gathered additional observational data that led them to believe that perception, thinking, and movement were functions of the brain tissue itself. Franz Joseph Gall (1758–1828) originated the field of thought known as *phrenology*, which posited that the outer part of the brain controlled more complicated mental processes, which were reflected in the shape and size of the skull itself. His was the first model to suggest that brain functioning was differentiated into separate brain areas.

> The thinking behind Gall's phrenology seemed completely logical: (1) Our mind's traits are biologically determined in the cerebrum, which (2) has specialized compartments such as memory and pride that grow proportionately to their use, (3) causing the surrounding skull to adapt its shape (4) and rendering it a medium for measuring the intellectual, emotional, and moral proclivities of the mind. How many of our current beliefs and understandings are logical conclusions built on incorrect assumptions?

This superficial review of the origin of thinking within the human body demonstrates how knowledge is cumulative. Advances in the ability to study the body, including the brain, led from one to the other. Today's incredibly sophisticated tools for studying the brain have led to far more complex understandings.

Modern neuroscience does view the brain as the biological basis for that which we label as thinking, or the mind. Everything we know about our external world, and about our bodies and brains, is determined by and, to an unknown extent, limited by what our neural circuits allow.

How the Brain Is Organized

Estimates of the number of cells in the human body vary widely; a commonly accepted range is 50 to 70 trillion. Among those cells that constitute the brain, there are an estimated 80 to 100 billion *neurons*. The brain also contains another class of cells, referred to as *glia*. Different sources estimate that the number of glial cells varies from a ratio of 1:1 with neurons, to 90:1, a range from 100 billion to 9 trillion. (My interpretation of numbers this large has changed since my youth. Back then, billions and trillions were more likely to appear in a mathematics classroom. Now we hear these numbers used routinely in reference to money markets and government debt and spending. Our understanding of the numbers of stars and solar systems and galaxies has likewise ballooned since the 1950s and 1960s.)

Much of our brain is involved with involuntary and unconscious activity that sustains and regulates our bodily functions. The intent of our conscious thinking is to *create meaning* from the vast, complex amount of information we gather via our sensory systems. We can use our attempts to understand this complex organ called the brain to begin to understand how we think. Trying to think about this in a meaningful way involves classifications similar to those we use in our attempt to understand the world. We think directionally (north, south, east, west) and subdirectionally (Near East, Middle East, Far East). We think according to economic status (developed, underdeveloped) or structure (capitalist, communist, socialist). Religion can define parts (the Muslim world), as can affiliation (the Allies, the Axis), continents, language, and race. All these classifications serve to simplify the complex so it can be understood.

> My wife and I visited Managua, the sprawling capital of Nicaragua. Fortunately, we were accompanied by friends who were both fluent in Spanish and familiar with the layout of the city. Like the individual neurons of the brain, the streets did not have names and the buildings did not have addresses. Location was determined by proximity to significant landmarks. Our hotel was located near a prominent radio tower. Our hosts would direct the cab to the tower area, then narrow the search to the exact location desired. A map of Managua with named streets would have been helpful. Given the number of neurons in the brain (streets in a city), and the fact that each brain (city) is organized differently, it is hard to imagine mapping each individual neuron of the brain.

We use a number of criteria in our quest to find meaning. With our brain, we are able to develop categories, or labels, based on such information as visual differences, location, function, and relationships to other labeled categories. These kinds of criteria lead us to a gross conceptualization of brain organization.

The brain is one of the two parts of the *central nervous system* (CNS); the other part is the spinal cord. These two parts are continuous but are labeled as separate entities where the CNS leaves the skull through an opening called the *foramen*

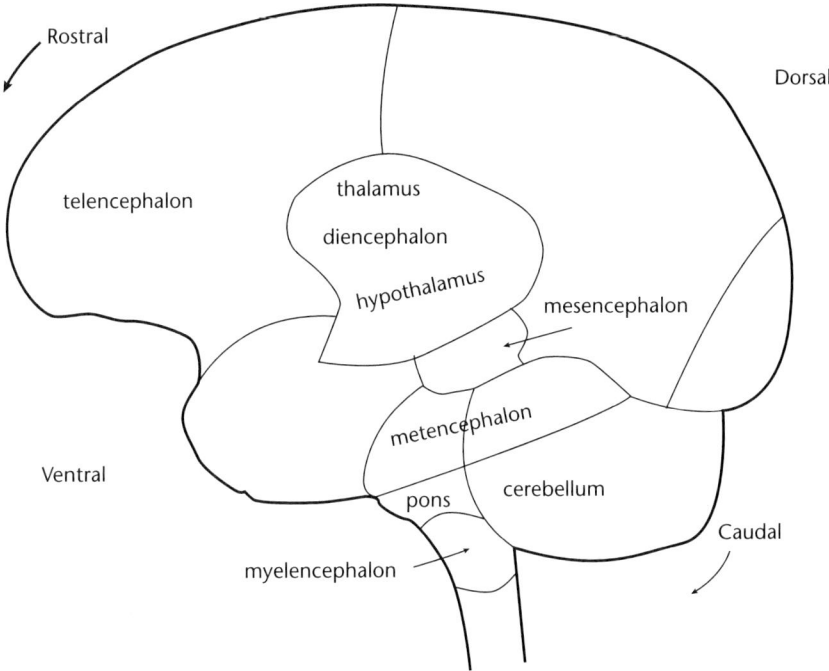

FIGURE 2.1 Gross Brain Organization

magnum. Scientists have further divided the CNS into the spinal cord, the *brainstem* (conceived as our older, primal area), and the two *cerebral hemispheres*. Gross locations within the brain itself are thought of by using concepts of direction. The term *rostral* refers to the front of the brain, located behind our face and eyes, while *caudal* refers to the back. *Dorsal* and *ventral* refer, respectively, to the top and bottom areas. Look at Figure 2.1 and imagine you rotate the front (rostral) area toward you and the back (caudal) away, until you are looking directly at the front, between the two eyes. The *medial* is the area nearer to the midline from the front to back, while the *lateral* is the area toward the outside, or ears. The midline is where the brain is separated into two hemispheres.

> Observation of chimpanzees at the Yerkes National Primate Research Center has led scientists to conclude that the chimps predominantly use their right hands to communicate by gesture. It's speculated that these gestures originate in systems within the left hemisphere, since brain hemispheres largely control the opposite body half. The left hemisphere is home to many language functions in humans, leading to speculation that ancestral gesturing could be the precursor of language in humans. The observations about the

> chimps involve knowledge derived from sensory experience and, as such, are a form of *empiricism*. The scientists' combining of multiple observations into a new level of knowledge are a form of *rationalism*. Together they represent one way of thinking about thinking.
>
> The connection between gesture and language has been conceived of in another way. When comprehending speech, Broca's area (located in the cortex and associated with speech production, gesture, and language interpretation) interacts less with other brain areas when the speech (auditory) is coupled with gestures (visual). This may represent a kind of brain economy, where the least amount of brain activity is utilized to complete a function (Branan, 2010).

The two hemispheres of the brain are connected by a bundle of cells called the *corpus callosum*. Much of our understanding of the roles of the two hemispheres is derived from studying patients whose corpus callosum has been severed, typically as the result of a surgical procedure performed in rare cases of severe, uncontrolled epilepsy. In one experiment, these patients were briefly shown a picture to the right or left of the visual fixation point, so that it was processed by just one hemisphere. Patients shown a picture through their right eye, and therefore processing it in the left hemisphere, could describe what they saw. Patients processing the stimuli through the left eye and right hemisphere reported seeing nothing. Scientists conclude that the left hemisphere contains centers for translating stimuli into language, while the right does not. Note that the left eye/right hemisphere subjects could "see" the object but could not express it via language: When asked to point to the picture they saw from among a whole series, they did so without error. Studies have revealed other differences in visual processing between the two hemispheres. The right is holistic and best recognizes complete objects, while the left is more analytic, recognizing details. Each stores encoded visual memories in its unique way, but in intact brains the two hemispheres process visual stimuli simultaneously.

In addition to these directional demarcations, there are numerous additional ways to categorize areas of the brain. One is into five areas from rostral to caudal (Figure 2.1). The *telencephalon* is the front part, including both hemispheres. It is thought to be the most recently evolved brain section. The outer layer of the telencephalon is called the *cerebral cortex*, which plays a critical role in thinking, language, emotions, intellect, and memory. It is made up of gray matter (neurons). The neural tissue is folded and compressed to fit inside the skull. The "bumps" of tissue on the outside are called *gyri*, while the hidden valleys are *sulci*. A deep *sulcus* is called a *fissure*. The number of layers of neural tissue in the cortex varies. Those areas that evolved more recently (neocortex) are thicker, while those that are older from an evolutionary perspective have fewer layers. The *hippocampus* is an older area involved in learning and memory and has three cell layers. Most of the cortex is neocortex, consisting of six layers.

Behind that is the *diencephalon*, an area divided into the *thalamus*, from which many connections are made with the cortex, and the *hypothalamus*, which controls such homeostatic functions as body temperature. Next is the *mesencephalon*, also referred to as the *midbrain*, which houses functions related to our reflexes. Farther back is the *metencephalon*, divided into the *cerebellum*, which plays a role in both thinking and motor functions, and the *pons* (remember your Latin: *pons* means "bridge") that connects the cerebellum to the rest of the brain. Farthest back is the *myelencephalon*, also referred to as the *medulla* or *medulla oblongata*, which contains groups of neurons connecting to the spinal cord.

Another gross categorization of the brain is based on the time when some parts evolved relative to others. The *hindbrain* refers to older, more primitive parts of the brain that control vital functions such as breathing and heart rate and includes the myelencephalon and the metencephalon. The *forebrain* includes what is elsewhere classified as the telencephalon and the diencaphalon and is considered the most recently evolved. Yet another area defined by age of evolution is the *brainstem*, an older area that includes the *myelencephalon*, the *metencephalon*, and the *mesencephalon*.

Up to now we have been considering the gross organization of the brain as viewed from the outside. Another way of thinking about how the brain is structured is to look at it internally. There are a number of different approaches to do this. One simple differentiation is by color. Early anatomists described the brain as consisting of *gray matter* and *white matter*. Today these color differences are better understood as the bodies of brain cells are better understood.

Neuroscientists think of the brain cells called neurons as consisting of three main parts: the *cell body*, the *dendrites*, and the *axon* (Figure 2.2). Through cell-staining techniques developed in the nineteenth century, it was found that gray

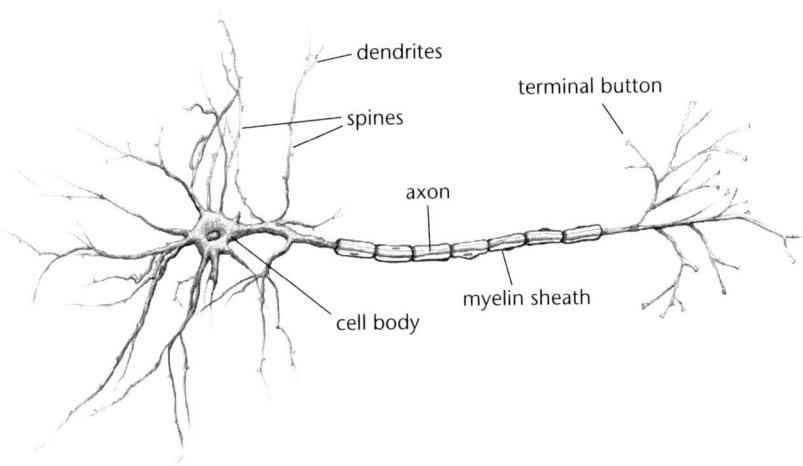

FIGURE 2.2 Neuron

matter consists of groups of neuron cell bodies. Groups of neurons that form a functional area in the CNS are called *nuclei* (not to be confused with a homonym that refers to the central part of a cell). The white matter, on the other hand, is made up of axons and dendrites. What the early brain researchers interpreted as white was actually the color of the *myelin sheath* surrounding most axons.

The two classifications of brain parts by color can be further divided by their structure and function. Structural groupings share similar cellular organization, or *cytoarchitecture*. Scientists have also grouped the CNS class nuclei into functional systems. A large number of nuclei have a specialized function in motor activity, coordinated by the cerebellum. Other nuclei have a role in processing sensory stimuli and are considered part of the visual, auditory, tactile, olfactory, or gustatory systems.

Another classification of the brain areas is by more general kinds of functions. For example, in the gray matter, the hypothalamus has a homeostatic function that includes such diverse tasks as body temperature, drinking, and eating. Another example is the *limbic system*, which is involved in learning, memory, emotion, and higher level executive functions. A third example is the *reticular formation*, a collection of more than 100 neuronal groups deep inside the brain that run from the upper spinal cord to the telencephalon, helping regulate the vital functions of breathing and heart rate, as well as dreaming and consciousness.

White matter also can be grouped into functional categories. For example, *association pathways* are axons that connect different areas of the cortex within each hemisphere. *Commissural pathways* are axon groupings that connect the two hemispheres (the major one being the corpus callosum). *Projection pathways* are groups of axons that connect different areas of the brain.

The cortex is subject to a number of systems of classification. One is by four lobes (Figure 2.3). The *frontal lobe* is associated with reasoning, planning, parts of speech, movement, emotions, and problem solving. (The *prefrontal cortex* is the anterior portion of the frontal lobe.) The *parietal lobe* is involved with movement, orientation, recognition, and perception of stimuli. The *occipital lobe* plays a role in visual processing. The *temporal lobe* is associated with perception and recognition of auditory stimuli, memory, and speech.

Another cortex classification system (Figure 2.4) was devised by Korbinian Brodmann (1868–1918). This system identifies about 50 different areas, each distinguished by the manner in which the neural cells are arranged in groups or layers. While more recent scientific findings have led to further subdivision of these brain areas, Brodmann's numbering system is still used. By comparing Figures 2.3 and 2.4, the reader can see that Brodmann's areas generally fit within the lobe structure.

One final classification system of the cortex is based not on structure or organization but on function. The cortex is devoted to three tasks: processing sensory input, managing motor functions, and completing *multimodal*, or *association*, functions. The latter are carried out by three *association areas* (Figure 2.5). The

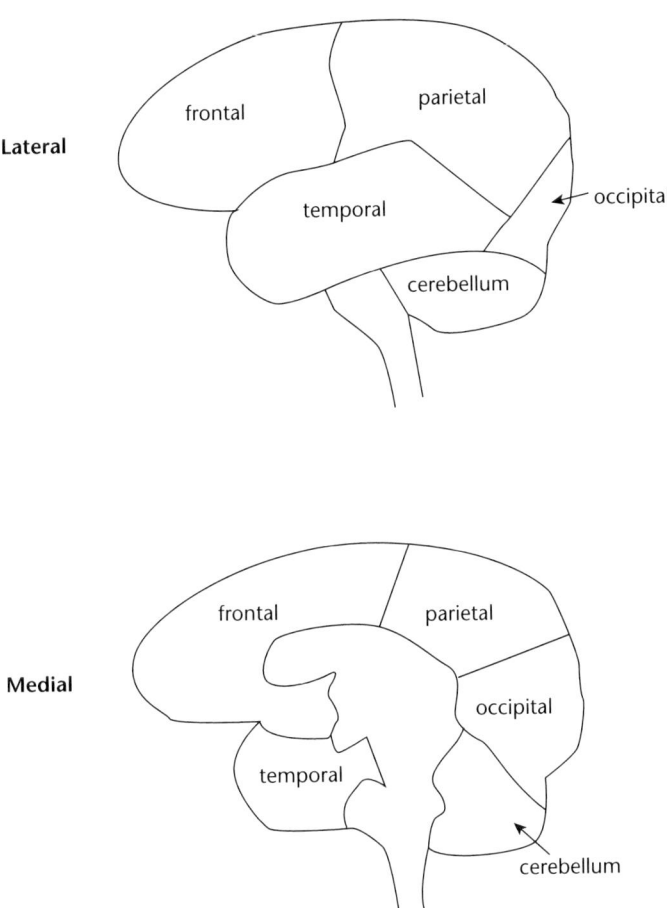

FIGURE 2.3 Brain Lobes

prefrontal association cortex permits us to appreciate the consequences of our behavior. Damage to that area via such insults as fetal alcohol syndrome is thought to contribute to criminal and related psychopathic behavior. The *parieto-occipital-temporal association cortex* processes sensory input from multiple sensory systems. The *limbic association cortex* is located within both the frontal and temporal lobes and consists of multiple areas that are interconnected in very complicated ways. The *amygdala* are almond-shaped structures located in the *medial temporal lobes* in both hemispheres and play a role in storing memories of emotional experiences.

The cortex has a high degree of redundancy, based largely on the twin nature of the hemispheres. The *occipital lobes* are located in the back of the brain yet largely process vision. The *temporal lobes*, at the bottom middle, process aspects of language, as well as hearing and visual object recognition. The *parietal lobes*,

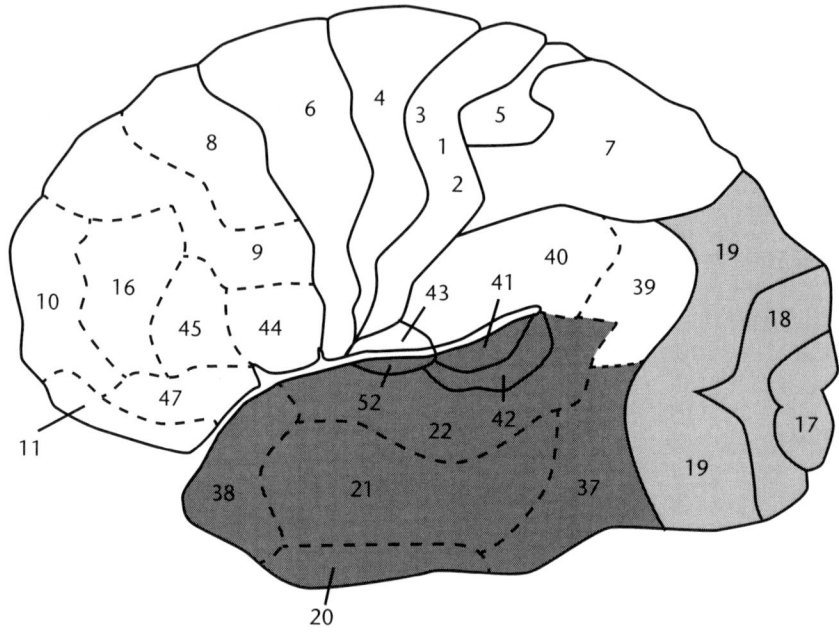

FIGURE 2.4 Brodmann's Areas

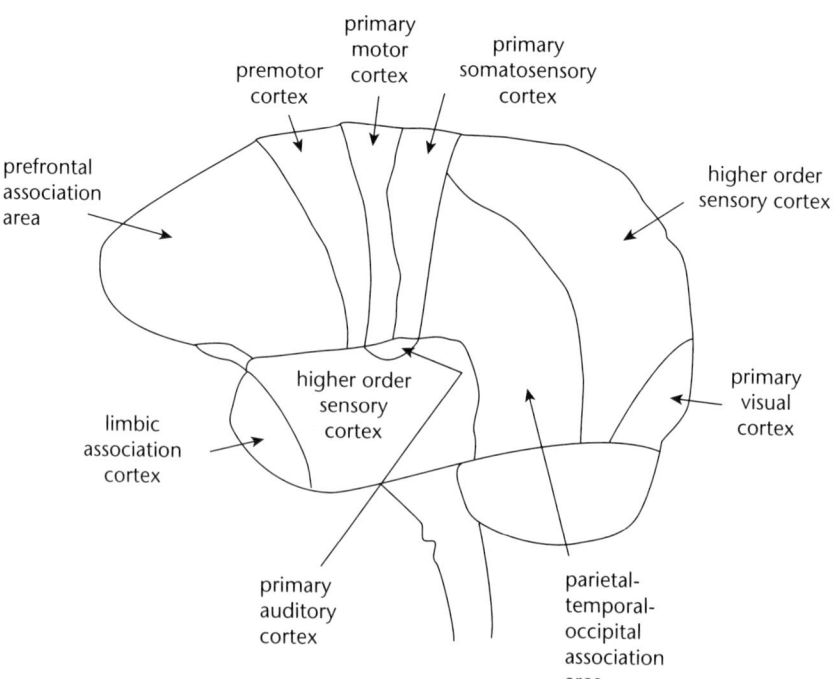

FIGURE 2.5 Association Areas

on the top back, process tactile sensation and our sense of space. The back part of the parietal lobes are involved with complex thinking, such as high-level problem solving.

The *frontal lobes* are most implicated in what we commonly conceive of as *thinking*. The front-most area, the *orbitofrontal cortex*, supplements and regulates the more primitive emotions emanating from the limbic system, creating the more complex emotions required in social functioning and risk/reward decision making. Most of the remaining frontal lobe functioning involves novel, creative, abstract thinking. The *lateral prefrontal cortex* and the *posterior parietal cortex* are believed to be heavily involved with conscious thought processes.

> Child welfare experts and child psychologists have been perplexed by the unexplained magnetism that draws victims of childhood abuse back to their perpetrators when the perpetrator is a primary caretaker. I have observed this phenomenon repeatedly in my practice. This seemingly destructive behavior defies the presumed innate impulse to survive. Psychologist Regina Sullivan of New York University observed that baby rats were attracted to nearly any odor, even those associated with aversive stimuli. Further examination found that the amygdala of these rats had lower levels of the neurotransmitter dopamine, which might have inhibited the normal fear response. Thinking about these findings as they might apply to abused children, psychologist Gordon Barr of Children's Hospital in Philadelphia speculates that attachment to even a threatening caretaker enhances survival, as compared to no attachment. The long-term impact on the victim's brain and fear response in later life is thought to be negative (Westly, 2010).

Given the astronomical number of brain cells and connections, and the variety of sensory stimuli to process and functions to support, there has to be some means of coordinating such a cacophony of electrical and chemical activity. The thalamus is a kind of central air traffic control or relay station that supports the flow of information among brain sites.

How We Know about the Brain

Our understanding of the way the brain goes about its work is only as good as the sensory information we have available to process. As the human cortex has increased in volume, so has the human ability to create external devices and structures that complement and multiply the ability to understand phenomenon of ever-increasing complexity. Examples of this scaffolding range from pencils to record information, thereby exponentially increasing memory, to the Hubble satellite telescope to look far into space to capture information regarding the rate of expansion of the universe. Following is a simple outline of the progress made in creating technologies to obtain more data about the brain.

Observation of cadaver brains by Leonardo da Vinci provided some visual inputs about the brain's structure and organization but no clue about how it functions. British physician Richard Caton published an article in the *British Medical Journal* in 1875 in which he reported evidence of electrical activity in the exposed cerebral hemisphere of rabbits and monkeys. Further research led to the invention of the electroencephalogram (EEG) by German physiologist and psychiatrist Hans Berger in 1924. By studying the electrical activity recorded by multiple electrodes placed strategically on the skull, neurologists are able to clinically diagnose different categories of seizures. Other uses for the EEG include diagnosis of an organic basis for encephalopathy and delirium, determination of brain death, and provision of neurofeedback in the treatment of psychological factors in stress-related illnesses, addictions, and ADHD.

As the wavelength of light decreases, the amount of energy it emits increases. X-rays, consisting of electromagnetic radiation, were first observed by accident in 1895 by German scientist Wilhelm Roentgen. The radiation passes through soft tissue but is absorbed by bones and metal. The results are captured on film, giving a crude depiction of internal structures. In studying the brain, the use of early X-rays was limited to diagnosing damage to the bony skull, since the brain tissue itself is soft.

Psychosurgery is an invasive procedure first done by Swiss psychiatrist Gottlieb Burckhardt in 1880. In the 1930s, Portuguese neurologist Egac Moniz introduced the leucotomy, renamed the lobotomy when introduced in the United States by Walter Freeman and James Watts. This procedure involved cutting the connections to and from the prefrontal cortex and was used in the treatment of depression and psychoses. Watts later developed a relatively less invasive technique, the transorbital lobotomy, in which an ice pick–like instrument entered the brain via the eye socket. Today, psychosurgery for psychiatric disorders has moved away from destroying brain tissue, instead implanting electrodes to induce deep brain stimulation. Psychosurgery did not make significant contributions to our knowledge of brain functioning.

The 1970s witnessed the advent of the computed tomography (CT) scan. The X-ray provided only a flat, two-dimensional picture. By contrast, the CT scanner provides a series of successive images as the subject moves slowly through the scanning ring, creating the illusion of depth. This advance led to the diagnostic capacity to differentiate between symptoms caused by head trauma and similar ones resulting from psychiatric disorders.

Utilizing the body's natural magnetic field responding to radio frequencies, magnetic resonance imaging (MRI) was developed in the 1980s and had the ability to distinguish among soft tissues of varying densities. Able to slice on three or more planes, the MRI creates a true three-dimensional image from which a computer can create a type of relief map of the entire interior of the brain.

Also in the 1980s came positron-emission tomography (PET), advancing imaging from still pictures to action movies. A radioactive tracer, often an analog of glucose, is injected into the blood while the scanner tracks both the blood flow and the breakdown of glucose in specific sites. A computer then creates a three-dimensional picture. This technique documented the difficulty the brains of persons labeled as schizophrenic have in communicating among distant regions.

Without radioactive tracers, the *f*MRI monitors the consumption of oxygen by brain cells, a measure of their activity levels. Typically, subjects undergo the procedure while performing a specific task. Starting in the 1990s, researchers have been able to pinpoint the areas of the brain activated by that task.

In the 2000s, the activity of various brain regions as identified by *f*MRI could be viewed in an interactive way by diffusion tensor imaging (DTI). While the *f*MRI could not create a clear image of the fatty white matter, the DTI could by detecting the flow of water through it. For the first time, brain imaging moved from a static to a dynamic mode.

From the CT scans of the 1970s to the DTI of the 2000s, the activity of the brain was interpreted by inferential clues—from the flow of blood and water to the consumption of glucose. More recently, technology has been developed to directly view the firing of neurons. Magnetoencephalography (MEG) detects changes in the magnetic signals produced by an active neuron. The result: The order and pattern of activation of brain regions associated with specific tasks can be traced.

The evolution of thinking about the brain, from a source of nobility for the spirits to a highly interactive organ with multiple feedback loops, has depended on advances in technology unimagined not long ago. Future advances will likely be even more exciting. There are major initiatives underway that will lead to further understanding of the brain through new technologies. The Brain Research through Advancing Innovative Neurotechnologies Initiative (BRAIN), announced by the Obama administration, involves an initial expenditure of $100 million in 2014 to develop technologies to record signals among brain cells and brain areas. The European Union's Human Brain Project is a 10-year, $1.6 billion endeavor to create a computer simulation of the brain. The Human Connectome Project, coordinated by Harvard University, seeks to create a wiring map of the brain. Some of the newer technologies required to achieve the goals of these projects will be considered in chapter 4.

The Developing Brain

The process by which a single egg, fertilized by a single sperm, grows into a living creature called a human being is so complex that we are prone to label it a miracle, something beyond human capacity to understand. Increasing knowledge of cellular biology and genetics renders the subject even more, not less, wondrous. From one fertilized cell comes a brain that can regulate the functioning of all the other bodily organs in ordinary folk, as well as in superb athletes, gifted musicians, and geniuses in physics, astronomy, and medicine. Here is a very simplified, condensed version of the story.

Some 18 days after conception, cells divide rapidly in a process called *mitosis*, forming a structure called the *neural plate*. The cells grow rapidly along its edges, and the neural plate folds over to form the *neural tube*. This tube closes as cells multiply, forming a cavity that will become the *ventricular system*, which continues through the spinal cord as the *spinal canal*.

During the first 12 to 20 weeks of gestation, mitosis is most productive, creating the most neurons. Neurons differentiate into gray matter along the spinal canal. Some will migrate outward to form what will eventually become the cortex. White cells will then develop to connect the neurons near the ventricles to the cortex. Further differentiation results in *long-axon neurons*, white matter that connects brain areas, and *short-action neurons*, which connect within the nuclei.

It is estimated that 250,000 new brain cells are created per minute in the fetus, differentiating and making complex connections with other neurons. How can tiny cells "know" to divide, to specialize, and to connect? The way we think about this question and its answer(s) depends on our sensory input and how we store and process it. Given the limited amount of sensory input I have provided so far, a number of explanations could be constructed by our thought processes. There could be an unseen force that controls the process through messages sent from the heavens, space ships, or gods residing within the earth. The whole developmental process might be a re-enactment of our evolution from single-celled creatures. Or there might be forces at work far beyond our capacity to comprehend.

Scientists seek meaning from this complexity, uncertainty, and apparent chaos. They search for additional information based on a key role that they now think is played by *deoxyribonucleic acid* (DNA). Every nucleus of every cell in our body, including every one of these highly differentiated neurons, contains the exact same DNA.

Evolutionary biologists estimate that birds diverted from their human ancestors over 300 million years ago, yet both species seem to rely on the same genes for vocal communication. These genes are thought to be factors in the vocal learning abilities of a limited number of other species, including whales, elephants, and bats. Such discoveries could potentially lead to the transplant of a human stuttering gene mutation into a zebra finch and a study of subsequent brain activities.

At this point, we might think we are confronting a paradox. Highly differentiated cells, such as brain, skin, and bone cells, contain the same DNA? More knowledge, in the form of processed sensory input, provides clues to understanding this. It turns out that DNA (genes) produce a protein that controls the structure and function of each cell. Further, the DNA recipe to build specific body parts (limbs, hearts, stomachs, and brains) is virtually identical in every creature.

Scientists often refer to DNA as "orchestrating" or "directing" cell division, specialization, and organization. These metaphorical terms might be at once edifying and misleading. The notion of orchestrating/directing might imply a being or force behind them that could be thought of as theistic, extraterrestrial, random, or otherwise. Our thinking seeks to make meaning. Meaning is a construct. Einstein, for example, pursued a theory of everything that would unify all other theories. Such a pursuit may say more about the mind in general, and Einstein's in particular, than about the stimuli we process from the environment.

Neurons divide and migrate at a higher rate at the *cephalic* end of the neural tube, where the brain will develop. This rapid production of neurons creates more cells than are needed, a redundancy that enhances survival and is corrected by a paring-down process that leads to more efficient operation. Only about half the neurons created in utero survive into adulthood. Many are removed through *apoptosis*, cell death mediated by multiple extrinsic and intrinsic mechanisms. The excessive number of cells compete for a limited amount of *trophic factors*, signals required to stay alive. In addition to a paring of the cells, there is a similar process to reduce the excessive number of connections among neurons. This occurs at critical times in the post-natal period, when specific kinds of learning (sensory, motor, intellectual) are happening. This culling of excessive connections represents the increased neuronal efficiency that accounts for learning. The reduced number of connections are more stable, strong, and reliable. At birth, the CNS has far more neurons than it ever will have again. Brain growth after birth consists only of the growth of *glial cells* and the development of *myelinated sheaths* around axons.

Connecting Diverse Neurons

Until recently our understanding of how the brain works was neuron centered. Brain scientists today can classify neurons into 150 different types based on the structure of their dendrites, making them the most diverse cell type in the body. Yet all nerve cells have common parts (see Figure 2.2). The cell body contains the nucleus and controlling DNA. Dendrites are extensions of the cell body that receive input into the cell from other neurons, while the axons send outputs to the dendrites of other neurons.

Neurons are different than other cells in that they are *polarized*, able to propagate, and conduct an electrical impulse. The electrical charge is generated in the *axon hillock* and travels down the axon by "jumping" from node to node between the myelin. This electrical signal is called the *action potential*, which is of the same amplitude within a single neuron. The intensity of the stimulus is conveyed by the frequency of the action potential. The quality of the stimulus is determined by the kinds of neurons involved, the neural pathways traversed, and the interpretation by various areas of the brain, especially the cerebral cortex.

> Until the early 1980s, there was general belief that brain cells did not divide and grow. Research using canaries, and subsequently rodents and monkeys, found that brain cells could divide and migrate to different brain areas and grow into specialized cell types. In 1998 these findings were confirmed in humans, as was the brain's ability to reorganize neural networks, create new networks, and render others obsolete, all in response to experience. This *plasticity* of the brain can be exploited to therapeutic effect when (1) it is induced by changes in the nature and amount of sensory stimuli; (2) the stimuli are accompanied by guided, focused attention; and (3) older, habituated thoughts, feelings, and behavior are inhibited by intentional repetition of more functional ones. Sensorimotor psychotherapy emphasizes increased awareness of the somatic responses to targeted stimuli and intentional training of more adaptive thoughts, feelings, and behavior. The following vignette illustrates the application of these principles.
>
> M, a 21-year-old male, referred himself for psychotherapy at the suggestion of his primary care physician. His adolescence was marked by rebellion and substance abuse. After getting a respectable job, he expressed a desire to address long-standing symptoms of anxiety. He was taking increasing doses of benzodiazepines, which his physician would only continue to prescribe if he agreed to psychotherapy. M's family history revealed he is the third child and the only male and that his father was physically and emotionally absent as the result of alcoholism. The parents divorced during his teen years, concurrent with his acting-out behavior. He reported experiencing anxiety from a young age, reactive to parental conflicts. His father now has multiple health problems arising from his chronic alcoholism yet continues to drink to excess. M has recently developed an interest in martial arts and goes to the gym on a regular basis.
>
> As M described a recent encounter with his father, I had him focus on his somatic reactions. He described increased heart rate, tension in his chest, and labored breathing, common symptoms of panic. I inquired about the

> thoughts accompanied these bodily changes. M identified powerlessness and a sense of shrinking in size. He appeared to be withdrawing his body into a fetal-like pose. At this first session, I had him stand and demonstrate stretching and breathing exercises he had learned at the gym while continuing to visualize the conflict with his father. We repeated this four more times; then I suggested he direct his attention to this same stretching and breathing activity during his next meeting with his dad. At our next session, he described a reduction of anxiety/panic symptoms, both when in his father's presence and when thinking about him. Subsequent sessions continued the practice of directing attention to physical experiences that were associated with thoughts of competence and control. A focus on new, in-the-moment responses to previously aversive stimuli is thought to encode new neural circuits that can override the older, less functional ones.
>
> The use of benzodiazepines to treat the symptoms of anxiety does not address the underlying cause of anxiety and runs the added risk of addiction after longer-term use. M was able to discontinue the anti-anxiety agent and manage his symptoms by continuing to use cognitive-behavioral techniques.

Neurons are surrounded by fluid containing, among other things, *ions*, charged particles that include chloride, potassium, and sodium. When not stimulated, the inside of the neuron is more negatively charged than the outside. When stimulated, the inside of the neuron becomes either more positively charged (depolarized, or inhibited) or more negatively charged (hyperpolarized, or excited). The resulting action potential is transmitted from node to node to the *presynaptic axon terminal*. The binary on-off nature of action potential can lead to the notion that neurons are like switches. In reality, they are filters that are tuned along multiple stimulus dimensions. This tunability to varying firing rates allows them to encode many different types of information.

Pyramidal neurons are named for the shape of their cell body, or *soma*. They are the most numerous of all the excitatory cell types in the cortical structures of mammals. The ability of these cells and their synapses to change function, referred to as *plasticity*, leads neuroscientists to think that they play a critical role in learning and memory. Nelson Spruston (2008) states that their structure endows them with computational functions necessary for cognitive processing, while their impairment leads to cognitive deficits such as those associated with Alzheimer's disorder and schizophrenia.

> Cell phones emit radiation. The amount varies according to different models, the distance the phone is held from the head, the distance from towers, and whether the phone is receiving (generating less radiation) or transmitting

> (generating more radiation) a signal. The amount of radiation exposure from cell phones is correlated with an increase in glucose metabolism in the brain. Whether this increase causes any negative physical or behavioral effects is unclear. Until such effects are better understood, it is common sense to avoid exposing young children to cell phones. Their young brains are thought to be more susceptible to radiation. Texting reduces exposure by increasing the distance between the phone and the head. Even small variations in distance affect the amount of radiation exposure

Each of the brain's 80 to 100 billion neurons, roughly equal to the estimated number of galaxies in the universe, makes up to 10,000 connections with other neurons, bringing the estimated number of nerve connections, depending on which neuroscientist you consult, up to one quadrillion. The axon of one neuron joins the dendrite of another at a tiny space called a *synapse* (Figure 2.6). An electrical signal arrives at the end of the transmitting neuron, stimulating the release of chemicals that quickly cross the synapse and connect with receptors on the surface of the receiving neuron. The receptors, in turn, feed the signals to a complex of proteins that process and store it. There are probably 1,461 genes that govern these synaptic proteins, more than 7% of the human genome's 20,000 protein-coding genes.

Within the limbic system, there are proteins called *neurotransmitters*. The purported role of specific neurotransmitters in depression has consumed much

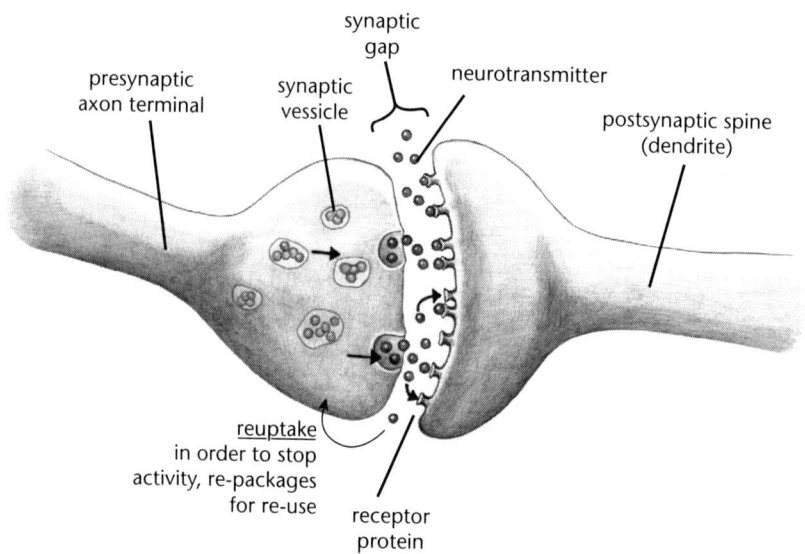

FIGURE 2.6 Synapse

psychiatric research over the past 50 years and has accounted for huge profits among drug manufacturers. It might be instructive to examine the thinking regarding the role of neurotransmitters and how that thinking has led to a medical-pharmaceutical complex.

To do that, we must first understand how neurotransmitters function in the brain. The electrical charge that reaches the axon terminal of neurons involved with emotions causes the release of calcium ions. As a result, the synaptic vesicles fuse with the presynaptic membrane, releasing the chemicals we call neurotransmitters. Neuroscientists have classified about 60 kinds of neurotransmitters operating in complicated ways that appear to be strictly regulated but, at present, poorly understood. One of the groups of neurotransmitters, the *biogenic amines* (*monoamines*), include the *catecholamines dopamine* and *norepinephrine* and the *indolamine* 5-HT, *serotonin*. These neurotransmitters operate within small cell groups in the brain, but their effect is magnified by neural projections to multiple brain areas. When a neurotransmitter is released into the synapse, it interacts (binds) with receptors on the post-synaptic membrane, affecting the electrical activity in the receiving dendrite. In order to end the synaptic action, neurotransmitters not bound are quickly reabsorbed for future use by the synaptic vesicle, through a process called re-uptake.

Neurotransmitters are thought to be implicated in a subcategory of depression called unipolar depression. The hypothesis is that depression is the result of neurotransmitter dysfunction within the limbic system. The so-called anti-depressant drugs are thought to facilitate transmission within synapses of the monoamine pathways. There are three categories of anti-depressant drugs. First were the *tricyclics*, which inhibit the re-uptake of all the monamine, thereby increasing the amount of neurotransmitters available at the synapse. Though widely used from the 1960s through the 1990s, these drugs had many shortcomings, including patient tiredness and drying of the nasal and oral tissues—and it turns out after longer-term evaluation of their use, possible increased depression and suicidal risk among a subset of patients.

A second class of anti-depressants consists of the *monoamine oxidase* (MAO) *inhibitors*, which prevent the breakdown of the monoamines by the enzyme MAO. From the late 1950s through the 1970s, these drugs were used sparingly because of the potentially serious effects from altering the metabolism of the dietary amino acid tyramine. Patients taking MAO inhibitors had to strictly limit their intake of foods high in tyramine, including cheese.

The most recent class of anti-depressants includes Prozac, which was released in 1987 after some 30 years in development. It was the first of a group of drugs that blocked the re-uptake of serotonin, making more of it available for binding. These drugs are called *selective serotonin re-uptake inhibitors* (SSRIs). While touted as having fewer side effects than tricyclics and none of the dietary limitations of MAO inhibitors, SSRIs have no positive clinical impact on depression in a significant group of patients and have been implicated in severe anxiety and decreased libido in others. In addition, some researchers and regulators have expressed concern that SSRIs might actually increase the risk of suicide among children and adolescents. The result has been "black box" warnings and general confusion among both professionals and patients. This subject will be discussed further in chapter 6.

New research suggests at least one reason why roughly one-third of depressed patients do not benefit from SSRIs. Neuroscientist Jennifer Warner-Schmidt and colleagues at Rockefeller University realized that some proteins in the brain that interact with SSRIs could be influenced by anti-inflammatory drugs (Cunningham, 2011). They showed that mice given ibuprofen along with the SSRI citalopram (brand name Celexa) failed to demonstrate the same positive clinical outcome achieved by those receiving SSRIs alone. Further, re-examination of data from studies of treatment-resistant depression in humans showed that subjects who had concurrently taken anti-inflammatory medications with citalopram demonstrated significantly less symptom relief. Just how and in what dosages painkillers such as ibuprofen, acetaminophen, and aspirin interfere with SSRIs is an ongoing investigation. The co-morbidity of pain and depression and the resulting frequency of taking both anti-inflammatory and anti-depressant medications is a promising area for further study.

The scientific criteria for proving the efficacy of a medical intervention are strict and very difficult to attain. As chapter 6 will explore further, powerful intervening variables that can affect the outcomes of science include financial and professional-advancement incentives.

> Often the best form of self-help and maintenance for your brain is regular aerobic exercise. According to the American College of Sports Medicine, exercise can reduce the risk of Alzheimer's disease by approximately 40% and can decrease depression. These benefits are in addition to lower risk of stroke (27%), colon cancer (over 60%), and recurrence of breast cancer (50%), as well as reduced incidence of diabetes (50%) and high blood pressure (40%) (Kravitz, 2007).

Beyond Neurons

Our current knowledge identifies two brain systems, the neuronal and the glial, that operate differently yet have an intimate association that accounts for the remarkable human capacity to learn and master, keys to survival. The focus of neuroscientific research has broadened in recent years to the study of the vast majority of brain cells, the glia (the Greek root for "glue"). In the past, pathologists considered these to be little more than packing material that held the brain together. Beginning in the nineteenth century, scientists used microscopes to identify the neuron, and despite their scattered locations in the brain neurons became the preoccupation of researchers, largely because of the technologies then available.

One type of glia cell, the astrocyte, named by early anatomists because it looks like a star, was thought until recently to transport nutrients and wastes to support the neurons. This function was inferred from the observation that astrocytes attached to blood vessels with some of their appendages and connected with neurons and synapses with others. However, this belief came into doubt with the discovery of the same neurotransmitter receptors on both glia and neurons. The significance of this was not fully understood until technology advanced beyond micro-electrodes to video and laser-illuminated microscopes in the 1980s and 1990s. Scientists could now observe that when they stimulated a neuron to fire an electrical impulse, the glia fired in response. In addition, the glia released neurotransmitters, starting a chain reaction with other glia.

> For unknown reasons, and in rare cases, astrocytes can become toxic and selectively kill neurons involved in controlling movement. Brian Kaspar, a neuroscientist at Ohio State University, is studying this phenomenon in amyotrophic lateral sclerosis (ALS), also known as Lou Gehrig's disease (ALS Association, 2011).

Philip Haydon (Pascual et al., 2005), now at Tufts University, discovered in 2005 that astrocytes responded to the release of the neurotransmitter called glutamate from one synapse by releasing a different neurotransmitter, *adenosine*, which then affected the strength of neuronal activity in both neighboring and distant synapses. Compared to the speed of neuronal electrical activity, this chemical communication among glia is slow, spreading like a wave through neural tissue in up to 10 seconds. While rapid brain response is required to react to and survive a pain stimulus, other brain functions, including learning, occur over longer periods of time. Until recently, theories of learning were based on the strengthening of synaptic connections. Now brain imaging reveals that learning complex abilities such as reading, playing the piano, or hitting a golf ball leads to structural changes in brain areas where there are no complete neurons—the "white matter" consisting of bundles of axons coated with myelin.

R. Douglas Fields (2004), chief of the Nervous Systems Development and Plasticity Section at the National Institutes of Health, has studied *oligodendrocytes*, glia cells that cling to axons and coat them with the myelin insulation. He has discovered that these insulation changes can increase the speed of electrical impulses through axons up to 50-fold. Like astrocytes, oligodendrocytes can sense the impulses sent through axons via the release of neurotransmitters through axon membranes. This speeding up of information transfers among brain areas involved in mastering complex cognitive tasks is thought to be a critical element in learning. Likewise, the breakdown of the mylenization process has been implicated in multiple sclerosis and Alzheimer's, and speculation exists that glia cells play a role in, and could lead to treatment of, both depression and schizophrenia.

> Recent research has focused on the developmental period labeled middle childhood, roughly from when a child in our culture enters kindergarten until puberty. During that period, the pituitary gland at the base of the brain signals the adrenal glands to start producing androgens, including dihydroepiandrosterone, or DHEA. This process, referred to as *adrenarche*, is not fully understood but appears to enhance the functioning of neurons and their dendritic connections. DHEA and other androgens may also divert glucose to aid in the maturation of the insula and anterior cingulate cortex, areas of the brain that interpret social and emotional cues. One can observe the effects of adrenarche by comparing the socio-emotional awareness of a sixth grader to that of a child in kindergarten.

Imaging techniques can trace the thickening, from caudal to rostral (back to front), of the myelin insulation from childhood into young adulthood. This knowledge has led to newer interpretations of the developmental period we call adolescence. The thickening of myelin has two consequences: It speeds up the electrical transmission and at the same time inhibits the growth of new axonal dendrites. Increased speed, then, comes at the expense of flexibility. What are the implications for learning? As the brain develops, it learns more quickly but is less flexible. Thus, the first 13 years of life are critical to language acquisition. As the involved brain area develops more myelin, it consolidates the knowledge it has gained but makes further gains more difficult. The practice in American schools of waiting until early adolescence to introduce a second language is contrary to the optimum language acquisition window of opportunity.

The wave of myelin thickening from back to front is considered an evolutionary adaptation that is unique to humans and can lead to different explanations of adolescent behavior. Behavior interpreted as irrational and self-defeating can be reframed as adaptive. Risk-taking behavior in teens can be seen as the product of the cortex's less developed myelin coating. The teen brain is also at peak sensitivity for both dopamine and oxytocin, each implicated in the reward circuits, while neuronal activity in the cortex is less restrained by myelin insulation. Social connections are especially rewarding, so peer relations are paramount. Studies show that adolescent risk taking increases significantly when peers are present. One price is increased rates of fatal car crashes, often involving alcohol, among teens. Yet there is an adaptive advantage: Risk taking renders the young adult better prepared to leave the safety of home to encounter the uncertainties of new territory.

The Brain and Trauma

One of our greatest psychological challenges relates to our memories of past experiences and how we process those memories in assessing the present—in other words, learning from the past to guide our assessment of current sensory stimuli.

Consider the following scenario. A young child is bitten by a dog. Prior to this incident, the child had learned to interpret the visual stimuli of a dog as cute and cuddly and had experienced excitement. After being bitten, the child will remember the pain associated with the sight of a dog and will likely feel anxiety. Hopefully, this child will continue to have experiences with dogs and learn to distinguish between small and large dogs, black and white dogs, beagles and retrievers, and, perhaps most important for survival, between dogs that growl and bare their teeth and ones that wag their tails. Every day we have new experiences that change, to some degree, the neural connections associated with various stimuli.

When we have an experience well outside the normal, involving a threat to our very survival, our brains function differently. Normally, our limbic system activates the autonomic nervous system (ANS) to create an adaptive survival response. However, if the threat is extreme and continuous, the ANS is flooded by corticoids, affecting the way this particular memory is stored. The amygdala is involved in processing and storing highly emotional memories, while the hippocampus creates a time perspective, giving events a beginning, duration, and end. During a traumatic event, the work of the hippocampus is impaired, so the time perspective does not occur. As a result, any stimuli associated with the traumatic memories (sights, sounds, smells, tactile stimuli, or tastes) will lead to a sudden flooding of the memories as if the event were happening currently—the classic "flashback." The survivor has lost the sense of the event being over and of having survived.

> An incest survivor related to me that she found herself at a physical location where her father had repeatedly sexually abused her. She tearfully related being able to see her father sexually touching her, feel the sensations on her skin, and smell the associated stimuli. The present was overcome by the past. It is no wonder that survivors of sexual trauma have such a challenge to experience the pleasure associated with consensual sexual activity. Any touch or intimate sensation can be processed as a threat.

Stress leads to increased production of the neurotransmitters dopamine and norepinephrine and the hormone cortisol, which activate the amygdala to alert the nervous system to prepare for danger. In the process, memories associated with fear are strengthened. Prolonged exposure to stress increases the synaptic connections within the lower, more primitive brain structures, while at the same time shriveling these connections within the prefrontal cortex. The resulting impairment of executive functioning includes reductions in concentration, abstract thinking, short-term memory, judgment, and inhibition of inappropriate thoughts and emotions.

Clinicians who are working with survivors of combat trauma are struck by the wide range of psychological tolerance for traumatic experiences. How we interpret this variability says a lot about the way different clinicians think and about the role of emotions in thinking. A common belief is that recruits in the all-volunteer armed forces are over-represented by lower income and minority populations. The reality is that the military attracts somewhat more recruits from middle-income families than their proportion of the whole population, somewhat less from lower- and upper-income families. African-Americans represent about 17% of the force and 13% of the total population. Hispanics constitute 9% of the military and 15% of the population. Nearly half of the youth of recruitment age do not meet the minimum physical and mental health standards for admission (the leading cause being obesity). ("Who is Volunteering. . . .," 2005) I am not aware of any reliable data regarding recruits' prior exposure to trauma and have no reason to believe that they would have any more exposure than others in their age cohort.

Unlike most other forms of trauma, traumatic combat experience is anticipated. Armed forces are trained by exposure to the sensory stimuli associated with combat: loud explosions, live ammunition, sensory overload, and chaos. Such training has limits, of course. Witnessing the severe injury or death of women, children, or a buddy cannot be simulated. Training also includes recognizing the signs of severe depression and psychological trauma in oneself and one's fellow combatants and the resources available to address them: the chain of command, medics, chaplains, and the mental health professionals who make up the Combat Stress Team.

A reality in providing timely and expert services to combatants suffering from traumatic stress is the lack of professionals with the requisite training. This expertise is attained through specialized education and supervised experience. The work is emotionally demanding, and the burnout rate among professionals is high. Training and maintaining an expert workforce is a never-ending challenge.

> Cognitive processing therapy (CPT) is a highly structured intervention consisting of 12 or 13 sessions that has been applied to military survivors of traumatic stress (Resick, Monson, & Chard, 2008). Symptom-rating scales

are obtained pre- and post-treatment to measure outcomes. Worksheets are employed to address the beliefs and emotions that arise from traumatic experiences. In keeping with the cognitive-behavioral paradigm, the sequence is: activating event (sensory stimuli), belief (thought or interpretation), and consequences (emotion and behavior). The following vignette illustrates its application.

C is a veteran of the Vietnam conflict, where he served as a medic. He sought help because of recurrent flashbacks of the death of his best buddy, whose life he was unable to save after a grievous injury. At the beginning of treatment his scores on both the trauma symptom checklist and the depression inventory were well above the level of clinical significance. In two sessions, he was asked to write a description of the activating event, including as much sensory detail as he could remember along with the accompanying thoughts and feelings.

C described in detail the helicopter flight to the scene of his buddy's combat injury; the sight of the gaping abdominal wounds; the sound of the victim's labored breathing and expressions of pain; the feel of the internal organs as he tried to replace them in order to transport; the stench of the bodily wastes, burning flesh, and sweat; and his buddy's imminent death. His associated belief was that he should have been able to save his friend's life. His emotion was recurrent, intense guilt that had persisted for 30 years.

Future sessions and homework focused on posing questions that gently challenged his beliefs and considered alternative interpretations, again using worksheets. Automatic thinking patterns that can produce faulty conclusions were examined. C had never talked about the death of his friend or his resulting beliefs and emotions. Instead, he had unsuccessfully tried to avoid the thoughts and feelings by self-medicating with alcohol. By finally revealing his memories and beliefs in a supportive environment, he was able to confront the reality of his situation: There was nothing he could have done to save someone with such horrific injuries. Further, he concluded that abusing alcohol was dishonoring the memory of his heroic friend.

Post-treatment ratings of symptoms of both trauma and depression were well within the sub-clinical range. A follow-up two years later confirmed sustained recovery.

The Brain/Body Connection

While it might be tempting to think we have advanced from the mind/body dichotomy made popular by Descartes in the 1600s, it remains pervasive today. Medicine is organized into specialties that magnify the separation. Psychiatry and neurology are distinct from internal medicine. Until very recently, health insurance plans maintained different benefits for conditions and services believed to be physical versus mental. In the United States, separate systems of care exist for supposedly physical and mental conditions.

This dichotomy ignores the fundamental fact that the brain is as much an organ as the eyes, the stomach, the spinal cord, and the liver. The brain interacts with the body to monitor and regulate functioning to promote optimal health. Stress originating in the brain's processing of stimuli can cause headaches, heart irregularities, and sleep disorders. This interaction is two-way and dynamic. The immune system, hormones, nutrition, and hydration all affect the functioning of the brain.

Cytokines are released through the body's immune system in response to infection. They bind to neuron receptor sites in brain structures that affect emotions. In turn, the neurons respond by producing *neuropeptides*, which cause fatigue, reduced concentration, and behavioral withdrawal. Sometimes we have asymptomatic chronic inflammation; that is, there are no symptoms such as a sore throat or cough but our immune system is active, resulting in persistent symptoms of depression. C-reactive protein, a marker for low-grade depression, increases the risk of more serious depression. Persons diagnosed as having depression or bipolar disorder have higher levels of inflammation; those with the most persistent inflammation do not respond to either anti-depressant medication or talk therapy. However, inhibiting cytokines seems to help the depressive symptoms to remit. Research on mice suggests that a higher level of the enzyme IDO, which is elevated in certain inflammatory conditions, correlates with symptoms of depression. Conversely, lowering those levels reduces the behavioral manifestations of depression in rodents.

> The discovery of the correlation between inflammation and depression is important but requires further study before it can be translated into effective clinical application. The correlation is not causative. One theory is that the hormone IDO is elevated by inflammation and, in turn, might contribute to depression. As noted earlier, there is evidence that anti-inflammatory medications might interfere with the action of anti-depressants. There are many other possible explanations. Coming up with effective remedies requires slow, deliberative thinking.

Hormones associated with sexual feelings and behavior also affect mood. Men with lowered levels of testosterone are more likely to complain of depression and self-doubt. Women approaching menopause experience a drop in estrogen, which can contribute to depression and a sense of hopelessness. An underactive thyroid increases the risk of a mood disorder seven-fold, while an overactive thyroid can unleash a chain reaction resulting in classic anxiety symptoms: racing heart, sweating, and irritability.

The maxim "You are what you eat" applies to the psychological, as well as the physical, self. We know that calcium is critical to the process of electrical activity that allows neurons to communicate with one another. Low levels of omega-3 fatty acids correlate with depression in women, possibly by diminishing levels of serotonin. Some seasonal allergies cause minimal symptoms of rhinitis (runny nose) but also contribute to severe headaches, nausea, and heart palpitations, symptoms usually associated with anxiety. Lower iron in the blood affects cognitive functioning in women, even if they don't reach the threshold for anemia. Taking iron supplements improves attention, memory, and learning.

Water also plays an important role in cognitive functioning. Even mild dehydration can cause shrinkage in brain cells and resulting enlargement of the brain's ventricles. A study of young children found that giving them a glass of water before a test improved scores. In the elderly, who often have a diminished sense of thirst, dehydration can cause symptoms often associated with dementia: confusion, forgetfulness, and slurred speech.

Indeed, focusing our thinking about thinking too narrowly, on only the brain, limits our understanding. Thinking, a component of interpreting stimuli, is the result of complex electro-chemical activity among billions of neurons and glial cells in multiple sites within the brain, interacting in a system of continuous feedback loops with the body and the environment. Unfortunately, current technologies do not allow us to fully understand the totality of this complex phenomenon.

In the next chapter, we will examine the other component of interpretation—emotion. Thinking about emotions is also instructive of how we seek meaning in complex topics.

3

THINKING ABOUT EMOTIONS

The intuitive mind is a sacred gift and the rational mind is a faithful servant. We have created a society that honors the servant and has forgotten the gift.

—Albert Einstein

Let's not forget that the little emotions are the great captains of our lives and we obey them without realizing it.

—Vincent Van Gogh

We are now going on a brief side trip to explore interesting terrain that shares location and features with our chief destination—cognition.

The study of psychology includes objective phenomena, which we call behaviors, and subjective experiences, which have been divided into two categories—rationality and emotion, or thinking and feeling. Plato and Aristotle noted the distinction between these two subjective experiences and believed that it was the capacity to be rational that distinguished humans from other animals. (Unlike Plato, Aristotle believed that the mind had three, not two, functions: cognition, emotion, and conation—or will, which we explore in chapter 5.)

The dichotomy between thinking and feeling illustrates the cognitive process of classifying and labeling experiences in the most economical manner. We interpret certain experiences as thinking, others as feeling, and view them distinctly. Consequently, psychology has pursued them as two separate areas of study. Modern neuroscience, though, is finding this simple dichotomy to be messy in terms of brain functioning. While the neocortex plays an important role in what we experience as thinking, and the amygdala and limbic systems have been implicated in what we call emotions, thoughts and emotions are not processed by separate systems. Rather, each is the product of complicated interactions among multiple brain sites. The dichotomy, as it turns out, is false. There is no such thing as pure logic, devoid of emotion. To enhance our survival, we need both.

> The false dichotomy between rational thought and emotion is evidenced in politics and religion and in the interface between them. Robert P. George of Princeton University is an emerging leader of conservative Christianity. He characterizes the divide between conservative and liberal thought as a debate about the nature of the self, a battle between reason and passion. Like Aristotle and St. Thomas Aquinas, George contends that there is an objective moral order discernible by human logic and that individuals possess the free will to obey it or not. Thus, reason controls emotion. George contrasts his view with that of the Scottish enlightenment thinker David Hume, who argued that the world contains facts but not values. George paraphrases Hume as saying that reason is the slave of the passions (Kirkpatrick, 2009). The consideration of those things called thoughts and those things called emotions becomes a debate involving complex thought and deep passion.

Perhaps not surprisingly, there is no unanimity among the experts on a definition of emotions. Some researchers focus on the biological manifestations and might study hormonal levels, brain changes, muscle activity, or skin electrical conductivity in laboratory animals and humans. Others explore the conscious experiencing of emotions, including subjects' self-reports. Like other words and concepts, the meaning of emotion and feeling is observer dependent. Underlying these different approaches is a fundamental philosophical question: How can we objectively study and confirm subjective experience?

> An example of a clear differentiation between emotion and logical thinking is the phenomenon of *phobias*. Many people experience strong, instantaneous fear responses to such creatures as snakes and spiders, even though we rarely confront any that are dangerous today. For our distant relatives, however, they constituted a mortal threat. A much more present threat in modern culture is the automobile, but do you know of anyone with a car phobia? Some evolutionary adaptations can take a long time.

Prepare yourself for more dichotomies. *Ontology* refers to the nature of the subject of study, a specification of the concept. If we examine a tree, for example, we might select specific characteristics or its similarities or differences with other living things classified as trees. In studying emotions, we might specify biologic manifestations or cognitive reports of subjective experience. Once we decide what we will study, we need to determine how we know what we are learning, a process known as *epistemology*. Philosophers have created a further dichotomy, dividing the epistemic into *empiricism*, knowledge obtained from sensory inputs (experience), and *rationalism*, knowledge acquired through cognitive processing or the use of reason. Thus, we observe that the leaves of certain trees assume different colors in fall. Further observation can determine the changes in ambient air temperature, the chemical composition of nutrients in the soil, the amount of rainfall and resulting moisture levels of both the air and soil. Utilizing this empirical knowledge, scientists can construct theoretical relationships between patterns of leaf colors and measures of temperature, nutrition, and moisture. Similarly, psychologists can use empirical methods to measure subjective and objective aspects of emotions, then develop theories about their stimulation, neurological processing, and evolutionary origins.

Language provides words to represent phenomena, although the phenomenon itself cannot be defined. Consider the two words "red apple." In kindergarten, we were taught to interpret certain processed visual stimuli as red and to distinguish it from others identified as green and blue, plus various combinations of the three. There is no way to know if my interpretation of the stimuli I label "red" is the same as yours. Nor does it really matter. We can get by perfectly well with proximity. "Red" is subjective, in that it involves the interpretation of visual stimuli by a mental process. "Apple" is thought of as objective because it exists in reality and can be experienced by our senses. We can see that it has a certain shape on the outside and meaty flesh and seeds when cut open. We can feel the texture of its skin, smell the skin and the internal juices, hear the crunch when we bite and chew, and taste the flesh as sweet or sour. The words "red apple" represent our interpretations of multiple sensory phenomena. Emotion can be thought of similarly. It is a word with associated definitions, not the phenomenon itself.

In 1884, William James published an article in *Mind* entitled "What Is an Emotion?" At a time when psychology was beginning its separation from philosophy, and before the advent of psychological and neurological research, James argued that "the perception of bodily changes as they occur *is* the emotion." In other words, an emotion is the cognition of our behavior in response to stimuli via the somatosensory system. The cognitive-behavioral formulation is thus conceived of as

stimuli → behavior → interpretation → emotion

In this conceptualization, emotions provide a way to organize our understanding of our actions. Further, this theory suggests bodily states as the cause of emotions. While this conceptualization has been surpassed by others, based on additional psychological and neurological research, it represented an intellectual achievement in its day.

Antonio Damasio (1994) defines emotions as specific and consistent collections of psychological responses triggered by certain brain systems when we experience objects or situations, either through direct sensory stimulation or from memory. They are part of the bioregulatory devices necessary for survival.

> The American Psychiatric Association created the *Diagnostic and Statistical Manual* (DSM) in 1952 to standardize the classification of those abstractions called "mental disorders." By 1980, the third version (DSM-III) had moved away from a heavily psychoanalytic conceptualization of disorders (e.g., eliminating the concept of "neurosis") to a supposedly more explicit, operationalized diagnostic criteria and entities. The goal was to increase inter-rater reliability (the likelihood that one professional would render the same diagnosis of a given patient as would others) to facilitate replicable clinical research. The newer diagnostic groups were based on a more careful description of observable phenomenon but did not lead to a better understanding of underlying etiology and intervention. APA President Carol Bernstein, MD (2011), termed this a "paradox."
>
> The APA tested new diagnostic criteria as it developed the DSM-5, the implementation of which has been delayed by the Federal Government until October 2015. Hoping to address "a failure to capture the rather messier reality faced by clinicians and researchers alike," the DSM-5 approach was to create large subcategories of disorders based on scientific evidence of a similar etiology, a kind of "megastructure." The DSM-5 has been disavowed by many—including Thomas R. Insel, MD, director of the National Institute of Mental Health—for lacking in validity and scientific integrity, among other things. The fate of this latest effort will be subject to an ongoing debate that will be illustrative of our collective efforts to create new meaning by combining previously developed concepts with newer information and understandings—a manifestation of the real-life drama of the human quest for cognitive order amidst the chaos that results from the limitations of our thinking.

Neural mapping of the limbic system suggests that emotions have evolved from and are elaborations of general vertebrate arousal patterns unique to mammals. Neurochemicals such as dopamine, serotonin, and noradrenaline increase or decrease brain activity associated with body movements that we label emotion. A different neurological explanation of emotion implicates the left prefrontal cortex, which is activated by sensory stimuli that cause a positive approach. Experiments confirm that selective activation of that area is correlated with more positive appraisals of stimuli.

In *The Ravenous Brain*, Daniel Bor (2012) notes that all animals are constrained by a value system (good or bad) born of emotion (pleasant or painful). The more highly evolved human emotional system expands that value system, shaping more sophisticated behavior and enhancing survival within the context of a complex and hierarchical social environment.

The American Psychiatric Association's *Diagnostic and Statistical Manual-IV-TR* (2000), recognizes four categories of anxiety disorders: panic, phobia, obsessive-compulsive behavior, and generalized anxiety. Alternatively, neuroscience identifies two types of anxiety with distinct brain activity. "Defensive avoidance" includes fear, panic, phobia, and flight behavior and operates in the amygdala. "Defensive approach" describes generalized and anticipatory anxiety and is centered among the septo-hippocampal circuits. The outward behavioral signs of most stress appear similar, despite different underlying neural mechanisms. The DSM-5 (2013) makes a distinction between *fear*, the response to real or perceived threats, and *anxiety*, the anticipation of future threats.

> The autonomic fight-or-flight response within the sympathetic nervous system is triggered by a perceived threat to survival. The adrenal glands prepare the muscles, heart, and immune and nervous systems for aggression, escape, and severe injury. The anterior pituitary adrenal cortex system elevates levels of glucocorticoids in the blood, while the hypothalmic-adrenal medulla system increases blood levels of epinephrine and norepinephrine. When this process is triggered by harmless sensory stimuli that the brain associates with a prior real threat, the result is posttraumatic stress.

Gerald Clore and Andrew Ortony (1998) add that emotions are not unitary constructs but rather have four major components: cognitive, motivational-behavioral, somatic, and subjective-experiential. There are no sensory receptors specific to emotions; both cognition and emotion depend on the same sensory organs/systems. It is cognition, through a complex feedback loop, that gives meaning to the emotional experience. Further, emotions are conceived as having two contrasting functions: preparation for rapid action, activated by sensory stimuli, and flexibility of action, mediated by cognitive processes that verify the stimulus, assess it in context, and make an appraisal and decision regarding action.

Words that are used interchangeably with emotions include "feelings" and "moods." Different psychologists make different distinctions among these terms. Emotions are sometimes thought of as having an object, as being about something. A feeling can refer to an objectless affective state. Others view emotions as automatic and regulatory, while feelings are the sensing and recognition of the emotion. A mood is a frequently occurring or continuous feeling. This lack of precise and generally accepted definitions is significant, and problematic.

Kenneth Heilman (Heilman et al., 2012), professor of neurology and health psychology, University of Florida, outlines the "three-dimensional" model of emotions, which includes *valence* (pleasant versus unpleasant), *arousal* (activated versus lethargic), and *motor activation* (approach or avoidant behavior). Thus, fear involves unpleasant valence, activation, and either approach or avoidance. Depression is unpleasant, lethargic, and avoidant. Joy is pleasant, activating, and approaching.

> At first blush, the valence of anxiety would seem to be negative, or unpleasant, compared to its opposite, relaxation. But is that so? Maya Tamir of Hebrew University found that chronically anxious subjects preferred being anxious prior to performing mental tasks and performed better when anxious. Brett Ford of the University of Denver found that chronically anxious subjects chose to be anxious even when it was subjectively unpleasant. There is a difference between *wanting* to experience an emotion and *enjoying* it. University of Michigan researcher Kent Berridge notes that the subjective experiences of wanting and liking involve two separate groups of neurotransmitters. Indeed, an intense desire for anxiety is a state that resembles an addiction, reports Harris Stratyner of Mount Sinai School of Medicine. Thus, the binary opposites of valence are not supported by the underlying neurological processes. This finding could be a factor in the resistance of some patients labeled schizophrenic to take tranquilizing medications, or in the reluctance of abuse victims to leave their perpetrator (Schwartz, 2011).

David Carmel, a postdoctoral researcher at New York University, was lead author of a study (Carmel, Nasrallah, & Lavie, 2009) that concluded that people are better at detecting words that contain negative emotional meaning than those that connote positive emotions. Subjects were exposed to a word for fractions of a second, too brief for them to consciously comprehend it, then asked to guess whether the word was emotionally neutral or had affective content. Subjects were most proficient at choosing words with negative emotional valence. One empirical conclusion could be that rapid processing of negative emotions enhances survival, a phenomenon referred to as the *negativity bias*. Are physical pleasure and pain emotions? Are hunger, thirst, and sex—sometimes labeled "drives"—emotions? It depends on your definition. Is jealousy an emotion or a variation of anxiety concurrent with certain thoughts about someone else? How about disgust, love, or stupidity?

> A study of the perception of physical pain by Sean Mackey of the Stanford School of Medicine found that physical contact with a loved one (youngster with mother, lover with lover) significantly reduces the subject's rating of the intensity of the pain. Further study by *fMRI* showed that visual exposure

> to the loved one via a photograph sparked activity in the reward centers of the amygdala, hypothalamus, and medial orbitofrontal cortex, while reducing activity in the major pain-processing areas, the left and right posterior insula. The researchers think that maternal affection and romantic attraction are more than merely a distraction from physical pain and involve a process within the same pleasure pathways activated by cocaine and other pleasure-inducing substances (Park, 2010).

The Biochemistry of Emotion

In *Molecules of Emotion*, Candace Pert, PhD (1998), included both pleasure and pain in her definition of emotion and explored their biomolecular basis. Her research began with the *opiate receptors* found on the surface of cells in the body, including the brain. These receptors are molecules made up of proteins, which are strings of amino acids. One neuron can have millions of receptors on its surface, which function as a sensory system at the cellular level. Instead of sensing sights, sounds, touches, smells, or tastes, receptor cells sense information via molecular properties when binding with elements called *ligands*. This molecular information is sent from the cell's surface to its interior, where it changes the state of the cell. There are a great variety of ligands and receptors. However, only those that match precisely will bind, in a process called *receptor specificity*.

Scientists have identified different kinds of ligands and have categorized their chemical differences into three groups. Neurotransmitters are among the smallest and simplest ligands, generally existing in the brain to carry information across the synapses between neurons. Steroids, which are created from cholesterol, are hormones that include those for sexual functioning (testosterone, progesterone, and estrogen) and those that express and motivate responses to stress (corticoids). It is the third group of ligands, peptides, that became the focus of Pert's research.

By the mid-1900s, science focused on brain wave patterns and the electrical activity within the brain because that was what the existing technology, the EEG, was able to measure. Pert was among a group of researchers who brought focus on a kind of second nervous system, the ligand-receptor interface. This molecular interaction was far more ancient than the electrical system, even pre-dating the important role of neurons and a separate organ labeled a "brain." Unlike the localized functions of neurotransmitters within the synaptic cleft, peptides moved through the bloodstream and cerebrospinal fluid to influence cells throughout the body.

Pert first focused on the opiates, drugs such as morphine that had a dramatic effect on the experience of pain and pleasure and a significant clinical impact on a patient's self-report of reduced pain. Pert set out to understand how these drugs worked at a molecular level. In the process, she contributed to a knowledge base that would lead to advances in the understanding and treatment of an array of illnesses and conditions that crossed the boundaries of medical specialties. Her first breakthrough, in 1972, was the discovery of the opiate receptor. Identification of the receptor meant there must be substances in the body that bound with it—a natural opiate. By 1975, Scottish researchers studying pig brains identified a substance they called *enkephalin* that bound to the opiate receptor. This endogenous (produced inside the body) ligand had the same effects as the exogenous (originating outside the body) drug morphine. American researchers labeled the substance *endorphin*, or endogenous morphine.

Peptides are tiny bits of protein that in turn are strings of amino acids held together by carbon and nitrogen. A chain of approximately 100 amino acids is referred to as a *polypeptide*; those with over 200 are labeled as protein. The first peptide replicated in the lab was oxytocin, which has been implicated in the female orgasm, uterine contractions in labor, and maternal bonding, as well as in the experience of pleasure in both genders. Peptides are produced throughout the organism and share the function of distributing information at a molecular level in all the organs, including the brain. Research has determined that all vertebrates, from the lowly hagfish to the *Homo sapien*, have opiate receptors in their nervous systems. The scientific implication is that peptides and opiate receptors are likely of great importance to the evolution and survival of the organism.

Studies of cadaver brains found a high concentration of opiate receptors within the limbic system, commonly thought to play a key role in the experience of emotions. Pert further established that opiate receptors were highly concentrated in the *periaqueductal gray area* connected to the limbic system. It is this area of the brain where the perception of pain is interpreted. The mapping of opiate receptors seemed to accord with the electrical pathways of brain sites associated with emotional experiences. The assumption was that neuropeptides must be communicating with their receptor sites across the synapses.

This theory was challenged when one of Pert's postdoctoral fellows, Stafford Maclean, devised a new autoradiographic technique that could locate where neuropeptides were produced, which in many cases was at significant distances from the receptors. Further study and analysis led to conclusions at great variance with the existing understanding that the vast majority of neuronal communication occurred at the synapse. Pert and others theorized that peptides circulated throughout the body, finding receptor sites in multiple remote locations. She believed she had discovered the basis for the mind-body connection. In her view, peptides and other "informational substances" were the biochemicals of emotions.

Emotions play an important role in memory. We are more likely to remember experiences associated with emotion, be it of positive or negative valence. The evolutionary perspective is that emotions help us remember what is important: both those locations and experiences we associate with pain and fear and those that we link to pleasure and safety. Because peptides circulate simultaneously throughout the brain and body, they produce a coherent response that we interpret as separate thoughts, emotions, and behavior.

The late Robert Plutchik of Albert Einstein College of Medicine proposed a three-dimensional circumplex model to explain relationships among concepts of emotion. (www.google.com/search?q=plutchik%27s+wheel+of+emotions+pdf). The top circle identifies eight primary emotions arranged as four opposites. Like the colors on a color wheel, the model digitizes the analog experience of emotion, both our own (via somatosensing) and that of others (primarily via visual and auditory stimuli). The vertical dimension represents intensity. The exploded model allows identification of dyads consisting of a combination of the two adjacent primary emotions. Plutchik further postulates that emotions serve a critical role in a process whose ultimate effect is the reestablishment of a state of equilibrium. Note the return to the linear cognitive-behavioral model: stimulus → thinking → feeling → behavior.

Within the context of clinical utility, I find Gloria Willcox's "The Feeling Wheel" (http://med.emory.edu/excel/documents/Feeling%20Wheel.pdf) most helpful to patients in describing their emotional experiences. This model identifies three fundamental categories of emotion: mood, comfort, and aggression. Mood is joyful or sad, comfort is anxious or peaceful, and aggression is angry or in control. The latter dichotomy is predicated on the assumption that we experience anger when we interpret stimuli as out of control and threatening as opposed to interpreting the environment as safe and in control. The model also allows for variations on these fundamental types, based on context and cognition.

The Campbell Soup Company, among many other purveyors of consumer products, has learned the important role that emotion plays in consumer choices. Their research found that consumers' memories of an advertisement had no significant relationship to sales. Using biometrics to measure minute changes in skin-moisture levels, heart rate, depth and pace of breathing, and posture, they were able to identify aspects of a soup label that stimulated an emotional response that preceded the decision to purchase. Steam pictured emanating from the soup bowl prompted subjects to report feeling more emotionally engaged and therefore more likely to put more soup cans in their shopping carts.

When we make a consumer choice, often it is not the product we desire but rather the emotional state we associate with it. We don't want the sports car, the stylish clothes, or the romantic vacation. We want the emotional experience we expect to come with it. David Nowell, PhD, has devised a tool to assist us in understanding our preferred emotional states. The Preferred States Inventory can be downloaded for a small fee at www.DrNowell.com. Knowing our preferred states not only can help us make better consumer choices but also better social and vocational ones.

Some categories of emotion include a cognitive element in their definition. Thus, shame might be a mixture of anger, depression, and anxiety, accompanied by thoughts and memories associated with a specific experience or series of experiences. Grief is depression, with associated thoughts and memories about a lost object (a significant person, pet, or job, for example).

A psychiatric/neurological disorder that offers insight into the interplay of emotions and thoughts is the *Capgras delusion*. Named after a French psychiatrist, this rare disorder is characterized by the conviction that a loved one (parent, spouse) has been replaced by an impostor. The patient recognizes the loved one as identical in all physical attributes but experiences emotional incongruity with the memory of the loved one. Neurologist V. S. Ramachandran (2005) discovered a further twist: The delusion existed only through visual stimuli. The patient believed his mother was an impostor when he saw her in person. However, when he heard her on the phone, he instantly recognized her as the real thing. Ramachandran notes that the visual and auditory systems have different connections to the amygdala. The auditory stimulus triggers an emotional response of recognition, while the visual, due to some unexplained malfunction, does not. Ramachandran cites this as underscoring the role our emotional reaction plays in understanding our environment.

> One of the most vivid descriptions of extreme anxiety comes from Stefan Fatsis (2008) in *A Few Seconds of Panic*. This 40-something sports writer recounts his pre-season experience with the Denver Broncos as a would-be placekicker. After weeks of conditioning and learning the basics of kicking, he was suddenly and unexpectedly ordered by Coach Shanahan to attempt a 30-yard field goal under game-like conditions: behind an offensive line, facing an onrushing defensive line with split seconds to execute in front of his teammates, coaching staff, and fans. Time became distorted, cognition blurred, somatosensory feedback overwhelming. Fatsis was "totally freaking out."

Language and Emotion

Biochemistry is one avenue for creating meaning from emotions; language is another. In *The Stuff of Thought* (2007), Steven Pinker examines emotions expressed through swearing. Culture defines what is interpreted as offensive. In contemporary American culture, "the seven words you can't say on television" reference sex and bodily secretions. In other cultures, such as the orthodox Jewish community in which Pinker was raised, negative religious references are defined as obscene. Regardless of the variation in definition, obscenity serves a universal purpose, says Pinker. For one thing, swearing is a means of expressing emotions, especially those with negative valence. Moreover, dirty language evokes previously learned meaning and emotion in those who hear and process it.

Pinker adds another level of insight. The listener, generally aware of his/her emotional reaction, interprets it as being stimulated by the person swearing and believes the swearer not only intended to elicit a negative response but knows the listener realizes this intent. It is this ability to interpret such complex emotional expressions that is believed to distinguish human cognition from that of other primates: I know that you know that I know, and on and on. Referred to as the *theory of mind*, this awareness develops in modern humans at about age four and has evolved as humans have become increasingly dependent on larger and varying groups of others for their survival. More on this awareness of ourselves and our relationship with others, otherwise referred to as consciousness, in chapter 5.

Puzzle solving illustrates another relationship between cognition and emotion. Mark Beeman, a neuroscientist at Northwestern University, reports on research showing that subjects are more likely to solve word puzzles after viewing a comedy routine. He postulates that amusement improves the ability to detect weaker, more remote patterns. Solving a word puzzle, then, results in a rush of dopamine as a reward. These findings have neurological equivalents. Brain imaging in subjects who anticipate a puzzle they have yet to see shows significant activation in the anterior cingulate cortex, an area strongly correlated with positive moods. Activation in this brain area is also associated with a widening of attention, making it more open to distraction and looser connections. Precipitous solutions, like creative insights, seem to be the result of sudden, new connections, as opposed to slower, analytic processes (Carey, 2010).

Positive emotional valence seems to engage a broader attentional state that has both perceptual and visual components, according to Adam Anderson (2005), a psychologist at the University of Toronto. Positivity allows one to see and think more broadly, making new meanings and creating order out of chaos.

Psychotherapy is almost always sought to alleviate negative emotional experiences. It is common, for example, to obtain a history of past traumas, such as sexual or physical abuse, involvement in life-threatening situations, or witnessing death or serious injuries. The danger is that the focus on the negative is so intense that it reinforces it. Successful therapy needs to incorporate positive experiences. From a clinical perspective, I find that even the most depressed and hopeless patient can access some kind of past contentment, relaxation, or joy, no matter how brief and fleeting. "What is the best thing that ever happened to you?" or "What is your most positive memory?" can be an opening to more positive ways to interpret the present.

Another perspective for thinking about language and emotion involves the brain areas associated with expressing each. The vocalizations of primates originate in activity in the brain stem and limbic systems, older neural structures associated with emotion. Human expressions of emotion, such as laughing, crying, or moaning, arise from subcortical areas. Steven Pinker's (2007) interest in swearing leads him to note that utterances after hitting your thumb with a hammer originate subcortically, as do the involuntary motor and vocal tics of Tourette's syndrome. On the other hand, language deemed as more intentional and ordered originates in a region of the cerebral cortex called the left perisylvan.

Some studies suggest that the right hemisphere plays a more important role than the left in the comprehension of emotion. This assertion has been criticized on the grounds that a whole hemisphere is too large and unspecified to be ascribed such a function and that this asymmetry should have a more focused etiology (Wager et al., 2003). Such criticism assumes that comprehension of emotions has a specific brain site rather than being the product of a process involving interactive feedback loops among multiple agents.

Emotions and Behavior

An example of how differences in sensory processing influence emotions and behavior is demonstrated by research led by Yu Gao (Gao et al., 2010) of the University of Pennsylvania. A longitudinal study was conducted over 20 years, starting with a cohort of 1,795 three-year-olds. The galvanic skin response to a series of unpleasant stimuli was gathered for all subjects, along with nine measures of social adversity within their home environments. Twenty years later, 137 of the subjects were identified as having been convicted of significant criminal offenses. When the offender group was then compared with 274 non-offenders from the original study, the only statistically significant difference between the two groups was that the offenders had lower fear (galvanic skin) responses at age three.

Along with similar studies, this one confirms indirectly the interpretation that there is a correlation between a low-functioning amygdala, as measured by lower galvanic skin responses, and later antisocial behavior. The amygdala interprets danger before our consciousness does and transmits the danger signal to the orbitofrontal cortex, which processes it for decision making. If the orbitofrontal cortex receives a diminished fear response message, the development of a conscience is apparently impaired.

Given these interpretations of research findings, what might a scientist conclude? One seemingly sensible conclusion might be that a child with a hypoactive amygdala needs to be exposed to more intensive doses of fear-inducing stimuli in order for the orbitofrontal cortex to make pro-social decisions. However, further examination of the research on the development of conscience suggests that it is a combination of both fear and empathy that produces such pro-social thinking and behavior. Gao concludes that the amygdala and orbitofrontal cortex of three- to five-year-olds can be significantly influenced by good nutrition, exercise, empathic connections, and clear expectations regarding appropriate behavior.

> Neuroscientific findings suggest that there is a "magic quarter second" between a sensory stimuli and an emotional reaction, during which it is possible to experience cognition. It is this magical moment that forms the foundation of cognitive-behavioral therapy. One variant of CBT is *stress inoculation*. The following vignette illustrates the application of cognitive-behavioral principles in a clinical setting.
>
> S, a nine-year-old male, was referred by his parents for behavioral concerns associated with Prader-Willi syndrome. PWS is a congenital condition whose symptoms include muscular hypotonia, global developmental delays, cognitive disabilities (average IQ of 70), compulsive eating with associated life-threatening obesity, immature sexual development, and behavioral challenges, including temper tantrums and compulsive behaviors. For S, the parents identified compulsive overeating and temper tantrums as the targets for change.
>
> Stress inoculation is a cognitive-behavioral intervention intended to teach cognitive skills in order to establish and maintain self-control of anger. It conceptualizes anger as beginning with stress and individuals with poor temper control as lacking the cognitive resources for coping with stress. In the case of S, I decided to broaden the role of stress to include his eating disorder. (Note that treatment of medical and psychological conditions invokes the scientific method: After a comprehensive collection of relevant data, a hypothesis is created; an intervention is designed to test the hypothesis; an objective measurement of the outcome is obtained which either confirms the hypothesis—symptoms remit—or creates additional data from which an alternative hypothesis can be created and tested—treatment fails. The TV show *House* portrays this scientific process, albeit in sometimes annoying, obnoxious variations.)
>
> Seemingly working against the success of this intervention were the genetic (and therefore supposedly unalterable) underpinnings of the symptoms, the lack of any professional literature to support the intervention's viability with persons with PWS, and the patient's limited cognitive abilities as measured by IQ testing. Offsetting these apparent liabilities were two highly motivated, cooperative parents and a patient with an unending desire to please.
>
> Phase One of treatment involved cognitive preparation. First, S was taught to identify the somatic precursors of the stress associated with anger and hunger. For him, they included tension in his stomach and clenching of the jaw and fists. Then, he was provided with a pocket notebook and

small pencil that he was to carry at all times to record the specific visual and auditory stimuli that triggered the stress response. Given his cognitive limitations, his mother and teacher were enlisted to transcribe his verbal reports.

In Phase Two, S rehearsed specific cognitive and behavioral techniques designed to enhance his coping skills. Provocation by siblings and peers was cognitively reframed as a game: The intent of the provocation was to enrage him; if he got angry, the provoker won; if he didn't get angry ("keeping your cool"), he won. Magnifying the reward of victory was the notion that it would be the provoker, not he, who would look foolish. S conceptualized the sensation of hunger as a monster in his tummy, demanding his obedience. This invoked the developmental imperative to resist being told what to do. He also was taught emotional control skills via relaxation training. Tensing and then relaxing fist and stomach muscles with the therapist added a fun element to the intervention.

Applying these skills to his daily experiences constituted Phase Three. A key skill for S was self-talk. We rehearsed repeatedly a script for responding to the earliest signs of stress: "OK, S, I can feel my stomach get tight and my fists clench. This means I am getting tense. The reason I am tense is that X is trying to get me angry (or get me to eat). If I get angry (or eat), he/she wins. But if I keep my cool, I'll win, and X will lose. I'll be a cool dude, and he/she will look like a fool. So I'm going to keep my cool, and be cool. I am a winner."

He reported in weekly on his successes and challenges via the notebook. We would review every provocation, reinforcing successes, and rehearsing "even better" behavioral responses. The notebook, as well as parental and teacher feedback, confirmed a dramatic improvement in his ability to resist provocation, either social or gastronomic. Emotional and behavioral stability has been sustained into adulthood.

It is not just youngsters labeled delinquent or developmentally disabled whose thinking is ruled by their emotions. The judges who adjudicate their cases function under the same psychological processes. A primary responsibility of the judiciary is to interpret the law. This legalese is often confusing, rife with ambiguity, and open to multiple interpretations. Steven Pinker (1994), referencing L. M. Solan's *The Language of Judges*, states that judges "try to find a way around the most natural interpretation of a sentence if it would stand in the way of the outcome they *feel* is just" (emphasis added). Pinker is one of the most renowned psychologists of our time. He is not referencing this use of *feel* as if it were interchangeable with *think*. Like all of us, judges make decisions that conform with their neural networks, thereby producing a response in the reward center of the brain, at least in part a function of dopamine. Remember taking one of those fiendish SAT or Graduate Record tests and being confronted with a question that your existing neural networks could not process? The emotion associated with the inability to interpret is of a decidedly negative valence. In those cases, I found emotional relief from a random guess, then quickly moving on to something I could (hopefully) interpret more easily.

Yet another approach to thinking about emotion is to consider the notion of *attachment*, which refers to the degree of emotional attunement between a mother (or other key caregiver) and the young child. Freudian theory focused on the infant's relationship with an object, the mother's breast. English psychiatrist John Bowlby had experience working in a residential facility for emotionally disturbed, delinquent youth after World War II. He wrote about a pattern he discerned between the early emotional deprivation that the youngsters had experienced and their subsequent anger, impulsiveness, and lack of concern for the consequences of their behavior. His thesis was that the lack of stable, consistent emotional attachment in the early years inhibited the development of empathy, resulting in young psychopaths. The correlate, of course, was that a solid mother-child bond led to healthy emotional development.

American developmental psychologist Mary Ainsworth (Ainsworth et al., 2014) became interested in Bowlby's theory after two years of observing mother-child interactions in Uganda. She set out to test the hypothesis in a controlled setting by devising the Strange Situation experiments. At Johns Hopkins University, she observed 23 white, middle-class mother-infant pairs in their homes multiple times during the children's first year. When the babies were one year of age, she observed each pair in the laboratory, using the Strange Situation protocol, which consisted of a series of 3-minute episodes over a 30-minute period. In the first episode, the mother and child were in a room with toys. In the next, a stranger entered the room. Third, the mother left the child alone in the room with the stranger. Fourth, the mother returned, and the stranger left. Fifth, the mother left the child alone. Sixth, the stranger returned. Finally, the mother returned. The psychologist's observations focused on the child's behavior during the two episodes when the mother prepared to leave and during the two when she returned.

The researchers discerned three patterns of behavior among the children, from which they constructed three categories. About two-thirds of the children cried mildly as the mother left but were easily comforted when picked up and soothed upon her return. These cases were labeled as *securely attached* and categorized as Type B. Another 20% didn't cry when mom left and showed no response upon her return. These children were categorized an *anxious-avoidant attachment*, Type A. The final 15% cried intensely when mom left and couldn't be soothed upon her return. Ainsworth interpreted this behavior as implying an *anxious-ambivalent attachment*, Type C.

Like most psychological research, this one speaks to the nature of human cognition as much as it does the subject under study. Bowlby discerned a pattern, and Ainsworth concurred. She attempted to prove the truthfulness of the pattern through controlled observation. She made meaning out of the children's behavior by constructing three categories and assigning a cause-and-effect relationship between the assumed quality of the mother–child bond and the observed behavior.

> D is a young mother of an infant who referred herself for psychotherapy due to escalating anxiety since becoming pregnant and giving birth. The thoughts associated with the anxiety were that she lacked the capacity to be a stable mother figure.
>
> Removed from the care of her parents at age five, D was raised by a series of reasonably stable foster families. She retained memories of her family of origin: much time spent alone in her room listening to alcohol-fueled verbal and physical conflicts between her parents. While her subsequent foster care did not include any trauma, there were the sudden, unexpected moves from home to home and school to school that are a too-frequent occurrence for children dependent on such care. She graduated from high school and obtained steady work, where she was considered pleasant, reliable, and competent. She fell in love and married a stable man. Their relationship was mutually fulfilling until she began her (planned) pregnancy, at which time her thinking became more and more focused on the belief that she would be inadequate to fulfill the maternal role.
>
> After introducing her to the cognitive-behavioral paradigm, I had her chart her daily experiences leading to distress: sensory input (baby crying) → interpretation (I am inadequate/failing) → emotion (anxiety) → behavior (crying). Underlying her belief in her inadequacy was her interpretation that removal from her family of origin and from foster care homes was because of some unspecified void in her character.
>
> Exploring alternative interpretations occurred on two levels. First, we considered all the possible explanations for why a baby cries, referencing child care resources. Together we normalized what she had seen as abnormal. Second, we reframed the impact of her childhood experiences from inadequacy to resilience. She had survived instability and had been able to experience more success academically, vocationally and romantically, than many of her peers with more stable upbringings. This positive self-appraisal required repetition and reinforcement and led to a reduction in anxiety and an improvement in maternal functioning and satisfaction.
>
> A history of poor attachment need not determine fate. Psychotherapy and other kinds of corrective experiences help people make sense of their histories by creating a coherent personal narrative.

Creating a cause-and-effect relationship in the study of psychology, as in all science, represents the quest for meaning. When the phenomenon under study is complex, creating causation requires ignoring or minimizing the influence of other contributing factors and assuming a model of central control. The attachment theory that emanates from this research ignores or minimizes the role of temperament as a contributing factor in the observed behavior. The concept of temperament grows out of the intuition that babies demonstrate a range of seemingly fixed emotional tendencies: Some seem placid, others are cuddly, and yet others are irritable. Most mothers will intuit that their infant's emotional personality is a contributing factor to the mother-child bond. Calm, cuddly babies contribute to a stable emotional attachment as much as do calm, loving mother figures. Human development is a dynamic, complex system with multiple feedback loops among contributing influences within the brain, the body, and the environment. Our cognitive abilities are strained in attempting to make this complexity meaningful. We simplify by creating binary concepts (nature vs. nurture, attachment vs. temperament) that ultimately limit the very meaning we seek.

The binary concepts of nature and nurture are being challenged by the study of identical twins, who share identical DNA (Miller, 2012). While some of the pairs have been raised separately, most have grown up in the same household, yet significant differences can be measured in their physical and mental development. One explanation is tied to neither nature or nurture. *Epigenetics* refers to chemical processes that influence how our genetic processes are expressed. Each gene can be rendered stronger or weaker, even turned on or off, by a *DNA methylation*. Some identical twins report the same interests in music, politics, and beliefs, including belief in their ability to communicate telepathically between themselves. Others exhibit markedly different interests and aptitudes, including significant differences in intelligence as measured by standardized tests.

Yet another example of the difficulty in conceptualizing emotion is to compare efforts to develop computer software that recognizes speech versus those programs that attempt to identify emotions. The algorithms that underlie speech recognition are based on a sequence of sounds and with repeated use can adjust to the accent or other vocal variations of a particular user. The output can be judged to be right or wrong based on a straightforward comparison to an input. If I say, "The woman wore a hat," and my software types "The woman war a hat," we can easily agree this is an error.

However, software that attempts to recognize emotions depends on either visual or auditory inputs. Visual processing involves establishing a database of pictures of hundreds of faces expressing a series of emotions. A subject's facial expression is scanned and analyzed, pinpointing 12 key trigger areas like eye and mouth corners and then comparing them to the database. The computer calculates which emotion is expressed by the face's correlation with the database images. Recognizing emotion through speech analysis is based on three characteristics that researchers have correlated with a particular affective state: frequency factors, such as pitch; energy descriptors, such as loudness; and temporal features, such as rate, duration, and pauses.

There are two features of this research that shed light on how we think about emotion (Franapanagos & Taylor 2005) (Ekman, 2003). First, different studies identify different core emotions. A face recognition approach identified anger, sadness, fear, surprise, disgust, and happiness, plus combinations of these emotions. One speech analysis study conceptualized emotions as being discrete (only one can be experienced at a time) and identified anger, fear, sadness, boredom, joy, and no emotion. Another succeeded in identifying fear, anger, joy, and sadness, but not confidence or sarcasm. Daniel Bor (2012) asserts that fear, disgust, and anger are the three primitive emotions. There is no consensus on what constitutes the set of basic emotions. Moreover, the identity of each emotion in the database was defined either by the person expressing it (subjects were told to exhibit a specific emotion on their face or in their voice when reading a sentence) or by consensus among a panel of persons who put each picture or recording into a predefined category. Thus, the definition of a specific emotion relies on either individual interpretation or consensual validation.

> Lack of consensus among the experts in a field is not limited to psychology and neuroscience. Mathematicians do not even agree on the definition of a polyhedron. Again, meaning is observer dependent.

These challenges in developing emotion-recognition software touch on a related question: How do people recognize emotions in another person? This query leads us to the work of Paula Niedenthal (Carpenter, 2011), former director of research at the National Centre for Scientific Research at the Blaise Pascal University in Clermont-Ferrand, France, and currently at the University of Wisconsin–Madison. She has focused her research on the smile—how the face creates it, what emotional states it represents, and how an observer interprets it.

A smile is produced by the contraction of the zygomaticus muscles in the cheeks, resulting in the corners of the mouth being drawn upward. The recognition of a smile by an observer can be accomplished in three ways: by comparing the geometry of the face in question to that of a smiling one; by considering the context and comparing it with situations in which a smile would be expected; and, most important according to Dr. Niedenthal, by mimicry. When someone smiles at us, we will usually smile back. This finding brings to mind the concept of mirror neurons and the notion that the brain areas active in the smiler are similarly activated in the observer. Dr. Niedenthal reports that different brain areas are activated by different categories of smiles. Perceiving a smile from a happy person activates the brain's reward centers. When parents perceive a smile from their own babies, a different brain pattern is elicited, this one within the orbitofrontal cortex. However, this area is not activated when parents perceive the smile of a non-related baby.

This research is an example of *embodiment*, the notion that cognition is the result of interactions involving multiple feedback loops in the brain, the body, and the environment—a model that will be explored further in the next chapter. For now, we will consider how embodiment manifests itself in the recognition of a genuine versus a false smile. Subjects were shown pictures of smiles and could easily distinguish between those that were genuine and those that were false. When subjects placed a pencil between their lips, restricting the action of the zygomaticus muscles so that they were unable to mimic the smiles in the pictures, their ability to distinguish between genuine and false smiles declined significantly. This finding supports the model of cognition that includes the body as essential to the dynamic process.

Emotions and Psychotherapy

The typologies we create depend on the context in which they are used. Psychotherapy differentiates between *primary* and *secondary* emotions, and between those that are *adaptive* and *maladaptive*. Leslie Greenberg (2002), a proponent of emotion-focused therapy (EFT) in the Department of Psychology, York University, Toronto, describes a primary emotion as the immediate, internally generated, "gut-level" response to stimuli, which is recognized and assessed within therapy to determine if it provides adaptive enhancement and organizes action. Maladaptive emotions are those learned in an earlier developmental and social context but no longer appropriate. Secondary emotions are responses, perhaps defensive, to the primary emotions. Examples include feeling ashamed of one's anxiety or feeling angry about sadness. They are maladaptive to the extent that they interfere with therapeutic interventions to regulate, modify, or transform the primary emotions. Greenberg identifies five principles that underlie the understanding and change of emotions within the clinical context.

- *Emotional awareness* is more than just thinking about a feeling or connecting a word to it. Greenberg describes it as "feeling the feeling in awareness," then articulating it in language. A skilled therapist helps a patient to safely approach, tolerate, and accept an emotion, thereby achieving emotional awareness. Avoiding or distorting emotions often leads to maladaptations such as destructive secondary emotions, obsessive or intrusive thinking, and self-injurious behaviors such as cutting, anorexia, or substance abuse.
- *Emotional arousal and expression* within therapy is more than mere venting. It addresses emotions that have been avoided and has been found to be a critical component in successful treatment of trauma survivors. However, arousal of

strong emotions is successful only within the confines of a strong therapeutic relationship. The ability to regulate emotions is believed to originate in a stable, safe, and soothing early attachment experience. The therapist emulates a healthy early attachment through empathy and validation of patients' emotional expressions, thereby promoting self-soothing and self-regulation.

- *Emotional regulation* has been advanced in clinical settings through the treatment of borderline personality disorder—characterized by a pervasive pattern of unstable, rapidly changing emotions, thoughts, and behaviors—and is often found concurrent with a history of childhood abuse. Marsha Linehan pioneered a cognitive-behavioral approach that included the teaching of emotional regulation skills such as self-soothing, grounding, breathing meditation, and mindfulness (Heard and Linehan, 1994).
- *Reflection on emotions* goes beyond awareness to make meaning of emotions within the context of one's life narrative. A common example from my practice involves people who have experienced various forms of abandonment during childhood or adolescence: death of a caregiver; absence of a caregiver via substance abuse or mental illness; unexpected, lengthy separations. Such early experiences can give rise to anxiety, sadness, and/or anger. Persons are likely to re-experience these primary emotions whenever the inevitable sense of abandonment occurs within an intimate relationship, such as when a partner is late or preoccupied. Through the cognitive function of language, the patient can organize, structure, and incorporate the past and present experiences into a meaningful story.
- *Emotional transformation* replaces a negative, maladaptive primary emotion with one that enhances current functioning, using a number of therapeutic techniques that involve replacing one emotion with another. Imagery can be a powerful tool, as can the therapeutic relationship in which alternative emotions are modeled. Such therapeutic interventions give rise to yet another dichotomy in thinking about emotions: *experienced* versus *expressed emotions*. Researchers distinguish between the subjective reports and the observable manifestations of an emotion. Thus, a subject may label her internal experience as anger, while independent raters might interpret their observations of her emotional state as sadness. This approach involves the implicit assumption that the terms "anger" and "sadness" represent distinct phenomena that cannot co-exist.

Emotions and Stress

Stress has been implicated in numerous physical disorders, including gastric ulcers, various digestive disorders, and cardiovascular disease. From these correlations came the cause-and-effect notion that stress causes disease and the next logical step: to reduce anxiety via medication and/or psychotherapy. Kelly McGonigal (2013) of Stanford University cites research that casts a deeper understanding on the stress–disease connection. While patients with stress do experience more health problems, it is not the stress itself that is the determining factor. Rather, the connection to disease is between how patients *think* about their stress and the somatic consequences. If patients view stress as negative and contributory, it will have that outcome. Research subjects educated on the positive consequences of stress performed far better than those who weren't. For instance, telling a subject that more rapid breathing has the benefit of added oxygenation in the brain resulted in reduced anxiety and enhanced performance on a social stress test. McGonigal notes that oxytocin, a hormone associated with pleasure, is actually secreted as part of the stress response and promotes social-seeking behavior. In yet another study cited by McGonigal, persons aged 34 to 93 who experienced major stress increased their risk of dying by 30% as shown in a five-year follow-up. But this was not true of all subjects. Those who acted on their oxytocin urges and spent significant time caring for others showed no increase whatsoever in death rates.

Stress need not have negative consequences. How we think and behave can transform stress into a positive personal and social experience, from debilitating symptoms to resilience and courage. Psychotherapy—which involves complex interaction and feedback among the brain, the body, and the therapist—can be the vehicle for such a powerful transformation. The therapist can serve as a kind of emotional coach, guiding patients in expressing their emotions. This technique is based on the concept of embodiment, with attention to the somatic manifestations of an emotion, such as posture, muscle reactions, and behavior. This approach harkens back to William James and his idea that we are afraid because we run.

The neuroscience of emotional transformation has been explored by neuroscientist Richard J. Davidson (Davidson and Begley, 2012), professor of psychology and psychiatry at the University of Wisconsin–Madison and director of the Laboratory for Affective Neuroscience and the Waisman Laboratory for Brain Imaging and Behavior. In the laboratory, he uses functional magnetic resonance imagery (*f*MRI), positron emission tomography (PET), and quantitative brain electrical activity to measure the role of brain areas in emotion. Persistent stress strengthens the axonal connections from the amygdala to the prefrontal cortex, resulting in impairment of executive functioning: impaired concentration and short-term memory, and a resulting increase in compulsive behavior. He suggests that negative, withdrawal-related effects in the right hemisphere can be transformed by activation of the approach-related system in the left prefrontal cortex. Mindfulness mediation and cognitive-behavioral therapy function to strengthen axonal connections from the left prefrontal cortex to the amygdala, allowing more inhibitory signals to calm the emotions.

Have you ever noticed that when your stress levels increase, you begin to arrange items, tidy up, or start checking that you did something? The neurological interpretation is that the amygdala is sending more electrical action to the prefrontal cortex. The psychological interpretation is that we are engaging in behaviors over which we have control in the face of stress, which we experience as a loss of control. We are trying to assure ourselves that we have at least some control.

It is hoped that by examining emotions, we can better appreciate the link between those abstractions we label "thinking" and those we label "feeling." Depending on our conceptualization, they are opposites, indistinguishable, or somewhere in between.

4
THINKING ABOUT THINKING

A human being is simultaneously a machine and a sentient free agent, depending on the purpose of the discussion.

—Steven Pinker,
How the Mind Works

If the brain were so simple that a single approach could unlock its secrets, we would be so simple that we couldn't do the job.

—Anonymous

The human understanding when it has once adopted an opinion . . . draws all things else to support and agree with it. . . . But far more subtly does this mischief insinuate itself into philosophy and the sciences, in which the first conclusion colours and brings into conformity with itself all that comes after.

—Francis Bacon,
Novum Organum

A young mother left her five-year-old daughter with a babysitter for the first time. The sitter was an adolescent girl of Mennonite faith. In keeping with her heritage and as a sign of respect to God, she wore a small white bonnet where her hair was gathered in a bun. A few days later, the mother and her daughter attended a community gathering, where the girl saw a group of Mennonite women, each wearing their traditional head covering. The girl exclaimed, "Mommy, look at all the babysitters."

—as told by Ellen Bush

Our metaphorical trip has covered territory called classical psychology in search of a definition of thinking, then has explored that complex terrain named the brain to begin to understand the neurobiology that underlies the subjective experience. A brief side trip offered a glimpse at that aspect of interpretation labeled emotions. Now we plunge into that other component of interpretation, referred to as thinking.

Understanding the interpretation of sensory inputs, like all interpretation, must be broken into bits in order to have meaning. One such model was offered by the late Edward Pols (1992), a philosophy professor at Bowdoin College. He digitized rationality into two distinct but complementary functions, *primary rational awareness* (processing of temporospatial stimuli within our size range, such as people, objects, and artistic creations) and *secondary rational awareness* (non-temporospatial entities such as theories, narratives, and sub-atomic particles). At the risk of oversimplification, I propose that, for our purposes, thinking does not create that thing we call reality; it creates our individual and collective interpretations of that reality as experienced through our sensory system.

Our knowledge of neuroscience is not yet advanced enough to explain the complete set of rules that govern thought processes. To begin our exploration of the intricate features of thinking, we turn again to Steven Pinker, author of *How the Mind Works*, *The Language Instinct*, and other books and articles that explore the complexities of psychology and neuroscience.

Few self-respecting 14-year-old boys come willingly for psychotherapy. J was no exception. He was brought to my office by his parents—angry, sullen, and determined to not cooperate. The presenting problem was an escalating pattern of oppositional behavior at both home and school. I intuited that he was very intelligent, and very persistent. He made no attempt to restrain his contempt for me or my profession.

I avoided direct inquiry, assuming it would only further inflame his resistance. Rather, I brought out a set of cards for teens from the Ungame, which is intended to promote communication. We took turns reading and responding to them. He gave cryptic responses to the first few, while I tried to model more thoughtful answers. Then he read his next card: If you could become anyone you wanted, whom would you choose?

"Does it have to be a person?" he asked.

"Not necessarily. It is up to you," I replied.

After a pause, he continued. "I'd like to be my cat. I wonder what he thinks about all day." What ensued was a lengthy consideration of animal versus human cognition, memory (his cat remembered where the food bowl and litter box were), and consciousness. My valuing his intelligence and ideas during that discussion was the beginning of developing therapeutic rapport. At future sessions, his parents reported that during the ride to my office, he complained bitterly about having to come. However, once inside he continued to actively explore psychological concepts and, with gentle prodding, began to apply them to his interactions with family, authority

> figures, and peers. He was able to mold his thinking, feeling, and behaving into a less oppositional format without having to admit to any faults or weaknesses. We agreed that he was ultimately in control of his behavior. He went on to college, where he studied psychology.

Pinker (1997) asserts that contemporary conceptions of the mind are archaic, arising from the psychoanalytic and behavioral theories that dominated the 1950s through the 1970s. As the best hope for understanding the complexity of our minds, he proposes a psychology of many computational faculties engineered by natural selection and examines two key concepts, intelligence and consciousness. In this chapter, we will examine his thinking about intelligence. However, he is not referring to IQ tests and what we think of more commonly as intelligence.

A word of caution. Do not confuse computation, which is a process, with a computer, which is a machine. The comparison of the brain to a computer is misleading. A computer transistor is either on or off. This *serial architecture* means an action has a single cause and effect, referred to as a *deterministic framework*. By comparison, a neural synapse is an incredibly complex system. The simple version is that within the synapse an electrical signal is converted to a chemical one, then back again to an electrical signal. As scientists study the details, they are learning that hormones, neurotransmitters, other chemicals, and even the pattern and pace of signal transmission affect the interpretation from one neuron to another. Synaptic activity is far more complex than a binary computer process, and a neuron is more than an on-off switch. Thus, there can be multiple causes and effects from this *parallel architecture*, resulting in a *probabilistic framework*.

Even in the simplest nervous system, like the 100 or so neurons of the worm *Caenorhabditis elegans*, a complete mapping of the interconnections of each neuron does not lead to an understanding of how the system functions. Multiply the worm's number of neurons by a billion, and you have a total that is equivalent to the number of neurons in the human brain.

We are beginning to understand the neuronal activity that produces the subjective experience of thinking, but we have a long way to go. What we have, so far, are theoretical models based on the characteristics of thinking as we currently understand them.

Intelligence

What are the characteristics of that thing we refer to as rational human thought? To address similarly complex questions in the realm of time and space, Einstein engaged in thought experiments. Pinker (1997) cites psychologist David Alexander Smith as doing the same in analyzing the concept of intelligence. Smith imagines what makes a smart alien from outer space. First, think about a dumb alien. It might bump into rocks and tip over or fall into lakes, rendering itself inoperable. It might see a bird take flight from atop a tree and decide to do the same, crashing to the ground. We would not judge such activities as intelligent. A smart alien, by contrast, would pursue goals by some set of effective rules. For example, it might first conduct tests to determine the effects of gravity and atmosphere before engaging in experiments in flight.

Pinker defines intelligence as "the ability to attain goals in the face of obstacles by means of decisions based on rational (truth-obeying) rules." Earlier behaviorists were interested only in what was directly observable and, therefore, measurable. B. F. Skinner (1904–1990) even questioned whether humans actually thought. Pinker, by contrast, is not so rigid. He believes that intelligence requires that we have *beliefs* and *desires*, concepts not readily measurable. He gives the example of two people who decide months ahead to meet in a distant city on a specific date, at a specific time, in a specific location. As Pinker says, "In what other domain could laypeople—or scientists, for that matter—predict, months in advance, the trajectories of two objects thousands of miles apart to an accuracy of inches and minutes? And do it from information conveyed in a few seconds of conversation?" Pinker describes the "calculus behind this forecasting" as *intuitive psychology*: "the knowledge that I *want* to meet my friend and vice versa, and that each of us *believes* the other will be at a certain place at a certain time and *knows* a sequence of rides, hikes, and flights that will take us there."

> It is not uncommon for people of a certain age to observe among our youth the increasing use of technology, a reduction in reading, and a drop in achievement scores and conclude that their intelligence is on the decline. At the same time, scores on standardized IQ tests have been increasing dramatically over the past century. Psychologist John Flynn (2013) asserts that these increased scores reflect the requirement for improved mental habits needed to create meaning in an increasingly complex world. These habits include coherent classifications of the concrete and abstract, the creation of connections among abstractions, and enhanced consideration of the hypothetical. Does this mean that youth are smarter than their grandparents? The Flynn Effect demonstrates differences as thinking evolves. IQ tests measure certain aspects of cognition, but there is an emotional component to a judgment of being smarter.

Pinker states that scientific psychology will have to explain how living tissue can express beliefs and desires. There is apparently nothing in our neurons that can explain it. Therefore, Pinker thinks the *patterning* of neural tissue is the critical factor. These patterns are essential for computation, and thinking is computation. Consequently, the fundamental activity of the brain is *information processing*, which Pinker refers to as *computational theory*.

What, then, is information? Pinker brings us back to that fundamental scientific concept of causation. *Information is the correlation between two or more things that is the result of rule-driven (versus random) processes.* I see two frogs copulating in my backyard pond. I see an egg sac develop. I see tadpoles emerge and develop into small frogs. I see this year after year. I read about this process in high school biology. I conclude that there is a rule-driven process here, not a chance happening. The awareness that there is an element of probability at work does not negate the apparent validity of the information. Perhaps some years more or fewer tadpoles will be produced. The addition of an element of probability only adds to the complexity of processes but does not prove they are random.

Information can be a physical thing. The marks left on a road by screeching tires provide information from which the speed and direction of a vehicle might be inferred. This information also exists as a symbol, a representation with meaning. It is transmitted via the retina, sent electrically down the axon, transformed to chemicals in the synapse, and back to electricity at the dendrite. It is processed and stored in the form of neuronal networks. The information in the form of a tire pattern has caused the creation of a neuronal network, which carries information. A system that carries and processes information is engaging in computation.

The goal of psychological study under computational theory is to discover the forms of mental representations (symbols) and the processes that access them, which Pinker (1997) refers to as demons, perhaps derived from the Greek *daemon*, meaning "genius." These processes of access also include basic logical and statistical operations apparently performed within the dendrites of millions of neurons.

I will try to illustrate the use of mental representation by the following example. You look at a short string of letters, *c-h-a-t*. If you are native English speaking, you immediately associate this combination of four symbols with a kind of light conversation. If you are exposed to the same four symbols while visiting friends in Paris and have a working vocabulary in French, you will associate them with a small, four-legged, furry creature that purrs and chases birds in the backyard. The knowledge attached to the word "chat" cannot be connected to physical qualities of the letters. When you first learned that "chat" in French means "cat" in English, you didn't have to relearn your knowledge about either word. Pinker theorizes that your knowledge of "chat" in English was connected to a node that has an address or location among the neural pathways. In the context of a different language, the four letters will have a separate node, one more closely connected to your knowledge associated with the English word "cat." You do not have to reconnect "chat" piece by piece to the qualities associated with "cat." According to Pinker, this is how we know that the mind contains mental representations specific to abstract entries for words, not just the shapes of the printed word.

The mental representation of a Parisian cat is illustrated in Figure 4.1, which is referred to as a *semantic network*, a *knowledge representation* or a *prepositional*

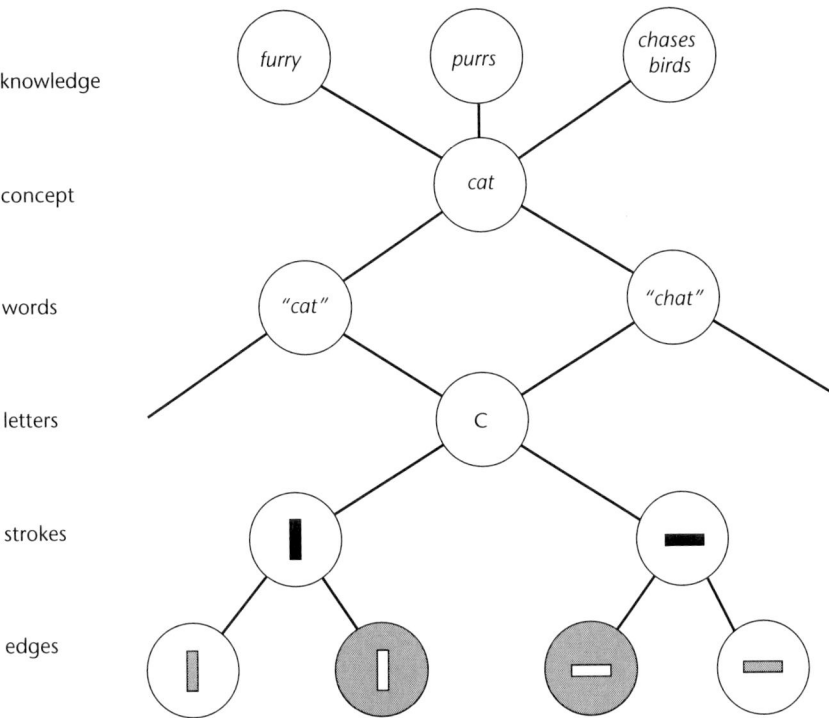

FIGURE 4.1 Knowledge Representation of "Cat"

database. Starting at the bottom, our retinal ganglion cells process visual stimuli by contrast and edges. Edges define strokes, and letters and numbers consist of the arrangement of strokes. The letters form two words, both of which are connected to the same concept, which in turn is associated with many facts, each of which has many more connections (fur to mammals, to similarities and differences with all other fur-bearing creatures, with all other mammals, with all other things, living or not). The combinations are exponential. Pinker estimates that our brain can compute a hundred million trillion different meaningful thoughts (let alone all the nonsense!).

That we have more than one kind of mental representation is demonstrated by the research of psychologist Michael Posner and colleagues (Carr et al., 1979). He timed the responses of subjects in identifying the same versus different letters. Subjects quickly pushed a button to report that *A* and *A* are the same and *A* and *B* are different. The same quick responses were reported for *a* and *a*, and *a* and *b*. The letters have the same visual forms. The response time increases, however, when the letters are flashed in pairs that have a different visual appearance: *A* and *a*, or *a* and *B*. When the second letter in different (capital or not) visual form is flashed seconds after the first, the response time returns to the same speed as when the letter had the same visual representation. Inductive reasoning suggests that in a few seconds, the mind converts the visual representation into an alphabetic one.

Pinker (1994) posits at least four formats of mental representation. First is the visual, as represented by Posner's study. Second is phonological, a stretch of sound syllables, like the way we silently repeat a phone number to ourselves until we dial and then forget it. Third is grammatical, a hierarchy of representations that determine how we construct sentences and communicate verbally, as Pinker explains in *The Language Instinct*.

The fourth form of mental representation is what Pinker calls mentalese, the language of thought. Mentalese differs from thinking in our native tongue. Pinker describes how communication by language includes ambiguities that the listener can fill in accurately via context. For example, the headline "Queen Mary Gets Bottom Scraped" is usually understood as a nautical, not a proctological, procedure. Mentalese, however, must be precise. One aspect of mentalese is the mind's creation of the gist of sensory input. Your visual system is processing the shape and order of the symbols on this page. From this input, your mind will distill concepts and knowledge. The other aspect of mentalese is the traffic of information in electrical and chemical form among brain areas. The hippocampus, encoder of long-term memory, and the frontal lobes, where decision-making occurs, are not directly connected to the areas that process raw sensory stimuli. There are intermediary regions that further process the stimuli before they reach the memory and decision-making functions.

These four (or more) forms of mental representation are essential to the modular organization of mental functioning, which places the representations of knowledge into separate formats (the cat is furry, purrs, and chases birds). The late Herbert Simon at Carnegie Mellon (2002) was interested in the way that complex systems, including the mind, are organized. He described them as being both modular and hierarchical. The army consists of divisions, that consist of brigades, then battalions, down to platoons. This book has chapters, then sections, paragraphs, sentences, words, and letters. Such structure of modules arranged in hierarchies isn't by chance. Elements arranged in modules attain a state of stability that permits their arrangement into hierarchies.

Let us return now to the neuron, a kind of building block of the brain. Each neuron has multiple connections to other neurons, forming neural networks. Mathematicians Warren McCullouch and Walter Pitts conceive of connected neurons as having "neuro-logical" properties (McCullouch & Pitts, 1943). To shed light on this concept, remember that a synapse is conceived as having three categories of strength: excitatory, neutral, and inhibitory. The incoming electrical activation level is multiplied by the synaptic strength. A receiving neuron adds up the incoming activation levels. If the resulting total activation level exceeds a certain threshold, the neuron fires more rapidly. Conversely, an activation level below the particular threshold results in a slower rate of firing. The increase or decrease in the firing rate is conceived of as either on (excitatory) or off (neutral or inhibitory). Computation is based on this binary model: 1 or 0. The difference between computation by a computer and by the brain is illustrated in Figures 4.2 and 4.3. In computers, one silicon chip is connected to another and communicates with a signal of *on* or *off*. Figure 4.2 represents a computer model of our family cat and a squirrel. Combinations of silicon chips that represent fur will produce a positive signal for both creatures; so, too, for having four legs and a presence in my backyard. Different signals regarding purring and eating nuts will differentiate the two mammals. A computer, because of its architecture of one chip connected to one other, has to compute each signal individually to find a match.

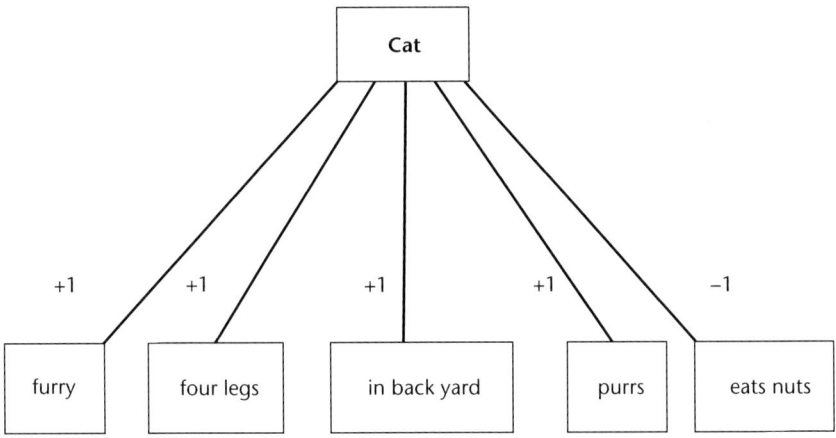

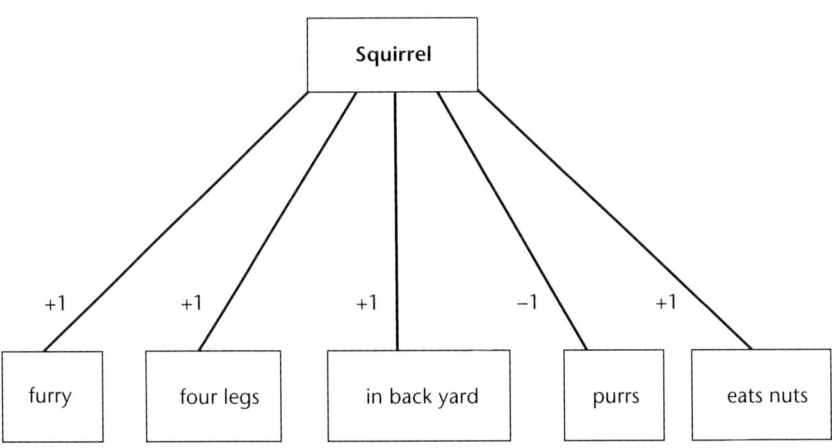

FIGURE 4.2 Computer Model of "Cat" and "Squirrel"

98 Thinking about Thinking

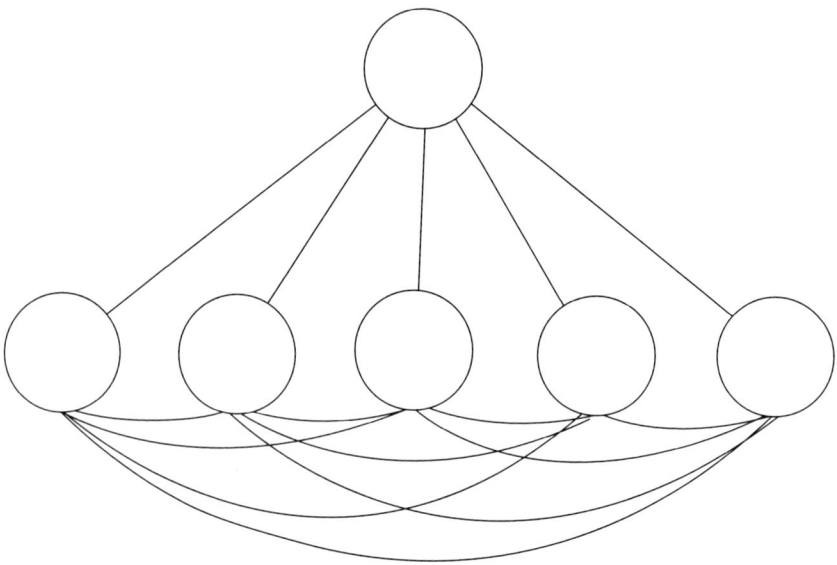

FIGURE 4.3 Neural Model of "Cat" and "Squirrel"

The brain, however, has multiple neural connections, so it can process the mental representations of each characteristic differently. Now we can begin to grasp the difference between mere computation and understanding. The computer can say which representations of characteristics equate to a cat or a squirrel. The brain goes beyond a simple "match" or "mismatch," beyond the dichotomous, and can consider the ways in which cats and squirrels are alike and the ways they are different. From this ability comes the capacity to weigh evidence, to consider probabilities, to make decisions.

The network represented in Figure 4.3 is referred to as an *auto-associator*. Pinker (1997) notes that auto-associators have five distinctive features. First, unlike a computer, these networks have content-addressable memory. Think the word "furry" and you connect with networks that include not only cats and squirrels, but many other classifications of living creatures, plus your grandmother's coat, your winter gloves, and, perhaps, the chest hair of a secret love with whom you spent a lustful weekend in Barcelona. In addition, the connections are redundant, so that if only part of a pattern is available to the network, the rest of the pattern connects automatically. We remember "cat" when associations are furry and purr, or litter box, or, in our house, Frankie and Iris.

A second feature of auto-associators is closely related. If you receive only a portion of the mental representation of stimuli, you can often fill in the missing data. A seven-year-old once gave me the following written rule for fishing: "If your just trying to cech fish and you haven't cot any yet get up and go fish another pool." My brain could compute and therefore understand this sage advice, while a computer could only respond with an error message.

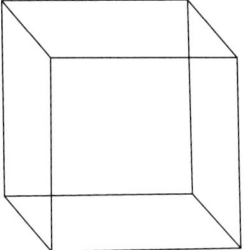

FIGURE 4.4 Visual Illusion/Ambiguity

The third feature of auto-associators is constraint satisfaction. Ambiguity occurs when we can associate the same interpretation of stimuli with different concepts. Such ambiguity occurs visually, as with the illusion in Figure 4.4. In this case, the choice of interpretation as to which square is in front of the other is inconsequential, so the mind is satisfied with either (and both) associations. In processing auditory stimuli such as spoken language, the interpretation can have consequences. Regional accents can give a word different meaning when interpreted in different parts of the country. "A-yuh" on coastal Maine equates to "yes" in the Midwestern version of English. Most people can quickly choose this interpretation after processing other language from the same speaker, plus the context in which it is used.

A fourth feature of an auto-association network is that it can automatically generalize, which gives the capacity to classify. Cats and squirrels have fur, which generalizes to mammals. Squirrels eat nuts, putting them in a class called herbivores, while cats eat mice, which puts them among the meat eaters.

Finally, Pinker ascribes a fifth quality to a neural network: the ability to learn from experience. These are not simple stimulus-response processes. The auto-association network can self-adjust in the face of new information, even creating internal representations between its input and output layers. Presumably, more complex thinking requires additional levels of internal representation.

The association of ideas was proposed long ago by such thinkers as John Locke, David Hume, George Berkeley, David Hartley, and John Stuart Mill. This doctrine proposed two laws governing human thought. These are *contiguity*, the notion that thoughts often experienced together get associated in the mind, and *resemblance*, the assumption that when two thoughts are similar, whatever is associated with the first is associated with the second. According to Pinker, association of ideas (represented today by a school of psychology called *connectionism*) attempts to explain most human intelligence as the product of simple neural networks. He disagrees with this explanation, arguing that only the "*structuring* of multiple neural networks into programs for manipulating symbols" (Pinker, 1997, p. 112) can explain uniquely human thinking abilities. He examines the capacities and limitations of simple neural networks and finds them wanting with respect to five aspects of normal thinking.

First, simple neural networks cannot account for the capacity of humans to distinguish differences from among identical stimulus generators. For example, if I am told that one of my Rhode Island Red chickens has been replaced by another, I will deem the flock to be different, even though I cannot distinguish one chicken from another. Pinker posits that the stripes on zebras evolved to give an advantage against predators, which are unable to distinguish one zebra from another. By contrast, he cites the high mortality rate of wildebeests returned to their herds after their horns were marked, concluding that the marking permits predators to distinguish one victim to pursue to exhaustion.

A second limitation of a simple neuronal network model is illustrated in language. The meaning of a sentence is derived from both the meaning of the parts and the manner in which they are combined. A combinatory point of view cannot distinguish between "Phil eats the chicken," "The chicken eats Phil," and "Phil and the chicken eat." For the listener to interpret these three simple sentences differently, he must assign roles to each combination of letters. Thoughts are built out of concepts, not stored whole. Such building of thoughts becomes incredibly complex and cannot be accomplished by the association of simple networks.

The human capacity to weigh variables is a combination of the ability to distinguish differences and the ability to combine and, as such, represents a third aspect of human thought that cannot be explained by simple neuronal networks. A more satisfying explanation comes from psychologists David Sherry and Daniel Schacter (1987), who suggest that organisms have evolved specialized memory systems engineered to meet the demands of their survival. Certain birds have the capacity to bury seeds in thousands of locations, remembering and retrieving them as their need for nutrition demands. (So much for the disparaging reference "bird brain!") The ubiquitous squirrels in my backyard have a similar, if more limited, ability. According to Sherry and Schacter, humans have evolved two separate memory systems to meet the demands they face. One is episodic memory, by which we record the who, what, where, when, and how of our immediate lives. Semantic memory, on the other hand, stores information about the more general operations of the world around us.

"Recursion" refers to the capacity to multiply the number of human thoughts into hard-to-comprehend totals, as in infinity. (Recursion as it applies to computer science will be considered in chapter 6.) This is accomplished through the creation of hierarchies, which merge one combination of concepts—a proposition—with another, then with a third, and so on exponentially: "I think. I think I know what you think. You think you know what I think you think," and on and on. This is the fourth aspect of thinking that is not possible via simple neural networks. Pinker envisions each simple thought structure being stored in long-term memory once but also connecting with multiple sites in short-term memory to create new thoughts.

Pinker cites two more cognitive abilities that cannot be explained by associationism—two opposite yet compatible modes of thinking: stereotypes and what he calls "intuitive theories." Stereotyping crudely creates whole categories by choosing similarities among selected attributes. Intuitive theories create systems of rules to define categories. These are distinctly different processes. The former simplifies by selection, while the latter creates rules that enhance understanding. Racial stereotypes restrict our understanding of individuals, while rules of grammar make communication more precise. Stereotypes might represent associationism in action, but the capacity to mentally symbolize and exponentially combine underlies the human capacity for abstraction, for establishing rules, and for creativity.

This, then, is Pinker's computational model of thought. While making associations or connections among our sensory experiences is a fundamental building block of cognition, thinking is far more than just the association of ideas. Humans have the capacity for precision, subtlety, and unending creativity. The sophomoric notions that all thoughts have already been thought, that all art has already been created, ignore the latest understandings of modern psychology and neuroscience.

Creating Memory

Thinking is the process of making meaning of stimuli. Meaning is relative; there can be no meaning in a cognitive (or emotional) vacuum. We classify a plant as a tree by comparing it to other vegetation with similar characteristics. We judge things tall or short relative to others, as we do with other characteristics: color, shape, age, and so on. Most people learn to expect certain results or consequences when they behave in particular ways in particular environments. (A deficit in this psychological process usually has dire social consequences and underlies some criminal behavior.) All of these judgments depend on memory, which compares the current stimuli with what we have processed before. Memory is created from previous stimulatory experiences stored in patterns of connections among neurons. Every stimulus that the brain processes alters in some way some existing neural connections. Even the act of remembering alters neural connections. Thus, we can never have the exact same memory twice. With up to a thousand trillion synapses, the average human brain is in a state of constant flux.

The early study of memory was guided by Aristotle's and Locke's notions that we learn by associating ideas. Ivan Pavlov discovered classical conditioning and later described two types of non-associative learning: *habituation*, when an animal ignores a trivial stimulus, and *sensitization*, or learning a stimulus that is important. These findings formed the basis of behavioral psychology, which focuses on observable phenomena—behavior. The internal processes that produced these behaviors were deemed by behaviorists to be unobservable and therefore not available to scientific inquiry.

Nobel Prize winner Eric Kandel's *In Search of Memory* (2006) describes his 40 years of research into the cellular biology of memory. His study, beginning in 1955, was guided by three principles derived from the research of predecessors such as Luigi Galvani, Hermann von Helmholtz, Edgar Douglas Adrian, Alan Hodgkin, and Andrew Huxley. The *cell doctrine* identified the neuron as the basic signaling unit in the brain. The *ionic hypothesis* centered on the transmission of information within cells via electrical means. Finally, the *chemical theory of synaptic transmission* focused on communication between nerve cells.

> The fluid nature of memory has implications for many aspects of society, not the least of which is our legal system. Witnesses are sworn to tell the "truth." The more they are questioned, the more they use their memory and the more the stored patterns of neural connections will be altered and the testimony will change. Even people we judge to be totally honest and forthcoming will have different memories of the same event at different times.
>
> Cognitive science has led to increased awareness of the unreliability of eyewitness testimony. Our brains do a poor job of encoding facial details. As both witnesses and victims relive the emotional aspects of the crime, their recollections are retrieved and re-encoded. This process allows our memories to morph to eliminate cognitive dissonance and correspond to our cognitive biases. *In Doubt: The Psychology of the Criminal Justice Process* by Dan Simon (2012) elucidates research into memory that raises serious concerns about our justice system outcomes. One example: 90% of subjects rated their memory recall as confident, while only 60% were accurate.
>
> Given the scientific evidence that memory can be unreliable, courts are beginning to respond. In December of 2012, the Oregon Supreme Court ruled that the burden of proof for the admissibility of eyewitness testimony be shifted from the defense to the prosecution to recognize potential contamination of memory by "suggestive police procedures."

Just as the experts do not agree on what an emotion is, there is also no unanimity about the number and nature of different memory systems. One duality concerns short-term and long-term memory. Short-term occurs in the frontal cortex, where the neural network interacts with other areas to make meaning and decide on appropriate action. After just a few seconds, the information may be encoded for long-term storage with the help of the hippocampus and other areas within the medial temporal lobe. Other information, like a phone number dialed for the first time, may not be processed for long-term memory.

A second distinction in thinking about memory is between recall and recognition. Recall is a partial retrieval of a stimulus from long-term memory, while recognition is a more complete one. We experience this distinction every day. We often recall people's faces but not their names.

A third dichotomy is between explicit and implicit, or declarative and nondeclarative memory. Explicit memories are those that you consciously know: your partner's name, the route to work, the number of states in the United States. Implicit memories are those that are experienced without consciousness: how to ride a bike, how to tie your shoes. These very different kinds of memory are processed in different brain areas. The hippocampus plays a necessary role in the consolidation and binding of explicit memory, which is then stored in the cortex area where it was first perceived. Implicit memory is processed in multiple areas: Motor skill learning involves the cerebellum and basal ganglia, perceptual learning the neocortex, emotions the amygdala.

In addition to these binary conceptualizations of memory, there are others. Semantic memory refers to our vocabulary and general knowledge. Performing routine tasks such as my hunt-and-peck typing or cooking breakfast relies on procedural memory. The recall of recent events is referred to as episodic memory, the loss of which can be an early indicator of dementia. Other categories of memory subject to decline during aging include source (where we first learn a particular piece of information), working (the temporary retention of short-term information), and prospective ("What did I come into this room to do?") Finally, there is thematic (the general emotional content of an event) and detail (the minutia of an event) memory.

> Psychologist Stanley Colcombe and colleagues (Colcombe & Kramer, 2003) at the University of Illinois-Champaign reviewed 18 controlled studies and found evidence that aerobic exercise led to improved memory functioning.

Try to remember the first three words of this sentence. Pretty easy for most of us. Now try to remember the first three words of the preceding sentence. (No peeking!) Not so simple. This illustrates the concept of working memory, which serves as a filter between our sensory inputs and our longer-term memory. Just how this works, like much of brain functioning, is a mystery. It seems to be far more complex than just conscious will, a concept we will explore in chapter 5.

Eric Kandel (2006) appreciated that multiple means of learning and memory resulted from varying patterns and combinations of stimuli. He sought the neural analogs of learning, the changes of synaptic connections caused by different stimuli patterns. His early research was with the giant marine snail *Aplysia*, selected because of its relatively small number (20,000) of brain cells and their grouping into nine clusters, or ganglia, allowing the identification of simple behaviors controlled by each. Along with Ladislav Tuac, Kandel discovered two important principles of learning. First, synaptic communication is changed by different patterns of stimulation. Second, the same synapse can be strengthened or weakened by such differences.

Studying the gill-withdrawal reflex in *Aplysia*, Kandel and Irving Kupfermann identified a specific motor neuron that controlled that behavior, leading to the realization that neurons and their synaptic connections do not vary. The same neurons and connections were involved in the gill withdrawal of every snail studied. Further, they found that during habituation, synaptic communication was weakened; however, it was strengthened during sensitization and classic conditioning. The duration of the memory storage correlates with the length of time a synapse is weakened or strengthened. Kandel began to conclude that chemical transmission might have an advantage over electrical in animal brains: the capacity to manage various forms of learning and memory storage.

Continuing his investigation of memory of a motoric response to stimuli in *Aplysia*, Kandel (2006) identified the role of *interneurons*, located between the sensory and the motor neurons, that release serotonin (the same neurotransmitter found in humans). These interneurons joined the sensory and motor neurons to form neural circuits of two types: *Mediating circuits* produce behavior directly through their structures, and represent a Kantian conceptualization of learning and behavior; *modulating circuits* are Lockean, modifying behavior through learning via changes in the strength of synaptic connections.

The fruit fly *Drosophilia* has been used since the early 1900s in the genetic study of learning. The commonality discovered between the underlying cellular mechanism of learning in both fruit flies and snails, and among many animal species, including humans, underscores the important biological principle that evolution does not require new specialized cells or structures to create new adaptations. Indeed, the biochemical mechanisms that support memory did not arise for that purpose, but rather were an adaptation of an efficient signaling system serving different functions in other cells.

Kandel's search for the mechanisms unique to long-term memory led to the role of proteins and genes. Nearly every gene of the genome is present in every cell of the body. Each specialized cell has a unique mixture of proteins that account for its functioning. Long-term memory is the result of the creation of additional synaptic connections. The important role of a regulatory protein CREB (cyclic AMP response element-binding protein) in both expressing and inhibiting gene activity led to two factors contributing to long-term memory: repetition and a highly emotional state. The former represents our intentional acquisition of knowledge and skills (learning vocabulary or mathematical facts, or riding a bicycle) while the latter includes intrusive flashbacks resulting from a traumatic experience. After a single exposure to threatening stimuli, the amygdala can retain memory of it throughout the organism's lifetime. Thus, treatment of posttraumatic stress can be very challenging. Learning, then, is not just cognitive. We learn emotional responses to stimuli, responses that are not conscious.

Neuroscientist have long debated between two theories regarding the encoding of memories from sensory inputs. One is that the representation of a single memory is distributed in pieces among millions or billions of neurons. Gaining more scientific support of late is a second interpretation: that a much smaller number of neurons hold a partial or "sparse" representation of a memory. Working with patients undergoing surgery to correct uncontrolled epilepsy, researchers have inserted microelectrodes deep into the brain and monitored brain activity for days at a time. From this came the discovery that a single neuron can be activated by a particular concept. Further, such cells responded to multiple representations of the same concept, even representations from different senses. Thus, a cell might be activated by a person seeing a picture of the Maine coast, hearing a verbal reference to it, reading about it, or smelling the sea.

Rodrigo Quian Quiroga, Itzhak Fried, and Christof Koch (2013) have referred to these as concept cells and theorize their functioning. For example, I first encountered Pemaquid Point in Maine many years ago. The light of that complex visual experience was converted to electrical activity in the retina and conveyed via the optic nerve to the primary visual cortex, located in the caudal region. Neurons there activated in response to only a fraction of the intricate detail of a total image. In order to make meaning, the brain can't just store a visual image; it must integrate that information with stored experience. Thus, I recognize concepts I have in memory: surf, blue, foam, rocks, trees, sea birds, seals, and, if I am lucky, whales and dolphins. I identify these concepts even though every experience with them involves some variance.

Concept cells are located in the medial temporal lobe and are thought to play an important role in converting short-term memories to long-term memories, allowing me to create new connections and memories when I re-experience Pemaquid Point each summer. I have stored the gist of that prior experience, not a fully detailed neural video. Gist has strong advantages over more detailed representations, allowing for fast and efficient creation of new connections and memories because far fewer neural actions are needed. Concept cells and their sparse representation may thus be critical to human cognition.

The Fallibility of Memory

Nearly all of our daily functioning revolves around the interaction of sensory stimuli with past experience, both cognitive and emotional, stored in memory. Given the unreliability of our memories, it might seem surprising that we function as well as we do. In *The Seven Sins of Memory*, Daniel Schacter (2001) delineates the most common shortcomings of our processing and retaining of past experiences. These include both errors of omission and commission. Schacter's group of omissions include transience (weakening of memory over time), absent-mindedness (interruption of the interface between attention and memory), and blocking (temporary inability to retrieve information). While all three can be a source of frustration and impairment, they can generally be managed with assistance.

The errors of commission are potentially more problematic, involving the presence of a degree of memory that is not accurate or not wanted. These errors reflect the very nature of the processing of memory: We select key aspects of our experience for storage, then recreate them through retrieval rather than by reproducing exact copies. These errors of commission are critical to understanding our most common errors in cognition, science, and psychotherapy.

Misattribution is assigning a memory to the wrong source due to sketchy recall of details of the experience. We cannot begin to process all the sensory stimuli around us. Each of us focuses on different aspects. In order to create meaning, we must put together the components we have retained into a coherent whole, a process called *memory binding*. The combination of selective storage and recall by reconstruction leaves much opportunity for error. Schacter cites the case of the Oklahoma City bombing of 1995 and the search for John Doe 2 based on the erroneous eyewitness report of a van rental. It was later determined by the FBI that the misattribution was the result of the witness combining two similar experiences on consecutive days involving persons renting vans. A similar binding error, called *memory conjunction*, occurs when subjects erroneously claim to have seen a picture of a face that combines elements of previously seen faces. Similarly, subjects are more likely to falsely remember words on a list if they saw similar words, such as claiming to remember *barley* when they actually saw *barter* and *valley*.

A related error occurs when witnesses view a number of suspects in a law enforcement lineup and are asked to point out the culprit. If the subject is not among those viewed, witnesses will tend to finger the one most similar in appearance, the one most familiar absent specific details. We can create associations where none exists.

Kandel (2006) notes that the late biologist Francois Jacob distinguished between two types of science. Day science involves experiments designed with precision, based on logic and pragmatism. Night science involves hypotheses based on loose associations, on exploring the possible connections among seemingly disparate processes or phenomena. Creativity is exploring new associations and connections asking the "what if?" questions. There is room for both day and night science, as long as we are clear about which we are employing at any given time.

In psychotherapy, most of a patient's presentation is based on reconstruction of past experience from fragments in storage. Rarely is there any opportunity to corroborate or validate the patient's version. The challenge for the effective therapist is to provide a safe environment in which the patient can explore different interpretations of remembered (reconstructed) experience in order to discover the meaning most relevant and helpful.

Schacter's second sin of commission is related to misattribution. Suggestibility refers to our tendency to incorporate misleading information from external sources into our personal memory. This error has particularly dire consequences that overlap the fields of forensics and psychotherapy. Schacter (2001) cites studies by University of California-Irvine psychologist Elizabeth Loftus and others documenting that suggestive questions produce distortions of memory. In one, the false suggestion that a store attendant wore a white apron was incorporated by participants into their narrative of a videotape of an alleged crime. An examination of eyewitness interviews in Britain rated one out of every six questions as suggestive. Even when witnesses recall that a detail has been suggested, their memory may be affected. More confident witnesses are no more accurate in their recall than those with less confidence. In (hopefully) extreme cases, coercive suggestive interrogation can cause false confessions.

Elizabeth Loftus reported on an early attempt to experimentally implant a mildly traumatic childhood event, being lost in the mall, in a teenager. Schacter references Ira Hyman and colleagues at Western Washington University, who were successful in implanting false childhood memories in a significant minority of college students. Their success depended on encouraging subjects to engage in rich, detailed visual imagery of the imagined event, thereby rendering it like a real memory.

Further, Schacter reports that the late Nicholas Spanos of Carleton University conducted studies on college students in which he suggested that hypnotic regression therapy (for one group) and "guided mnemonic restructuring" (for another) could cause them to "return" to the first day of their life and identify the color of the mobile above their crib. A control group received no such instruction. With no further intervention, all were asked to recall the mobile over their crib. None of the control group could, while about half of those in the other two groups did. Such recall is considered "patently preposterous" by Schacter and other experts in psychology and memory.

When I trained in psychotherapy in the 1960s, there was no mention of childhood sexual abuse. The subsequent sexual revolution modified the norms about what could be talked about, including in therapy. Suddenly there was a cohort of mostly female patients who reported victimization at the hands of siblings, parents, adult relatives, neighbors, priests, and others. This newfound freedom to uncover what was previously unspeakable had the therapeutic result of reducing stigma and shame while celebrating resilience and recovery. Like all new discoveries, especially those with high emotional content, this one was an opportunity for a few practitioners to go too far too fast in applying it to practice. Hypnosis and guided imagery were employed to help unlock supposed buried traumatic childhood memories. In reaction, parents and others who claimed to be falsely accused formed the False Memory Syndrome Foundation and sued the accusers for damages.

There was an epidemic of cases in the 1980s involving accusations of bizarre, horrifying acts of molestation of children in daycare settings. One receiving extensive coverage involved the Fells Acre Daycare Center in Malden, Massachusetts, operated by the Amirault family. Parents expressed concern following an incident in which a child engaged in sex play with a cousin (a not uncommon childhood event). Investigators conducted repeated and lengthy interviews of the preschool children, none of whom had spontaneously reported any untoward behavior by daycare staff to their parents. Questions posed were not open ended, but rather involved specific and repeated inquiry until an affirmative response was elicited. The defendants were not permitted to cross-examine their three- and four-year-old "accusers" and were convicted. Subsequent research on the suggestibility of children's memories by Maggie Bruck, PhD (Principe et al., 2013), was cited upon appeal, noting that the interview techniques themselves could be responsible for inaccurate recall. Subsequent research has confirmed that children's spontaneous reports tend to be accurate, while responses to specific questions are more likely to be distorted. Further, new information produced by additional interviews of young children is highly likely to be less than accurate.

At the time that the Amirault case was receiving widespread, sensationalized media coverage, emotions were running hot among child-serving professionals. One concluded, "Children do not lie," reducing a complex psychological and forensic phenomenon to a simple binary choice: either the children were telling the "truth" or lying. Such digitizing, while emotionally satisfying for some, ignores the analog complexity of the memory systems of developing young children, who have particular difficulty with source information, the specifics of when and where an event happened. Seasoned child therapists understand the necessity of moving slowly with their young patients, of looking for symbolic representations of their reported memories, and of the critical importance of their own self-awareness in the accurate interpretation of children's symbolic play. These qualities are beautifully displayed in Annie Rogers's (1996) *A Shining Affliction: A Story of Harm and Healing in Psychotherapy*.

Bias also plays a role in processing memories. Daniel Schacter (2001) notes five types of bias that influence our recall. *Consistency bias* refers to our tendency to reconstruct past experience so that it is similar to the present. Social psychologist Michael Ross (1989) refers to the "implicit theory of stability," our assumption that our current beliefs or experience are congruent with the past. He notes that subjects do not always have clear notions of their views on past social issues, but rather infer them from their current opinions, beliefs, and feelings in order to create cognitive harmony.

We are prone to the *change bias*, the belief that our past was significantly better or worse than the present. A study of college students' assessments of their romantic relationships showed that their recall of initial ratings of their partner's personal traits was significantly influenced by their current evaluation of the relationship. Two months after the initial assessment, those who professed more love for their partner remembered their initial ratings as higher than recorded. Conversely, those who expressed more negative feelings toward their partner recalled ratings lower than the actual. Both the change and consistency bias reflect the need for cognitive economy

Hindsight bias reflects the same need for cognitive consistency, so that our reconstruction of the past fits neatly with our interpretations of the present.

The danger is that the need to avoid cognitive dissonance interferes with our learning from experience. "I knew that would happen" blocks a more objective consideration from which we can derive important lessons. Herein lies the powerful potential, both positive and negative, of psychotherapy. In its most beneficent application, verbal therapy provides a safe, non-judgmental environment in which the patient can explore alternative interpretations of the relationship between the past and present, uncovering connections that cause undue emotional pain, distorted thoughts and beliefs, and self-defeating behaviors. Bad psychotherapy can be damaging, involving a kind of psychological imperialism that imposes the expert therapist's beliefs and biases on a vulnerable, suggestible subject.

We tend to interpreting everything, including stored memories, as they relate to our being. This *egocentric bias* reflects our encoding and recalling (however inaccurately) our own behaviors more strongly than those of others. Combined with our powerful tendency to view ourselves positively, this bias underlies much interpersonal conflict—relational, vocational, and social. Effective marital therapy avoids repetition of pre-existing conflicts over differences in recall and interpretation of the past, instead creating a safe environment in which both partners can begin to re-experience the sense of value and success that motivated their initial attraction.

The final memory heuristic cited by Schacter is the *stereotype bias*. Again based on the need for cognitive congruity and economy, memory is reconstructed to be consistent with current expectation. Racial, ethnic, gender, political, and vocational stereotypes help ease the cognitive burden at the expense of missing out on the rewards of a more fertile consideration of the world around us.

The underlying neuropsychology of all these biases is believed to reside in the bicameral structure of the brain. Our left hemisphere governs our cognition as expressed in language and symbols, while the right is more concerned with thinking in visual images and spatial locations. Based on his study of patients whose hemispheres were separated as a treatment for persistent epilepsy, Professor of Psychology Michael Gazzaniga, who heads the SAGE Center for the Mind at the University of California–Santa Barbara, postulates that the left brain provides explanations and rationalizations after the fact, creating order and meaning by integrating past experiences with current stimuli (Wolman, 2012). Such meaning is often at the expense of accuracy. The right hemisphere has been shown experimentally to interpret stimuli on a more literal basis, thereby providing a potential balance to distorted inferences created in the left. Consciously slowing our thinking increases the probability that our interpretations will be more balanced, both hemispherically and cognitively.

Schacter cites the most debilitating of memory disturbances, persistence. While transience, absent-mindedness, and blocking involve the loss of desired memories, persistence involves the opposite: obsessive, intrusive, unwanted memories that you want to forget. These are often related to heightened emotion at a time when attention is associated with activation of our survival instincts. Such memories tend to be focused on the emotionally charged stimuli, with impaired recall of more peripheral stimuli. Chris Brewin (Brewin et al., 2010), professor of clinical psychology, University of London, has conducted research demonstrating that persons suffering from clinical depression are more prone to negative self-rumination. Clinicians know that depression is by far the most co-morbid diagnosis in persons labeled with posttraumatic stress disorder. While trauma can obviously contribute to depression, it seems likely that persons with pre-existing depression will be more prone to a major depressive relapse. Conversely, the lack of prior depression might be a very significant protective factor for PTSD.

Persistence plays a role in another debilitating psychiatric condition, obsessive-compulsive disorder (OCD). We are not talking here about Aunt Millie, who gets upset if her bathroom towel is not folded in a certain way but otherwise functions well despite such quirks. Indeed, most of us have a few such idiosyncrasies, some of which may contribute to our successes in life. OCD has the opposite effect. Sufferers are unable to handle the most basic life functions because of persistent, intrusive thoughts about such things as contamination, hoarding, or checking. As with all psychiatric conditions, the underlying mechanism of OCD is not known, but it seems to be related to that of PTSD. In both conditions, the amygdala seems hyperactive, overproducing the stress hormone cortisol that stimulates the catecholamine norepinephrine, one of the chemical messengers active within the synapses. Heightened levels of norepinephrine in urine samples are correlated with more intrusive negative memories. Note that there is no cause-and-effect relationship; like all scientific discovery, this one just creates more questions to pursue.

Given the limitations of our perceptual mechanisms and those of our memories, it might seem wondrous that we can muddle through life as well as we do. From one perspective, such amazement is warranted. From another, these apparent deficiencies are a necessary condition for a three-pound organ to fulfill all that is required of it. Survival does not require perfection. Indeed, a perfect memory of all life experience would require far more storage capacity than is available. Thus, transience is adaptive, freeing connections that are not used. The less a memory is used, the less probable it will be needed in the future. The same probability schema applies to blocking and absent-mindedness and contributes to greater functionality by reducing the potential for cognitive chaos. Occasional lapses of memory are a small price to pay for being mentally productive.

Schacter elaborates on this "less is more" notion as it relates to the other memory limitations he cites. Our memory systems are most adept at deriving the gist of an experience, allowing us the benefit from it without being burdened with superfluous details. Distilling the gist from a stimulatory experience of which we process no more than 5% may yield vastly different results among participants, but it also underlies our ability to create categories and make meaning. Our functioning can be enhanced by sharing our memories and interpretations with others, thereby enriching our choices by creating a cognitive smorgasbord (a linguistic, visual, and gustatory metaphor utilizing both hemispheres). Exceptional classroom teachers of the humanities have this talent in abundance. This mastery of "gistness" is missing in persons labeled on the autism spectrum, who miss out on patterns and associations because of an over-focus on details. The ability to recite the names and telephone numbers of a small city may provide ample entertainment value but offers little functional advantage in managing our lives.

Likewise, bias and stereotypes lead to unwarranted assessments of people and groups but involve the same system of generalizations that is accurate enough to create meaning. The egocentric bias of overly favorable self-evaluation and the hindsight bias may be illusions, but they yield benefits in the form of better mental health. Thus, the old maxim: Happy people are out of touch with reality.

Perception and cognition involve inherently limited processes but still provide us with the tools necessary to navigate the multi-sensory cacophony that is our environment. While acknowledging our shortcomings, we also are capable of acquiring new cognitive skills to enhance our functioning. This is likely a uniquely human attribute.

> A common belief that memory declines with age is based on our observations that older folks are slower at retrieving names, titles, and other words and concepts. Psychometric testing confirms the slowing of retrieval, and scientific literature contains multiple references to aging as persistent mental decline.
>
> A common psychological defense to this apparently inevitable degeneration is humor. I've often heard older folks declare that they are not losing their memory; they just have a lot more to remember. Turns out this light-hearted avoidance of the dread of dementia is supported by recent scientific literature. In "The Myth of Cognitive Decline," Ramscar and associates (2014) interpret the slower results of older persons' performance on psychometric tests as the inevitable consequence of the accumulation of more and more items to recall. This slowing is the predictable result of learning on the processing of information, not cognitive decline.

Irony occurs when an idea or word leads to contradictory outcomes. The fluid nature of our memory systems contributes not only to the litany of inaccuracies and shortcomings but also to the possibility of improving our powers of recall. Proven mnemonic techniques to enhance memory involve the utilization of emotion, as well as transforming a strictly factual exercise into one that has multi-sensory dimensions. For example, one can better remember a list of objects by associating them with positive emotions, sometimes by means of humor and crudeness. Memorization involving humor based on incongruity enhances functioning. Visualizing facts or concepts and associating them with a creative story can also be helpful. Traumatic memories, on the other hand, involve emotions that impair functioning.

Brain imaging of successful participants in memory competitions reveals that they use different brain areas than the rest of us—specifically, the right posterior hippocampal region, an area involved in both visual memory and spatial navigation. Mental champions describe constructing elaborate stories with vivid visual referents and movement from well-known location to location when confronted with the challenge of conferring long lists of random data to memory. In *Moonwalking with Einstein*, Joshua Foer (2011) relates setting a U.S. record for memorizing the order of a full deck of playing cards in 1 minute and 40 seconds. He assigns a person, activity, and object to each of the cards beforehand. He flips three cards at a time, selects one of the three assigned meanings for each, and constructs a story that takes place in his childhood home. He begins at the front door: His friend Liz (two of hearts) vivisects (two of diamonds) a pig (three of hearts) and moves through the house with each trio of cards, ending at his parents' bedroom door, with himself (four of spades) moonwalking (king of hearts) with Einstein (three of diamonds). He creates a coherent, if bizarre, story by imbuing expected but randomly occurring stimuli with meaning by associating them with visual action, the memory of the latter being an essential element for survival from an evolutionary perspective. In 2011 Nelson Dellis set another U.S. record in the same event, 1 minute and 3 seconds, using the same technique. (The measured time is when a contestant actually has visual contact with the cards, after which he has five minutes to mentally arrange them in the correct order.) Dellis has established a best time in practice of 34 seconds, which he is hoping to match or best in competition (Foer, 2011).

There are often emotional components to memory, too. Remembering that 2 + 2 = 4 has little recognizable emotional content to an adult. However, the learning of this factoid was likely accompanied and enhanced by activation of the pleasure center in the neocortex of a five-year-old in response to praise by parents and teacher. Memories of the birth of our children or being caught at some illicit adolescent activity are accompanied by the emotions experienced. Traumatic experiences evoke the most intense emotions.

Memory allows us to compare current stimuli to past experiences, to make a prediction and to decide on a course of action (or inaction). Psychotherapy is an experience by which the patient processes the stimuli provided by his/her interaction with the therapist, making new neural connections and altering old ones, with the intended outcome of relieving distress. Executing a successful golf shot creates a memory that can be accessed to aid in a similar shot later. Repressing memories of failed shots is a time-honored strategy but can contribute to an inflated sense of competence.

Research on the treatment of survivors of psychological trauma has focused on altering the connections between cognitive memories of trauma and the associated intense emotional reactions. One intervention being explored is the use of propranolol—a hypertension medication that reduces common somatic manifestations of fear, including rapid heart rate and sweating—in patients exploring memories with therapists. After a number of such sessions, subjects report significant reduction in emotional distress associated with the memories, even when no drug is administered. Apparently the neural connections between the memory and the emotion have been altered. These findings await confirmation using placebo and double-blind interventions.

> M is a 27-year-old soldier who has had four combat deployments in Iraq and Afghanistan, where he was exposed to multiple traumas. He referred himself for therapy, expressing concerns about lack of motivation, weight gain, and feeling overwhelmed. Within the safety of my office, he began to remember both positive and negative details of his deployments. He expressed a need to remember and make sense of his years of highly emotional experiences. Underlying his quest for meaning was a seemingly universal query: Am I normal? Am I losing control? Soldiers in combat experience multiple exposures to abnormal sensory stimuli. Educating them to the way the brain processes such experiences reassures them that their reactions are normal and that they can recover.
>
> As M became more comfortable with his memories, he was able to articulate a line of thinking that is common, but often not expressed, among soldiers: Deployment provides a structure, purpose, and emotional stimulation that is lacking in normal military (and civilian) life. The deployment-induced cognitive-emotional state becomes the new "normal." With this acknowledgment, M has reframed his psychological task. He must examine the option of volunteering for yet another deployment and the implications it has for his intimate relationships and his post-military career.

Behavioral therapies also hold promise. Laboratory studies suggest that an induced association between a neutral and an aversive stimulus can be unlearned if training is provided within a certain time after the memory is retrieved. Such memory modification has been shown to persist for as long as a year. Applying this intervention to trauma survivors will require further study under rigorous scientific methods.

> Memory loss is a concern among those of us of a certain age. But is it possible to have too much memory? Russian neuropsychologist A. R. Luria (1987) first came in contact with such a case in 1928, when S was referred to him because of his ability to repeat verbatim what had happened in a long meeting. Luria tested him and found that S could remember long lists of words and sounds, including complex mathematical formulas without knowing the math, Italian poetry without speaking Italian, and just plain nonsense. Even more remarkable was that those memories never seemed to fade. S was able to exactly repeat complex material 16 years later.
>
> Currently, AJ is being studied because of her ability to remember nearly everything she has done since age 11. She describes being able to recall the exact dates and times of experiences, both significant and mundane: the breakup of a romantic relationship, an episode of a TV sitcom. The character played by Dustin Hoffman in *Rain Man* was based on a *savant* who had memorized some 12,000 books. Such memory abilities may come at a cost to other mental functions.
>
> As for me, I try to employ tricks to assist my memory. The results have been mixed. I have a set of rain gear that I use for golf and fishing. I could never remember where I left it: Was it in my golf bag? With my fishing gear? The front closet? The back closet? The basement? Then I had an epiphany: I have a very clear memory of the excitement I experienced when I came up with a foolproof location. Unfortunately my memory of the excitement overshadows the memory of the location. I haven't found my rain gear since.

The study of memory has included a model that considers probabilistic inference and assumes that the knowledge we store in memory is encoded via language. The Retrieving Effectively from Memory model proposed by Steyvers, Griffiths, and Dennis (2006) postulates that words, and groups of words, are stored in memory based on their specific features: phonologic (sound), orthographic (letters), and semantic (meaning). Statistical analysis, including Bayesian inference, is employed by the scientists to create rational models of memory retrieval, aided by advances in computer science.

> Classic logic, or Boolean logic, is based on a binary digital conceptualization: Something is either true or false. Bayesian probability theory is based on the notion that things are not necessarily true or false but, rather, uncertain, an analog model. This model involves defining a set of variables, creating a graphical model connecting the variables based on causal relationships, and estimating the strength of those relationships. For example, a Bayesian

> model of lung cancer would identify all known risk factors (family history, personal health factors, exposure to environmental contaminants, including tobacco smoke) and estimate the relationships and relative strengths of each.

Our understanding of brain functioning is often advanced by freakish instances of injury or insult to specific areas. One such case was that of EP, in whom the herpes simplex virus destroyed two walnut-size areas within his medial temporal lobes, including the hippocampus and adjacent tissue. As a result, EP suffers from both anterograde (can't form new memories) and retrograde (can't recall old ones) amnesia. He lacks the capacity to remember that he can't remember. In this cognitive vacuum, his ability to make meaning is severely limited. He has lost his sense of time. He is in the ultimate Buddhist state: living in the moment, perfect enlightenment, with no apparent awareness of the continuity essential to a sense of self. How do you think this affects his mood? Observers might experience a range of emotions about his fate, starting with sadness. According to his family, EP experiences only one emotional state: happiness.

> Subjects who read information in hard-to-read fonts will remember it better than those who read the information in easier fonts, report Connor Diemand-Yauman, Daniel Oppenheimer, and Erikka Vaughan (2011) in *Cognition*. Perhaps activation within the anterior cingulate cortex associated with narrowed attention enhances memory encoding, just as it does problem solving.

The brain requires disproportionate amounts of resources in order to carry out its functions. It constitutes a mere 2% of the body's mass but utilizes 20% of the oxygen we breathe and 25% of the glucose we burn. It has evolved in remarkable ways in order to fulfill an increasing number of complex tasks. You will recall that our vision works by recording just bits of the environment and constructing a whole from them. Similarly, our brains cannot store every bit of sensory stimuli that they process. There is some sort of selection process, like the selection of bits of visual sensations from which we construct a mental image of our environment. Memory requires us to fill in the missing data points, which lead to inaccuracy and unreliability. Like other aspects of our mental functioning, memory need not be perfect but sufficient to support our survival. While memory is critical to our meaning-making function so, too, is forgetting. It enhances our ability to associate by clearing out information that is no longer relevant to our current information processing.

How the Brain Thinks

Steven Pinker describes a model of thinking based on psychological research. Andrey Vyshedskiy (2008) explores thinking from a neurological model, including a process that distinguishes conscious from unconscious thought. Like Christof Koch's model of consciousness described in chapter 5, Vyshedskiy's model focuses on visual stimulation that has been the most studied to date because of our solid understanding of the basic architecture of the visual system.

During the visual process, the initial electrical activity is generated when light interacts with the retina. The impulse is sent via the optic nerve to the thalamus, which serves as a relay station for both visual and auditory stimuli. The lateral geniculate nucleus within the thalamus routes the impulse to the primary visual cortex, or V1, located within the occipital lobe. From here the visual information, in the form of electrical impulses, is sent in two directions. The first visual impulse is sent ventrally to the inferior temporal cortex, which processes it to recognize the object. The V2, V4 posterior inferotemporal, central inferotemporal, and anterior inferotemporal cortex interact to compare the neuronal network created by the new stimuli to those stored in memory. The second direction in which the impulses are sent is dorsally to V5, where the object can be located in space.

A mental image, states Vyshedskiy, is stored in a huge number of neurons, referred to as an ensemble, and recalled through the synchronous firing of action potentials. He represents ensembles schematically as triangles (Figure 4.5). At the bottom are the non-specific neurons, such as those in V1, which can be members of any number of ensembles. At the tip of the triangle are the neurons specific to a particular object, located in the temporal lobe. These neurons belong to just a few ensembles representing very similar objects. Those in the middle have intermediate specificity, such as representing certain shapes. Most of our experiences are multi-sensory and are represented by the pyramid (Figure 4.6), in which each face represents a different sense.

This triangular representation helps make some meaning of the neurological difference between recall and recognition. Together, they can be conceptualized as a self-organizing of the neuronal ensemble into a synchronously firing unit.

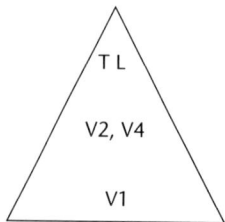

FIGURE 4.5 Triangular Representation of a Neuronal Ensemble

Thinking about Thinking 117

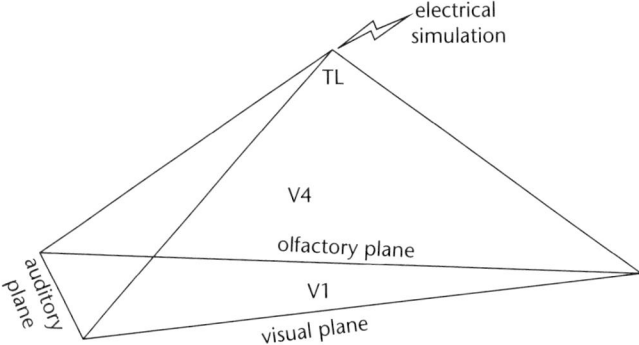

FIGURE 4.6 Pyramid Model of a Neuronal Ensemble

Recall begins when the visual stimulus activates neurons at the tip of the pyramid and then moves down to the less specific neurons ("I recall that face."). Recognition, on the other hand, begins at the bottom, with the stimulus activating neurons upward to the specific ("That is Ruth from my biology class.").

The emotional content of remembering 2 + 2 = 4 has faded for most of us, given a lack of continuing external reinforcement, which results in a weakening and eventual disintegration of that aspect of the neural ensemble. However, many of our everyday experiences involve both multi-sensory and emotional content. Vyshedskiy (p. 160) proposes a polyhedron model to conceptualize these more complex processes. The emotions associated with each sensory mode might be processed separately, then integrated via the neuronal ensemble. I have tried to conceptualize this process in Figure 4.7.

Now, let's apply Vyshedskiy's theory of conscious thought to the experience of driving your car. You are taking in visual stimuli of the highway itself, other

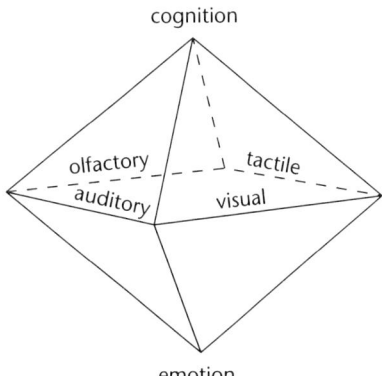

FIGURE 4.7 Polyhedron Model of a Neuronal Ensemble

cars, the movement of your vehicle relative to others, your speed as recorded on the speedometer, and a multitude of data not directly associated with your primary function: the dial on your radio, the image on a billboard, and the location of your cell phone. You also are experiencing auditory stimuli: the sound of horns honking, traffic conditions as reported on the radio, and the critique of last night's football game being debated by your passengers. Tactile stimuli include the feel of the steering wheel, the pressure generated by your foot on the accelerator and brake, the sensations generated by accelerating, braking, and turning, and the relative comfort of your seat. Finally, there is the smell and taste of the sandwich and coffee purchased at the local kwikstop.

Each of these sensory stimuli generates a neuronal pathway to that part of the brain that processes it, then to the part that stores encoded memories in neuronal ensembles. You are actively thinking about all of this sensory-induced activity, but most of it does not qualify as what we experience as conscious thought (more in chapter 5).

All is going smoothly in your drive, when suddenly your olfactory system interprets a new stimulus that takes priority over the coffee. Your interpretation is of heat and/or burning and is connected to emotions related to anxiety. The neuronal ensemble created by the new stimulus fires in synchrony with the memory and associated emotion and breaks through to consciousness, and your foot hits the brake.

As with a routine drive to work with our colleagues, the vast majority of our brain activity is not in phase with the attention rhythm and thus is regarded as non-conscious or unconscious. It represents thought, though, whether or not we are conscious of it. Consciousness is the result of synchronicity of firing among ensembles within the attention phase. Sensory inputs take the form of spikes, sharp microsecond rises in voltage that travel between and through neurons, from the million ganglion cells in the retina to the thalamus and then to the cortex, giving rise to conscious perception. The meaning of these streams of spikes are interpreted from the rates and their variability.

Researchers also look to the relative timing of spikes in proximate neurons. Horace Barlow, a neuroscientist at the University of Cambridge, suggests that each cell in the visual cortex may be activated by a specific physical feature of an object (color, shape, size, orientation). When combinations of these cells are activated at the same time, the brain detects a "suspicious coincidence" (similarity to patterns stored in memory) worthy of processing. This synchrony, with each spike representing one aspect of an object, assembles a percept from its components (Sejnowski & Delbruck, 2012).

Attention, a central component of cognition, seems to be the product of sequences of such synchronized spikes. Robert Desimone at Massachusetts Institute of Technology (Fries, et al. 2008) has identified a correlation between attention by monkeys to a stimulus and both the number and rate of synchronized spikes in their cortical neurons. Memory is enhanced not only by the rate of spike firing but equally by their relative timing. The hippocampus is important in creating memories of events and objects. Gyorgy Buzsaki at New York University has shown that the spiking of neurons in the hippocampus and the visual cortex with which it interacts are greatly influenced by synchronous oscillations of brain waves (Sejnowski & Delbruck, 2012).

Neurological models of thinking often focus on the patterns of electrical activity among different regions of the brain, largely because this is what our current technology permits. Research is beginning to go beyond patterns of activity to being able to decode that activity. Using *f*MRI technology, scientists have been able to analyze the pattern of activation the fusiform face area and the parahippocampal gyrus area and infer with 85% accuracy the category (face or building) subjects reported imagining (Haynes & Rees, 2006).

Yet another approach to decoding relates to visual processing, which takes advantage of both the advances in technology and in techniques to process its findings. It again starts with the *f*MRI, which does not directly measure the activity occurring in milliseconds within synapses and among neurons. This technology measures the change in color and magnetic force associated with the consumption of blood by specific brain sites. When synapses and neurons are active, they need to replenish the oxygen required for power via hemoglobin molecules. The *f*MRI detects these changes in blood supply that take place in a matter of seconds in an area about the size of a pea (a voxel). One challenge: to correlate the millisecond action in the synapses and neurons with the sluggish measurements from the *f*MRI.

Jack Gallant of the University of California–Berkeley has developed a two-stage process to decode visual images processed in the brain (Smith, 2013). First, he has volunteers look at thousands of images while in the *f*MRI, using the data to train an algorithm to predict the response for each voxel. Next he reverses the process, using Bayesian probability techniques to infer the image that most likely created the response in a particular volunteer. (Another example of how we all experience the world differently: It is not possible to use one brain to predict the response of another.)

While the number of possible images is huge, the types of scenes in the environment most of us inhabit is finite and includes people, animals, buildings, and vegetation. In an initial trial, three subjects watched two hours of short segments of Hollywood movies. Using data about nerve cells in the visual cortex from two decades of research on monkeys and humans, coupled with the *f*MRI blood data, a separate encoding model was created for each voxel. Again using Bayesian methods based on prior experience, the decoder estimated the most likely clip that subjects would watch, and that they had not previously viewed. Go to www.gallantlab.org to see a side-by-side comparison of the viewed and decoded clips. The results are far from perfect, given the sluggishness of the *f*MRI processing, but still represent a significant step toward decoding complex cognition and consciousness (Smith, 2013).

New technologies, including methods for recording the simultaneous spikes in thousands of neurons among different brain areas, will likely reveal important patterns from which scientists can create further meaning about how we think.

Making Decisions

We can conceptualize many types of thinking: among them, memory (both short-term and long-term), mathematical, philosophical, intuitive, and rational. However, the way we make decisions requires looking at thinking through a different lens.

Decisions are predictions (Kahneman & Tversky, 1973) derived from the interpretation of sensory inputs that are processed by comparing them with memory. Thus, decisions are dependent on the sensory inputs available, the limitations of the sensory, cognitive, and emotional processes, and the current state of the processing system that involves the multiple feedback loops among the brain, body, and environment.

Using classical dualistic categories, popular psychology conceptualizes decisions as being either rational or emotional. Neuroscientific understandings have turned this paradigm on its head. The brain has limitations and imperfections as it processes and responds to stimuli, so rationality is a myth. Instead, *rationalization* is the reality. Our responses to stimuli are not driven by thoughtful interpretation; they are determined by our emotional response to stimuli. Our explanations for our behavior represent nothing more than our groping to make meaning out of what we have done. In one study (Wilson et al., 1993) college students were allowed to select a poster that they could display in their residences. Subjects in one group simply chose a poster, while those in the second group had to provide an explanation for their choice. When given the opportunity to exchange their posters at a later time, subjects in the second group expressed more dissatisfaction with their initial choices by exchanging their posters at a much higher rate than those who didn't have to explain their choice. The researcher's interpretation: Providing an explanation interferes with one's ability to make a satisfying emotional choice. (Interesting implications for choosing a partner, asserts my mate.)

The prefrontal cortex has severe limitations in its ability to process information, which complicates decision making. It consumes large amounts of blood sugar in order to function. Experiments demonstrate that subjects performing a taxing mental activity who did not get glucose replenishment relied significantly more on emotion in subsequent decision making compared to subjects who got a sugar fix (Wang & Dvorak, 2010).

In addition, due to its limited processing abilities, the brain depends on a type of thinking that economist Richard Thayer labeled "mental accounting." Rather than rationally considering every dollar as identical, people will categorize their assets into separate, non-transferable groups. Consider this experiment. Subjects were presented with a scenario in which they either lost $10 in cash or lost a ticket to an event that cost $10. When asked whether they would purchase a second ticket, only 46% of those who lost a ticket were willing to buy a replacement, compared to 88% of those who lost cash. The interpretation is that people create different mental categories for their funds. Losing a ticket and buying a replacement effectively takes $20 from the entertainment account. The lost cash is not charged to the same mental account. The result is considered irrational by economists because it ignores a basic principle: Money is fungible, meaning every dollar is equal and can be substituted for another (Thayer, 1999).

Another decision-making limitation of the brain is its inability to ignore irrelevant information. Experiments show there is an anchoring effect by which random numbers play a significant role in the amount a person is willing to pay for something. In one classic experiment (Tversky & Kahneman, 1974), subjects were asked to estimate the percentage of African countries in the United Nations after being exposed to a random number generated by a roulette wheel. Those exposed to higher numbers on the wheel had significantly higher guesses than those exposed to lower ones.

The limitations of the prefrontal cortex are increasingly challenged by the massive amount of data available in our society. Popular psychology would conclude that more information leads to better choice, but experiments suggest otherwise. Psychologist Paul Andreassen had MIT business students choose a stock portfolio, then divided them into two groups. The first had very limited information—just the changes in the price of their stocks. The second had access to all available market data, plus the advice of experts. The group with limited information earned more than twice as much as the fully informed group (Sousa, 2012). The explanation: The highly informed investors, using the vast amount of information available, traded twice as often, believing that their knowledge led to better decisions.

Employment decisions by both the employer and the employee are predictions about the future and are subject to numerous irrelevant correlations. The same is true of college admissions. Both the admissions official and the prospective student are trying to project future performance and emotional satisfaction based on limited information. There are a very large number of factors that influence success at work or study, many of which cannot be anticipated. Therefore, decisions can only be based on what can be processed, no matter its relevance. Illusory correlations figure in many areas of human prediction. For example, psychotherapists' predictions (including my own) of patient outcomes following the initial assessment are often highly inaccurate and based on irrelevant data. The acronym YAVIS (young, attractive, verbal, intelligent, and single) was created to describe female patients rated by their male therapists as most likely to do well in treatment.

What are we to make of these counterintuitive findings about decision making? I would begin by revisiting the notion that thinking and feeling are discrete phenomena, as the cognitive-behavioral formula suggests: Sensation → Thinking → Feeling → Behaving. The label we apply to a feeling is an interpretation of somatosensory data (thinking) by the prefrontal cortex. For example, we might interpret muscular tension in our jaw or stomach as anger, psychomotor slowing and tearfulness as sadness, and tremulousness and sweaty palms as anxiety. These somatic experiences often seem to happen automatically and are the foundation for our interpretation of the situation. When we put our hand on the hot stove, we don't think, "I'm getting burned; I'd better move my hand." We remove our hand almost simultaneously with recording the sensory input, then think, "That was stupid; I'd better not do that again" or "Which blankety-blank left the burner on?" Trying to solve more complex problems, such as thinking about thinking, might begin with stimulation of the reward center with dopamine, but eventually such effort leads to prefrontal cortex fatigue from over-activity and resulting frustration. Our decisions are typically not the product of rational thought processes.

The ever-increasing amount of data that technology generates adds another complication. Our working memory can process a limited (usually thought of as seven) number of items. More requires long-term memory, which is harder work. Thus, we choose to process as few factors as possible, giving more consideration to those that are more recent and those that are more redundant. Finally, generalizing from one study (Paese & Sniezek, 1991), the more experience we have in making predictions, the more confident we are, even though our accuracy demonstrates little or no improvement.

The preceding consideration of decision-making has been based on a scientific paradigm: Choices are subject to objective measurement and fall into one of three digits: less, more, or equal. However, many of our choices involve values. What job to choose might involve consideration of living environment, moving, income, lifestyle, and self-worth. Deciding whether and/or whom to marry is equally as value laden. Ruth Chang (2014) transforms these decisions from being "hard" to being an opportunity for people to utilize their unique capacity to *make reasons*. Despite psychology's best efforts to subject human thinking, feeling, and behaving to scientific analysis, it cannot use reductionism to explain our value-based choices.

The Role of Thought in Survival

There is a notion that we are born with a *tabula rasa*, a blank slate of a mind waiting for experience to fill it with thoughts, ideas, and beliefs. While our environment no doubt provides us with sensory experiences that shape the content of our thoughts, there are also important cognitive processes that are the product of natural selection. This is the position explained by Wray Herbert in *On Second Thought: Outsmarting Your Mind's Hard-Wired Habits* (2010b). Herbert argues that human forms that have survived have done so by adapting to the threats in their environment. While the nature of those threats has changed, mental survival adaptations from our ancestors persist in the form of *heuristics*, cognitive shortcuts that are "hard wired" into our brains. These habits of thinking are essential to our day-to-day functioning as we automatically make the millions of decisions necessary to ambulate, eat and drink, navigate in human and vehicular traffic, and otherwise carry out the tasks necessary to survive. Like all habits, heuristics can be imperfect and seemingly illogical. The current understanding is that they originate in the older, more primitive brain structures and express rapid, impressionistic responses to stimuli. The slower, more rational processes are located in the neocortex areas and include interpretations of our heuristic responses, or rationalizations for our automatic, non-conscious behaviors.

> I have a mixed emotional response to the term "hard wired" as applied to the brain. Increasingly used by neuroscientists, the term does effectively convey a fixed internal processing mechanism. My negative reaction is to the simplistic computer analogy. As I have noted, neuronal interactions via synaptic activity are far more complex than digital processing. In addition, "hard wired" suggests a rigidity that is challenged by research findings about neuroplasticity. Indeed, the title of Herbert's book suggests that we can "outsmart" the hard wiring. To do so requires conscious will, a concept that will be explored in the next chapter.

Some heuristics are conceptualized as products of our primitive pasts, while others are thought of as products of more recent cultural influences. The latter has been labeled *cognitive scaffolding*, the layering of more complex social thinking and behaving on top of the primitive processes essential for survival. An example is the blurred and changing line between consensual sexual behavior and rape. Nicola Gavey (2005) explores the cultural contexts that limit some and encourage other women's choices in *Just Sex? The Cultural Scaffolding of Rape*.

Classes of living creatures either survive well enough to reproduce, or they become extinct. Heuristics are cognitive rules that we use automatically and that are sufficient to ensure survival. Herbert (2010b) utilizes pattern discernment to identify three broad categories of heuristics involving a mixture of primitive and cultural influences: those involving the human body's interaction with its environment, the manner in which we engage in numerical processing, and finally, our non-numerical cognition.

Our somatic sensations, as processed via the somatosensory system, influence our interpretations and thus are factors in our survival. Herbert cites examples of bodily sensations that appear to shape metaphors in our language. One is the connection between our need for warmth and our language for expressing emotional closeness or belonging. The theory is that our ancestors enhanced their chances of surviving by gathering together in groups, both for mutual protection and for staying warm. After one group of study subjects was primed to recall an experience in which they had felt a sense of belonging with others and a second group primed to remember a time they had felt rejected, all subjects were asked to estimate the temperature of the room. Subjects who recalled rejection guessed the temperature to be, on average, five degrees less than those who had recalled feeling valued. The researchers concluded that the subjects' emotional states influenced their interpretations of the environment. Herbert notes a similar connection between the survival need of cleanliness and the use of "clean" and "dirty" to describe positive and negative ethical behavior. He cites another study in which subjects were primed to think of cleanliness or dirt, then asked to make ethical decisions about a variety of scenarios. Those primed for cleanliness were much more tolerant and lenient toward themselves and others.

Herbert describes another somatic heuristic that derives from our intuitive physics, a subject that Steven Pinker considers as an influence on language (see chapter 6). Herbert relates intuitive physics to the way our innate sense of speed and momentum in the physical world shapes our understanding of our psychology. He cites researchers who discern a similarity between the physics concept of mass and the psychological concept of emotional importance. In physics, momentum equals velocity times mass. In psychology, emotional importance is the equivalent of mass, resulting in the *propensity effect*—the prediction of future outcomes based on the most recent trends, especially those to which we attribute special emotional significance. Anyone who participates in the weekly office football pool or March Madness experiences this heuristic. Teams that have won a few games in a row are thought to have momentum, and we are more likely to expect them to win their next game. Even if we had information with a more meaningful connection to the outcome of a game—such as the real injury status of players, the comparative skills of their replacements, or key match-ups between interior linesmen—we probably wouldn't know how to fairly evaluate it. Highly paid and well-informed network commentators do no better at predicting. Regardless of whether we have the relevant data and the capacity to process it, we all fall back on our "hardwired" sense of momentum.

Intuitive physics also comes into play in the connection between our interpretation of distance and our experiencing of emotions. Herbert cites a study by Yale psychologists Lawrence Williams and John Bargh. Half the subjects were given the task of graphing two points that were close together. The other half graphed two points with a greater difference. Subjects were then asked to read a passage containing a high degree of emotional content, such as violence or embarrassment. The group that graphed the close points reported significantly more intense emotion in response to the reading than those that graphed more distant points. The researchers interpreted this as illustrating the brain's evolutionary connection between distance and safety. On the savannah, our ancestors experienced emotional safety when far away from the potential danger of a threatening predator. Distance can be temporal as well as geographic. In other experiments, subjects primed to think in abstract, theoretical terms exhibited increased emotional control and physical endurance compared to subjects primed for practical, concrete, solution-based thinking.

Moreover, our assessments of choices and our decisions are often influenced by factors that have no apparent rational basis. We tend to opt for the simplest, easiest-to-process option, even when the simplicity is unrelated to the choice at hand. In a series of laboratory experiments, subjects were influenced by seemingly extraneous factors. For example, an amusement park ride with a hard-to-pronounce name, Vaiveahtoishi, was judged to be more risky than the identical ride named Chunta. Students were more likely to undertake an exercise regimen if the instructions were printed in an unfussy font as opposed to one that was flowing and harder to read. In the real world, investors are more likely to purchase shares of new stocks with palatable names. Our preference for the simple and familiar is thought to be an artifact of evolutionary processes that helped humans survive in a more threatening world.

The final cognitive bias Herbert considers is how we interpret our relation to a group. Anyone who spends a lot of time with teens, or can remember the experience of their own adolescence, will note the simultaneous drives to belong to the group through conformity and to individuate by being different. How can we account for such an apparent contradiction? As it turns out, researchers have confirmed that subjects will mimic others, even in response to subtle, unconscious clues, to connect to a desired group. Such cognitive effort comes with a price, however. Efforts to synchronize our movements, thoughts, or emotions with those of a group can deplete our cognitive resources, leading to exhaustion and the breakdown of self-discipline. Herbert also speculates that if a group is too tightly synchronized the exhaustion of one member can spread to others through contagion. The *mimicry heuristic* suggests that our successes and limitations may be more influenced by others than we care to think.

The second category of heuristics that Herbert cites relates to thinking in numerical terms, which can lead to illogical conclusions. Study subjects rated a hamburger labeled 75% lean as more tasty and less greasy than the same burger labeled 25% fat. In other studies, volunteers rated a 10% chance of danger as less fearful than a 10 in 100 chance. The increased use (and misuse) of statistics and percentages in health care may actually contribute to reduced compliance and adverse health outcomes. Even physicians who are educated in scientific methods misinterpret statistics, as elaborated on in chapter 6.

A related numerical heuristic is the connection between our interpretation of scarcity and value. Herbert cites a study whose subjects were primed to consider the unconscious link between scarcity and value by thinking about the worth of rare postage stamps. Half then listened to Muzak, the other half to classical music. The latter group interpreted the length of the music as shorter, or more scarce, than did the Muzak group, and expressed a willingness to work more for the experience of listening to classical music, reflecting a higher value. Subjects in another study were exposed to two different advertisements for bottled water: One had a background of snowy peaks, the other desert and camels. The group who viewed the ad showing desert and camels subsequently rated the availability of works by their favored artist as rarer, and their market value higher, than the group who viewed the water ad showing snow. Herbert's pattern discernment is that scarcity and value heuristics cut across different areas of human needs and preferences in a circular way, reinforcing our initial beliefs, thereby influencing our decisions for better or worse.

Our interpretation of value is also influenced in the marketplace by the numerical presentation of a price. A listed price sets in motion the *anchoring effect*, establishing a framework for computing value. There is a reason an item is listed at $19.99 rather than $20. (In chapter 6, the influence of the anchoring effect on consumer decisions will be explored further.) Anchoring goes beyond numbers, though. Herbert cites the example of a supposed pro-drug message when a certain recording is played backward. Listeners who are told the message is there will more likely report hearing it, even though it doesn't exist. Thinking is the process of creating order out of randomness, of creating meaning. We are more comfortable and experience positive emotional valence when we discern meaning, as opposed to ambiguity. This principle extends to our thinking about thinking. We overestimate what we think we know about the thoughts of others, as well as our own.

Researchers have conducted numerous studies that indicate a correlation between the physical sensation of hunger and the interpretation of relative scarcity and value. Subjects who had not eaten for four hours were less generous in charitable giving than those who had eaten. Subjects exposed to the smell of baking brownies were less generous givers than those who were not, even though all had eaten recently. In a classic study from the 1940s, poor children overestimated the size of coins while non-poor kids did not. Male subjects with little or no money in their wallets expressed a desire for women who were significantly heavier than did men with ample amounts of money. Male subjects surveyed before dinner expressed a preference for more full-figured women than did men after dinner. Though we can discern a pattern between hunger, sexual preference, and financial security, its significance is open to interpretation. Herbert (2010a) offers one: Poorer people in our society have higher rates of morbid obesity because their thwarted desire for money is replaced by the closely related, more primitive currency of calories.

Numbers influence our decisions in other ways. If we face a choice between two options with equal trade-offs (an apartment that is $500 per month and 15 minutes from work and one that is $600 per month and 10 minutes from work), we will choose one or the other half the time. However, if we include a third choice that is clearly inferior ($1,000 per month and an hour from work), we are more likely to choose the middle of the three options because we appraise it as relatively better than the third, something cognitive psychologists refer to as the *decoy heuristic* (Herbert, 2010a). The consumer movement of recent years is based on the notion that people should be provided with choices from which they can make more informed decisions. However, when I choose a toothbrush or a bottle of wine from a wall-sized display of options, I would be hard-pressed to describe my choice as informed or rational.

Consider dating and the choice of a mate within a consumer model (not an outlandish notion in this age of Internet dating services and speed dating). Herbert (2010a) cites a study by psychologist Constantine Sedikides demonstrating that college-age respondents making (hypothetical) choices of partners were strongly influenced by decoys who most resembled, but were inferior to, their actual choice. Given the choice between handsome but dim-witted John and average-looking but witty George, Mary must make the classic looks-versus-intelligence decision. Now introduce a third choice, Bill, who is better looking than George, less handsome than John, but equal to John in lack of wit. According to Sedikides's interpretation of her research, Mary will reject Bill as lacking on both looks and intelligence yet still be influenced by his addition to the mix: She will more likely choose John because Bill is more like him than is George.

Our brains also function by comparing past experiences, stored in memory, with current sensory stimuli. We seek to discern a pattern between the present and one or more similar past experiences. Then we make a decision based on our imagination of the emotional outcome. However, we do so with a bias toward the future. Studies by Daniel Gilbert (2006) at Harvard, among others, show that we value future time over the past. A group of subjects completed a boring and lengthy task. Half were asked to place a monetary value on the completed task; the other half were asked to put a price on doing the task in the future. The future value the subjects assigned was double that for the past work. In a similar vein, columnist David Brooks (2011b) sought "life wisdom" from readers over 70 years of age. He found that they undervalued the contributions of their parents (the past) and over-valued their expectations for their grandchildren (the future). An evolutionary explanation for this bias is that the future is more important to survival than is the past. Our survival is enhanced by expecting better outcomes and more positive associated emotions.

After body sensations and number processing, Wray Herbert considers a third group of heuristics that we utilize to create meaning from the overwhelming amount of sensory stimuli around us in order to survive. The first of these he calls the *design heuristic*, describing exactly what he himself has done in his study of the psychological research: the application of categories and labels to create order and meaning. That meaning doesn't have to be the correct interpretation. Rather, it is the simplest one that will result in our survival. Thus, we are at the very center of the created meaning.

> In clinical work, the bias toward self-centered interpretation is referred to as *personalization*. I explain it to my patients with the following scenario: I am driving down the road, when someone suddenly and unexpectedly pulls out in front of me. My first interpretation: "Why did that SOB do that to me (make me feel so scared and angry)?" However, I also have the capacity to interpret this event in a less emotional, less reactive way. Upon further reflection, it is extremely unlikely that the other driver was waiting to pull out in front of anyone, and especially not me in particular. It is more likely that he or she was distracted by the kids in the back seat or an earlier fight with a partner.
>
> This simple anecdote illustrates the difference between *Thinking Fast and Slow*, as elaborated by Israeli psychologist Daniel Kahneman (2011a). We have a strong bias toward the simplest, most available explanation, a product of our more primitive, emotion-driven brain structures. Slower to operate is the ability to think about our thinking, to consider alternative, more complex explanations, which are the product of the neocortex.

Survival of our ancestors on the savannah required a lot of exploring to find ample sources of food and water while still remaining safe. Thus, there is a tension in our survivor-shaped cognition between the need to explore and the need to focus more close at hand and be safe. Herbert explains this *foraging heuristic* of cognition as being driven by emotion. Exploring is motivated by anticipation of satiating needs, which has a positive emotional valence. On the other hand, focusing on limiting behavior to familiar circumstances calms the negative emotions of fear. Most people's daily lives involve a complex dance between these opposing impulses.

Another way to think about the brain's methods of processing and organizing sensory stimuli to create meaning is represented by the *caricature heuristic*. In order to conserve energy, the brain simplifies, creating stereotypes. We do this constantly as we interact with our environment. The process is driven by emotion, as our sensory processing leads to positive or negative emotional valence. In turn, we use our cognition to create meaning of the somatosensory experience we label emotion. Nowhere is this more dramatically acted out than in modern American politics. We have created two broad categories, liberal and conservative, in which we try to include all the ways to think about the political choices we face. Then we go through cognitive contortions in an attempt to create meaning from the mish-mash of contradictions within each. Our "slow thinking" has difficulty creating meaning from our "fast thinking." To conserve time and energy, we often let the fast thinking suffice.

Two related heuristics also enhance survival. Herbert describes the *cootie heuristic*, which refers to an evolutionary aversion to contamination. Paul Rozin, a University of Pennsylvania psychologist, has studied people's stated preference for foods and products they consider "natural" because they believe they are healthier and kinder to the environment and because they are more moral, evoking more positive emotional valence. Might this preference be a rationalization motivated by the emotional need?

The related *naturalist heuristic* stems from our inclination to return to the natural world. Those of us who live in rural settings have daily opportunities to process the sensory stimuli associated with nature. Those in urban and suburban environments also often seek more naturalistic environments in which to "recreate." Research supports the notion that exposure to nature replaces "executive functioning" with a less active mode that replenishes our cognitive functions.

> Psychologist and physician Leonard Sax has raised alarms about what he interprets as the increasingly impaired motivation and achievement of boys and young men in our American society. In *Boys Adrift* (2007), Sax asserts that the increasing gap in educational and vocational achievement between young men and young women constitutes a social crisis with potentially dramatic consequences. Contributing to this concerning trend, he argues, are the proliferation of video games (to which boys have a much greater affinity than girls) and trends in education away from multi-sensory interaction with the real world in favor of computer-based learning. Contrast a boy learning about frogs from the sterile visual images on a video screen, to another who is exposed to their natural habitat, a rich and diverse multi-sensory experience that contributes to more meaningful learning. The term "nature deficit disorder" was coined by Richard Louv, author of *Last Child in the Woods* (2005), to describe a kind of "cultural autism" experienced by a child who spends his time indoors.

Making moral choices is another area of psychological research that explores the interaction of emotion and decision making. (These two distinct categories lead to the same kind of cognitive convolutions as do "liberal" and "conservative" in politics.) The ways in which we study moral dilemmas in psychological research revolve around our understanding of causation. Moral dilemmas are frequently characterized as decisions where one person must be sacrificed for the sake of more lives. An example is the trolley dilemma: You are driving a trolley that loses its brakes and will kill five people in its path unless you switch it to another track, on which it will kill one person. Under experimental conditions, most people can make the choice quickly. Modify the dilemma so that the choice is to pull a lever that opens a trap door, dropping a fat man onto the track to block the trolley and save five lives. Again, most subjects decide quickly. Make one more modification, whereby subjects have to directly push a fat man in front of the trolley to save five people, and they are less decisive. Their explanation:

A mechanical act (pulling a lever) is more palatable than a personal one (direct contact). Herbert characterizes any fast decision to act or not as driven by an evolutionarily produced intuition, later rationalized with explanatory intent in order to make meaning.

Paul Piff (2013) is a social psychologist at the University of California–Berkeley who has studied the influence of wealth and power on thinking, emotion, and behavior. In both laboratory experiments and observations in natural settings, he has conducted studies from which he concludes that increases in wealth contribute to a reduction in empathy and generosity and an increase in thoughts of self-entitlement and behavior that is unethical and law-breaking. Even in a laboratory study in which the acquisition of wealth was rigged, subjects who acquired more (play) money attributed their success to a more intelligent strategy. Our self-centered bias leads us to over-value our abilities.

In our society, moral decisions are institutionalized by the judicial system. There are two kinds of judgments, involving different psychological mechanisms. The first is an accused person's guilt or innocence. In a recent local case, a young man was accused of killing a three-month-old child by shaking it violently. The jury convicted quickly, using an intuitive, emotion-driven moral heuristic. The more complex judgment was sorting out motivation: The accused was a soldier, with multiple deployments involving intense combat exposure, who had been diagnosed with posttraumatic stress disorder. Weighing multiple causative influences and their impact on others is done by our slower, more deliberative cognitive processes.

As far as we can tell, among the cognitive abilities that distinguish us from other thinking creatures is the awareness of the inevitability of our own mortality. At the same time, we seem to be driven by a desire to control our lives. The way we resolve this dilemma is referred to as the *grim reaper heuristic*. Research that examines the unconscious thoughts of subjects who have been inundated with sensory stimuli associated with death reveals unexpected results. Compared to controls who have not been so exposed, these subjects seem to more automatically access and express pleasant, positive content. While we can't control our death, we can control how we think and feel about it. As I grow older, I observe more of my peers engaging in "old fart" thinking, a nostalgia for the "good old days." Another apparently unique human emotion, nostalgia seems to be protective against our existential dread of death.

> Wray Herbert (2010a) cites a more depressing product of our awareness of death: our tendency to become more rigid in our beliefs when they are threatened. He creates a connection between such threat-induced fear and genocide and conceptualizes that our need to make meaning is threatened by alternative meanings or understood life purposes. A philosophy that counters mine heightens my awareness of my own mortality. The inability to

reconcile opposing beliefs creates such anxiety in some people that they are driven to exterminate the source of the perceived threat.

In contrast, Steven Pinker argues that the rates of violence and murder have declined dramatically over the millennia. In *The Better Angels of Our Nature: Why Violence Has Declined* (2011), he cites the development of effective nation-states and the growing equality between the genders as among the important influences driving this trend. In *Scientific American Mind* (January/February 2012), critic Robert Epstein expresses his interpretation that Pinker arrives at his conclusions by employing the confirmation bias.

The final heuristic that we have inherited from our distant ancestors is characterized by a void, or default. Often we decide to *not* decide. Given our understanding of the energy required to weigh all the options before making a decision, it is little wonder that in situation after situation we opt to not decide. So, what determines whether we engage in an energy-consuming mental process or opt for default? It is our motivator: emotion. Some decisions are affected by the context in which they are posed. Take organ donation. In New York State, one must make an active decision to be an organ donor by signing a card when applying for a driver's license, which only 25% of all registrants do. In France, where everyone is considered an organ donor unless he or she makes the active decision to opt out, over 99% take the default option (Herbert, 2010a). The notable discrepancy between France and New York State in organ donating does not likely represent differences in social or cultural attitudes; rather, it reflects the cognitive economy of the default option because it is less driven by emotion. The herd mentality of the stock market represents a contrasting scenario. Although it is common wisdom that investing should be for the long-term, when a threat to our financial safety presents itself in the form of a market downturn, our emotions kick in, motivating our primitive bias toward action. Such action is not always in our best interest, but it provides a behavioral outlet for the triggered emotion.

I never played soccer, but as a fan of my daughter's youth teams, I was intrigued by the penalty kick. In particular, I wondered how I would approach defending the net if I were the goalie. The ball is placed in a stationary position, 36 feet from the goal. The goalie has to protect an area that measures 24 feet wide and 8 feet high. The kicker lets loose without any interference, sending the ball in a split second to a predetermined corner of the net. In a study of more than 300 professional goalies in thousands of situations, behavioral economist Ofer Azar found a clear self-defeating bias toward action. Goalies who moved either left or right in anticipation of the kick were able to block about one in eight shots. Goalies who stayed put stopped more than one in three (Cohen, 2008).

Cognition follows sensory processing. It turns out our biases are not solely the product of cognition. Heather Sheridan (University of Southampton) and Eyal M. Reingold (University of Toronto) conducted experiments involving decision making among chess players. Tracking the eyes of both novice and expert subjects, they confirmed that players scanned squares that had previously yielded a helpful move at the expense of squares that might lead to a better solution in the current situation. We unconsciously seek out data that confirms our previous experience (Reingold & Heather, 2011).

While our thinking is influenced by evolutionary biases that contributed to our ancestors' survival, our more evolved neocortex gives us the capacity to think about how we think, consider the consequences of our decisions, and modify our behavior to further serve our best interests. Investors and soccer goalies receive intermittent reinforcement from their bias toward action. By teaching the known outcomes of our slower, more analytic thinking, soccer coaches can help young goalies be more effective, and behavioral economists can curb the selling impulses of fearful investors.

Working in concert with culture, evolution has shaped interpretations to various types of sensory stimuli and the consequent instinctual responses, processes that originate in our more primitive brain areas. At the same time, evolution has yielded an increasingly productive cortex that can engage in more deliberative, analytic reasoning—including creating meaning from our quick, instinctual responses. Our continuing survival is now dependent on our effective utilization of two contrasting cognitive styles, and the ability of the more deliberative one to make appropriate judgments and to outsmart self-defeating heuristics as needed.

Higher Order Thinking

Driving a car is conceptualized as the interaction of the five senses, the somatosensory system, affective processes, and motor behaviors. As such, it represents the three domains of learning: cognitive, emotional, and psychomotor. Thinking about driving a car is an example of what educators refer to as higher order thinking.

In 1956, educational psychologist Benjamin Bloom proposed a model of thinking about thinking as it relates to learning. It was revised in 2001(Anderson, Krathwohl, & Bloom, 2001). The least complex is memory, which we have defined neurologically as synchrony between a neuronal ensemble being experienced and a neuronal ensemble encoded in previous experience. The synchrony is most often partial, since two instances of sensory input are rarely totally similar. As one moves through the following categories, the mental tasks become more complex and more abstract: *remember, understand, apply, analyze, evaluate, synthesize.*

These levels of thinking are not purely cognitive, however. They involve a complex interaction among the things we experience and interpret as parts of our mental functioning. Take memory, which in Bloom's taxonomy is on the lowest level. The feats of participants in the World Memory Championship challenge our interpretations of ourselves and of what we experience as memory. The types of memory competitions are extensive and involve both visual and auditory inputs and instant to long-range recall. For example, the record for accurately remembering random binary digits in one minute is 240! The record for correctly reciting the calculation of pi is to 67,890 digits! Memory might be classified as "low" on the hierarchy of thinking, but extraordinary memory skills impress, nevertheless. (If it is any consolation, the 2009 world memory champion admitted on National Public Radio that he was terrible at remembering people's names.)

The neurology of higher order thinking is far from understood but is believed to be centered in the cortex, with connections to other brain areas. At this stage, researchers are just closing in on being able to read a single word encoded in the electrical activity of a brain area. We are a long way from deciphering the thought processes involved in the creation of a symphony, a painting by a master, or an understanding of thinking itself.

> Words acquire different meanings within different fields of study. Take the word "information." In psychology, we refer to the storage of information as memory. In the field of knowledge management, information is part of a knowledge hierarchy. On the lower step is *data*, an example being a statistic: the rate of inflation in a given time period. The middle level is *information*, or drawing a meaningful conclusion from data: comparing inflation rates over a series of time periods or in selected time periods. *Knowledge*, the highest level of the hierarchy, involves attaining a broader understanding from the data: identifying factors that correlate with higher or lower rates of inflation.

Thinking beyond the Brain

Both classical psychology and modern neuroscience focus heavily on the brain as a central processor of external stimuli, conceptualizing cognition as primarily involving computation and internal representation via neuronal activity. But what about all that other activity in the brain? Cognition and consciousness are relatively recent adaptations in the evolution of the human brain. Over time, our brains have evolved beyond being just an organ to control our bodies and direct action, increasing capacity to store and manipulate data. Andy Clark (1998), professor of philosophy and chair in logic and metaphysics at the University of Edinburgh, proposes a model of cognition whose domain goes beyond the brain and includes the dynamic interaction of the brain, the body, and the environment.

The field of artificial intelligence (AI) produces one kind of intelligence—symbolically coded solutions to symbolically encoded problems. The results can be quite astonishing. First was the success of Deep Thought in defeating human chess champions. More recently, the computer Watson defeated the biggest winners on the TV quiz show *Jeopardy*. (Whether that was a fair contest is disputable; the impressive performance of the computer is not.) AI programs also support face and voice recognition and scanning of handwritten zip codes. They are capable of manipulating symbols according to a set of rules.

Human intelligence is different. It is the product of evolutionary adaptations and selections, with the outcome of making the human body act in ways that enhance survival. According to Clark, intelligence is not rooted in the presence and manipulation of language-like data structures. Rather, it involves the tuning of our basic responses to the environment in order to sense and act, like David Alexander Smith's smart alien. For us to survive, that action must be fast.

The model of the mind as conceived by classical psychology is that of a central planner that is privy to all information created by the system, producing behavior to satisfy certain needs. Research in AI points out the fundamental flaw in such a conceptualization. Rodney Brooks, professor emeritus of robotics at MIT, has identified the representational bottleneck that such a model would encounter: The brain would have to convert sensory data into a single symbolic code, process it, then convert it again to formats necessary to execute motor action. Such a process would preclude the fast responses needed for survival (Brooks, 1991).

Clark instead proposes a model in which the brain is the controller not of all necessary information but of *embodied action*. The characteristics of such embodied cognition include (1) processes geared to immediate behavior production but not to excessive information storage, (2) minimization of processing to respond to specific stimuli, and (3) limitation of perception to that which is essential to survival.

To better understand Clark's model, let us return to our consideration of the processing of visual stimuli, first mentioned in chapter 1. As it turns out, we experience high resolution in less than 0.01% of the total visual field. We compensate by moving our eyes rapidly (about three times per second) from point to point within the visual field. (Such movements are labeled *saccades*.) Research has discovered that the patterns of saccades vary with the task being performed and that our eyes return to specific locations as needed to gather and confirm data. Furthermore, research on the cortical processing of primate vision reveals the complex interaction of multiple brain areas and specialized cells, resulting in interpretations of such visual qualities as resolution, color, motion, location, and object identification. Thus, we are not creating a complete internal representation of our surroundings. To do so would use a huge amount of energy and capacity and would be too slow to produce the action required to survive. Instead, we utilize our environment as its own model, visiting and revisiting it as needed. The notion that we are experiencing a full, detailed image of our surroundings is a subjective illusion. Perception involves a sequence of partial representations from which we create our individual interpretations of "reality." Human intelligence is based on environmentally specific strategies for processing stimuli and reacting to them.

One quality of human interpretation of stimuli is to attempt to identify a central cause for a perceived phenomenon. As we process sensory stimuli, we identify patterns. Because the basic economics of neuroprocessing require minimal energy consumption and fast results, we interpret phenomena as having a central cause, even when none exists. Clark notes that complex phenomena involve a great deal of self-organization. The flocking behavior of birds and the foraging behavior of ants are examples of what we might easily interpret, on quick observation, as being centrally caused. Further study, involving the processing of additional information via sensory input, reveals that the apparently organized behavior is not the result of central causation but of simple local rules involving air currents and wing patterns in the case of birds, or food sources and the presence of other ants in the latter instance.

To illustrate this theory of self-organizing without central cause, Clark cites the example of termites that construct elaborate condominium-like homes from mud, complete with archways, corridors, and rooms. At first glance, it looks like an example of detailed architectural planning. However, all termites make mud balls as part of their basic instinctual behavioral repertoire. At first, they drop them randomly. Each mud ball contains a tiny chemical trace left by the maker, and termites have an inherent tendency to prefer to drop mud balls where these chemical traces are strongest. As more mud balls are amassed, the chemical traces become stronger, promoting bigger piles, then columns. On proximate columns, termites will be more likely to deposit mud on the side nearest the adjacent column, attracted by the perception of the chemical traces. The result: arches, then passageways and rooms. There is no plan, no leader, no cognitive processing. The resulting mud structure emerges from a collective phenomenon that stems from chemical stimuli.

In *Dynamic Patterns*, J. A. Scott Kelso (1995) applies the notion of self-organizing systems to the brain and behavior, which he describes as complex adaptive systems. He cites the example of cooking oil in a fry pan. As the temperature increases, the difference between the cooler oil on top and the warmer oil beneath creates movement: The hotter oil rises, while the cooler sinks. This continues in cyclic fashion, resulting in a persistent pattern of convection rolls. The point is not that this emergent pattern has no cause. Clearly, the heat is the proximate cause. However, the organized state of motion has no external architect but is an emergent property of a collection of molecules responding in a self-organizing manner to the application of a force. One can observe a similar phenomenon in group psychology: the frantic rush of shoppers when the doors open on the Friday after Thanksgiving, the deadly actions of soccer spectators in some countries after a loss, or the sudden rush to judgment by "deliberative" bodies when inflamed by strong emotions. However, our brain is constructed to find associations within the sensory stimuli processed from the environment and to construct simple patterns. The simplest explanation assumes central causation.

Clark notes that classical psychology has focused on an individual organ, the brain, as the central cause of cognition. While the brain cannot contain complete descriptions of all external stimuli, as noted in our consideration of vision, it does have inner structures that allow it to reduce the computational load by interacting with the environment. Clark describes how the evolution of the brain has allowed it to exploit selected external stimuli and objects to increase intelligence and decrease computation. This interactive process with external structures is illustrated by the strategies we employ to solve a jigsaw puzzle. We first organize pieces by shape (edge pieces first) and color, manipulating each within our visual field. This interaction with the puzzle environment greatly reduces computational demands on the brain. Imagine trying to solve a 500- or 1,000-piece puzzle by thought alone! Other external structures that we utilize regularly include paper and pencil, letters and words, and, more recently, digital technologies. All provide us with the potential to perform more intelligently without being inherently more intelligent. Clark refers to this process as *cognitive scaffolding*, somewhat akin to the *cultural scaffolding* referred to by Nicola Gavey with respect to rape.

Our brain functioning is constrained by the evolutionary processes that depend on adaptations of existing neural architecture and resources. Clark is describing a new paradigm of *embodied, active cognition*, whereby the brain is empowered by exploitation of environmental resources, increasing its capacity to store knowledge and enhancing its ability to perform computations.

> Anecdotal evidence that we utilize embodied, active cognition can be found in disparate places. Actors report that they learn their lines more quickly when moving about the stage or set after their actions have been blocked by the director. There is also some evidence that cognitive-behavioral therapy is effective not because of changes of thinking alone but because of the resulting associated behavioral activation. Modifying the environment so that positive reinforcement follows activity and negative reinforcement is paired with inactivity enhances outcomes in the treatment of depression.

Consider the following range of cognitive tasks: a baby learning to walk, a golfer hitting a drive, planning for a wedding, and Einstein thinking about the theory of relativity. The study of how babies learn to walk uncovers a complex interaction among a multiplicity of factors across the brain, the body, and the environment. There is no genetic encoding of prior instructions enacted in a stage-by-stage process. Rather, walking emerges from a complex, continual process of feedback loops among neural, somatic, and environmental sources. The brain develops new synaptic connections from back to front. Motor functions are controlled in the rear area of the cortex, while language is more to the front. Hence, crawling, sitting, and walking typically precede a comparable level of language development. Equally as important as motor development to walking is the acquisition of balance and the closely integrated proprioception, or awareness of the location and integration of different body parts.

Likewise, there is no genetically based coding for learning to hit a golf ball, a skill acquired by means of repeated interaction and feedback loops involving visual processing, motor action, and a scaffolded structure—in this case a golf club. The role of implicit memory is critical. Think of carrying a cup of coffee while walking up stairs. The more you focus your conscious mind on keeping the cup steady, the more likely you are to spill the contents. Take your attention from the cup and transfer it to the rhythm of your movement, and you will probably not spill. Success at golf rests on the ability to *not* think consciously about mechanical details. The great American philosopher Yogi Berra proclaimed, "You can't think and hit a baseball."

Planning for your wedding would seem to require some additional cognitive process, some kind of internal representation for absent phenomena (flower arrangements, bridesmaids' dresses, a location for the reception and honeymoon). Likewise, Einstein's thought experiments required both verbal and visual internal representations of imagined activity (a moving train or spaceship, objects or beams of light moving in opposite directions).

One model of internal representation, developed by Marc Scheiber at the University of Rochester School of Medicine, is based on the study of finger movements in monkeys. His research challenges the classic intuitive model of the homunculus in the brain's motor region, in which distinct neuronal groupings arranged in sequence are thought to control individual digits. He and colleague Lyndon Hibbard (Scheiber & Hibbard, 1993) discovered that the movement of each individual monkey digit was tied to activity throughout the motor cortex hand area. In addition, they observed that additional motor cortex activity is needed for more precise movements, including some motor cortex activity to prevent movement in other fingers. In support of an evolutionary perspective, they conceptualize the action of opening and closing the whole hand (to grip a vine and swing) as basic, while that involved in moving individual fingers (as in playing the piano) as more complex, and evolved. Scheiber's findings support the role of *distributed internal representations* in cognition: Inner encoding in the brain is not specific to a location and time as suggested by the classic, intuitive model, nor is it encoded in discrete, serial code as with the computational model; rather, it is carried by a pattern of activation spread across groups of neurons.

Francisco Varela and colleagues (1991) note the active nature of perception as a reflection of our physical interactions with the world, along with emergent behavior in simple systems and reciprocal (versus linear) causation. Taken together, these themes represent the notion of cognition as *enaction*—repeated sensorimotor interactions between the person and the environment, not the internal mirroring of an objective external reality.

From these ideas Clark (1998) has developed a conceptualization of the embodied, enacted mind as involving what he calls *continuous reciprocal causation*, wherein the brain is not just a passive organ merely perceiving the world but is engaged in mutual modulatory complexity with the body and the environment. Clark identifies the ultimate scaffold for human intelligence as one humans created themselves: language. He sees language as transforming the computational task of the pattern-completing brain, allowing it to address and solve otherwise intractable classes of cognitive challenges. Further, he describes the dynamic synergy of the interaction between language and the brain as a reverse adaptation: The brain first experienced minor neural adaptations that made basic language development possible; then linguistic forms evolved that exploited pre-existing, language-independent processes of pattern recognition. Thus, the biological brain is empowered by the artifacts it creates. Written and spoken language is the most powerful of all such artifacts. In fact, it is this dynamic, synergistic process that describes the evolution of our understanding of cognition.

> The artifact of public language permits cognition to be collective, transcending the path dependence of individual cognition. Psychotherapy uses public language as its tool for expressing, and ultimately altering, personal cognition. A challenge for any clinician is the ability to bridge the gap between Wittgenstein's concept of private language and the assumptions and vagaries of public discourse. Though our capacity for linguistic precision is limited, it is this imprecision that can be exploited to obtain otherwise seemingly impossible results, as illustrated by this case example.
>
> L, a male in his 40s, had been unhappy with his weight since adolescence. He reported a pervasive family pattern of moderate obesity. He recalled being popular as an adolescent but thought his weight had limited his physical activity and intimate relationships. Nevertheless he had married, had two children, and enjoyed a professional career. In middle age, he began to experience health complications secondary to his weight: hypertension, elevated cholesterol, and blood-sugar abnormalities. His primary-care physician referred him for psychotherapeutic intervention after attempts to reduce weight through dieting failed.
>
> L presented as mildly to moderately depressed. His attitude toward his obesity was characterized by helplessness. He thought he had tried every possible intervention and was resigned to his fate. His participation in the initial session was superficial and passive.
>
> My experience has been that focusing on a persistent problem that has been resistant to change only deepens the thoughts of hopelessness and the feelings of depression. Therefore, after just 15 minutes, I suddenly changed the subject, asking him what experiences he associated with fun and freedom. After a brief moment to change his cognitive focus, he began to recall an experience in late adolescence when he had participated in a protracted paintball battle with friends. His mood lifted as he re-experienced the memories and emotions associated with that playful time.

> I reframed his experience as an adventure and inquired if he might like to have another adventure right then. L was confused but agreed. With minimal preparation, I suggested that we spend the rest of the session by my introducing him to this new adventure—hypnosis.
>
> Induction and deepening were uneventful, as they often are when the subject has not had time to worry and resist. I had L visualize himself at the location of the paintball game and stressed that he focus on the sensory experience—the sights, sounds, smells, and touch involved. Then I had him visualize a friend directing a paintball at him in slow motion. I directed him to imagine himself as smoothly and effortlessly floating aside to avoid contact. I repeated the suggestion many times over again, emphasizing the words "lightly" in describing his agile, graceful avoidant movements and making frequent use of the word "light" in describing the colors of the environment, the paintballs, and the feel of his imagined gun as he shot at his friends. Under my verbal suggestion, he ultimately won the imagined battle, and I reinforced his feelings of competence, of being in control of his actions. When he awakened, I simply suggested he call me in a few weeks to let me know how he was doing and ended our session.
>
> In psychotherapy, there can never be an attribution of causation between the intervention and the outcome. An intervention is far too complex to condense into a technique, a label. In this case, though, there was a correlation between our interaction and L's subsequent report of a successful and sustained loss of weight associated with increased physical activity. My speculation is that the altered cognitive state in hypnosis transcended both the private and public language associated with "light," allowing L to incorporate it in a different way into his cognition of himself.

Finally, Clark speculates that the artifact of public language has led to a distinctive quality of human thought—second-order cognition, which, in simplest terms, refers to "thinking about thinking." Humans are able to interpret sensory stimuli in order to act. We can analyze our interpretations and actions in order to make modifications that enhance our achievement of goals. Our thoughts then become objects for further interpretation and revision. In short, our biological brain has become empowered by the artifact it has created. Herein lies the potential power of psychotherapy. Second-order cognition allows us to critique our own thoughts and associated emotions and actions and to modify them, to become more attuned to our goals and desires.

More difficult to grasp are the limitations that this dynamic interaction between brain, body, and environment impose. Our brains are able to re-create detailed knowledge of our surroundings precisely because of that constant, dynamic interaction, which creates a subjective illusion of central control. Our brains confuse the forms and structures of the artifact of language with the structure of neural activity. In reality, the brain functions in a more fragmented and opportunistic fashion than our cognitive intuitions can conceptualize. Advances in such areas as brain imaging, artificial neural networks, and robotics are providing scientists with a much deeper understanding of the dynamic complexities of human cognition. Additional technologies will be required in order to meet the goals of the BRAIN Initiative, the Human Brain Project, and the Human Connectome Project. According to Rafael Yuste of Columbia University and George Church of Harvard University (2014), these will likely include:

- new nanotechnology methods of measuring more precisely the electrical activity both among small networks of neurons and across the entire organ;
- new imaging technologies that will, among other things, advance an appreciation of the persistent and seemingly spontaneous activity among neuronal groupings;
- improved microscopes that can picture neuron activity in three dimensions;
- optical methods to record membrane voltage directly, rather than indirectly through sensing calcium;
- quantum optics technologies to measure cellular electrical activity;
- computational optics technologies to probe into deeper areas of the brain;
- DNA technologies to assess neuronal activity;
- optogenetic and optochemical approaches for both research and therapeutic uses;
- advanced computational capacities to manage and share the explosion of data.

In the meantime, critical issues confront humankind in the fields of the environment, economics, politics, and medicine. As we will see in chapter 6, intuitive cognitive processing can be a significant obstacle to addressing those issues in an effective way. Turning our thinking onto itself was once thought of as a strictly philosophical endeavor. Then William James initiated a field of inquiry that morphed into psychology. Now neuroscience is taking us to new conceptualizations of our thinking, the environments within which we interact, and that thing we call the self.

Thinking is more than passive interpretation of sensory stimuli as represented internally. It involves a dynamic interaction among the brain, the body, and the environment in which constant feedback stimulates and modulates the process. This is not the paradigm of intuitive, popular psychology that we use to navigate through our daily lives. That paradigm may be sufficient for us to achieve the simple goals we set to enhance our short-term survival and enjoyment, but it is inadequate to comprehend the more complex matters that involve long-term outcomes. These issues require us to think more deeply about our thinking.

5
THINKING ABOUT OUR SELVES

The most wildly improbable organism of all is one that can fret over its improbability.
— John Horgan, *The Undiscovered Mind*

Somehow, we feel, the water of the physical brain is turned into the wine of consciousness, but we draw a total blank on the nature of this conversion. Neural transmissions just seem like the wrong kind of materials with which to bring consciousness into the world.
—Colin McGinn

I in my selfhood am that Satan, I am the evil one.
—William Blake

How much larger your life would be if your self could become smaller in it.
—G. K. Chesterton

Conundrums, paradoxes, and enigmas are not the result of basic contradictions in nature. Rather, they are a product of the limitations of our thinking. We become victims of the limitations of our own brains. Nowhere is this more evident than in attempting to solve the brain–mind conundrum: How can a material organ produce an immaterial, subjective sense of awareness and self-awareness?

Understanding Consciousness

Some argue that consciousness is beyond the capacity of the human brain to understand. Julian Jaynes, in his seminal work, *The Origin of Consciousness in the Breakdown of the Bicameral Mind*, posits that consciousness has evolved over the past 3,000 years and continues to evolve today. According to Jaynes, the Hebrews of the Old Testament and the Greeks of Homer's era lacked consciousness. Their behavior was the result of automatic, non-conscious neural activity in the left hemisphere that was modulated under stress by auditory hallucinations from the right hemisphere, the latter experienced as voices of a chieftain or god. Jaynes believes that consciousness evolved concurrently with the spread of writing. His notion of consciousness was more narrow than many and reflected a kind of meta-consciousness, awareness of awareness, thinking about thinking.

Consciousness actually constitutes only a small portion of the brain's activity. Most of the brain is concerned with the myriad functions that keep us alive: regulating vital functions such as breathing and circulation, digesting food and eliminating wastes, and processing motor functions that ensure our survival. We are not conscious of these, at least not until brought to consciousness by reading about it in a book.

The language that researchers and philosophers use when exploring consciousness differs, as is the case when searching for meaning in any endeavor. Consciousness as a mental state is analog. We digitize it with such bits as consciousness, sub-consciousness, pre-consciousness, semi-consciousness, and unconsciousness. Another digitization is the differentiation between consciousness and self-awareness. Consciousness might be thought of as awareness of your body and its distinction from the environment, while self-awareness might be recognition of that consciousness. Another conceptualization: Being conscious is to think; being self-aware is to know that you think and are able to think about your thinking (metacognition).

One solution to getting something immaterial (a thought) from something material (human tissue)—the subjective from the objective—is to declare consciousness an illusion. Susan Blackmore, PhD (2011), a visiting professor at England's University of Plymouth, does just that. Like William James, she notes the futility of trying to examine consciousness through insight, which James likened as turning up the gas to examine the dark. Blackmore creates a modern metaphorical equivalent: looking into the refrigerator to see if the light is still on. Rather than trying to examine how neural impulses turn into conscious experiences, she would have us reframe the question: How does this grand illusion called consciousness get constructed in the first place?

For now, though, we will pursue the evidence that the subjective experience we call consciousness can be traced to specific brain areas, measurable electrical activity, and synchronous electrical processes across multiple brain sites. We will end with a rudimentary understanding of how to decode electrical activity to identify a simple thought.

To start, here's an attempt at defining consciousness. Like all thinking, it is subjective. It is the interpretation of sensory, including somatosensory, inputs that we call awareness—both of what we consider self and what we interpret as outside of our self. The self is a complex construct of consciousness built on the separation from the non-self. It is the digital product of processes that take place within the somatosensory system (awareness of the body), the hippocampus, and other memory processes (awareness of our past) and the posterior parietal cortex (where we can distinguish between self and non-self).

Before delving into the concept of self, let us consider a more basic definition of consciousness. We can be considered conscious if we are not asleep or in a coma. In another context, we can be conscious of a sensory stimulus if we acknowledge and respond to it. For our purposes, our concern is with *phenomenal consciousness*: the awareness of subjective experience.

Neuroscientist Stanislas Dehaene (2014) says the challenge within the scientific study of consciousness is to identify the change of stimulus that the subject claims makes his perception shift from non-conscious to conscious. He calls this *access to consciousness*. We are conscious of only a very small percentage of the stimuli with which our brain is bombarded. One lab experiment exposed subjects to the visual stimulation of a word on a screen for just 30 milliseconds, after which they could translate the stimulus into language. However, when they were exposed to another string of letters after the word, they reported seeing only the string, not the word. This reported lack of awareness occurred when the delay between the word and the string of letters was less than 50 milliseconds. Delays of more than 50 milliseconds allowed the subject to see both the word and the string of letters. When the delay was exactly 50 milliseconds, subjects saw both the word and the string of letters half the time. This is but one example of experimental approaches that can measure a stimulus going in and out of consciousness.

Steven Pinker, in his computational model of the mind (1997), refers to three aspects of consciousness, as described by linguist Ray Jackendoff and philosopher Ned Block. The first is *self-knowledge*: I can see colors, I can feel warmth. (It is below zero outside in northern New York as I write this, so being able to experience warmth is near the top of my hierarchy of thoughts right now.) And I can connect those sensory interpretations to my mind, a part of this complex blob of tissue named Phil.

A second aspect of consciousness is *access to information*. Here Pinker distinguishes between two kinds of information processed by the central nervous system. One can be accessed by neural systems that produce verbal expression and organized thinking and decision making. This includes our interpretations of sensory inputs (the letters on this page, the muffled click of my computer keys). The other involves automatic processes, the internal computing that underlies our sensory interpretations and subsequent verbal and motor behavior (the transmission of electrical impulses from the retina and inner ear to specific brain areas and the eventual production of a verbal and motor response).

Information is stored in many locations involving multiple pathways (remember our French cat from chapter 4) and can be accessed by multiple routes. Still, there are limitations to our access to that information. Pinker identifies these limitations: space (the number of neurons and pathways), time (a solution needs to be timely or it has no value), and resources (working brain tissue consumes more glucose).

Linguist Jackendoff (1987) postulates three levels of mental representation. Using vision as an example, the lowest level is the electrical charge created within the retina when we see an object. The intermediate level involves the representations of edges, surfaces, and depth. The highest level is the recognition of the object itself. Similarly, our mental process of understanding spoken language goes from perceiving raw sound, to identifying words and phrases, to understanding content. Jackendoff thinks that access to information, the second aspect of consciousness, takes place at the intermediate level of mental representation.

Access consciousness has four features, says Pinker (1997). First is a *rich field of sensation*: colors and shapes, soft music and loud noises, gentle massage and piercing pain, the pleasing smell of baking bread and the stench of a latrine, the sweetness of chocolate and the bitterness of a lemon. We are unaware of the lowest level of representation for these sensory experiences. The highest level, where we draw greater meaning from context and experience, is not usually necessary or helpful in dealing with our immediate circumstances. Rather, the higher representation tends to be stored in long-term memory for processing later. The intermediate representation, then, is what we need to take action.

The second feature of access consciousness is the *spotlight of attention*. An experiment devised by psychologist Anne Treisman involved differentiating conscious and unconscious processing (Wolfe & Robertson, 2012). When subjects were shown a display of hundreds of Xs, among which there is one O, they can quickly find the O and push a button. Subjects respond equally as quickly to a green O among a page full of red Os. However, the task of finding a letter that is both green and O among a mixed display of green Xs and red Os requires a slow, *conscious* search. Calculating the conjunction of two features (color and shape) requires attention to one before further processing the other. Pinker notes that these conjunctions are combinatorial, meaning that the total number of possible conjunctions is astronomical and that "the combinations have to be computed, consciously, at one location at a time."

The *emotional coloring of experience* is a third attribute of access consciousness. We encode our awareness of stimuli as being either good or bad, pleasurable or painful. This duality has evolutionary significance. Generally, those stimuli that gave us pleasure enhance our odds of survival: food, water, sex, and mastery of our environment, among others. In current Western culture, this pleasure–pain dichotomy underlies our discussions of politics, religion, and sex.

Pinker identifies the fourth and final feature of access consciousness as an executive function that asserts control over the others, referred to variously as the *self*, *willpower*, or *I*. These concepts are subject to cognitive fuzziness and a disconnect between public and private language. Remember Antonio Damasio's description of the patient who was cognitively alert yet unable to make a decision due to damage in the anterior cingulate sulcus. We do respond to our environment in a meaningful way, not through the activity of a specific brain area to which we can attribute "will" or "self," but through the dynamic, complex activities and feedback loops among the body, the brain, and the environment.

The third component of consciousness, according to Pinker, is *sentience*. The distinction between sentience and access is tested by thinking about thinking. In my office, my patients and I are exposed to an immeasurable quantity of stimuli. Some of this is processed through the auditory system—the faint, constant bubbling of the aerator in my aquarium; the intermittent chiming of a mantel clock every quarter hour; our mutual verbal emissions. If therapy is productive, we are sentient of the bubbling and chiming but are not accessing them because the verbal interaction is more relevant. It is not entirely clear that sentience is distinct from access. Pinker refers to sentience as "an extra quality of some kind of information access."

The Neurobiology of Consciousness

One way to address the neurobiology of consciousness is to contrast it with unconsciousness. The level of consciousness is the result of projections from areas within the reticular formation to the thalamus and/or cortex. These projections are part of the *ascending reticular activating system* (ARAS). They are necessary in order for us to be awake but are not sufficient for us to have the subjective experiences of consciousness. (Being awake has both objective and subjective correlates.)

Daniel Bor (2012) believes the "best guess" for the mechanism of anesthetics is that they increase the production of the neurotransmitter gamma-amino butyric acid (GABA), thereby slowing activity throughout the cortex, which results in more harmonized, less differentiated patterns. He believes that consciousness requires the interactive exchange of information across the neural landscape, which is the product of highly differentiated electrical activity.

The term *qualia* refers to our awareness of subjective internal experiences. Most sensory inputs do not result in conscious subjective experiences. Ambulating and other motor activity involve an incredibly complex interaction of sensory, neurological, and muscular processes that move us about on two feet to planned destinations while maintaining balance, all with little or no conscious awareness of these processes. Perhaps more illustrative of such neural activity without qualia is the common act of driving a car for miles with no conscious awareness or memory, yet navigating safely.

The brain structures involved in Pinker's notion of access consciousness might be deduced by identifying those which act differently when one is awake versus when one is anesthetized. The lower levels of the cerebral cortex seem to be likely candidates. The late Francis Crick and Cristof Koch (2004), a neuroscientist at California Institute of Technology, suggest that because information about a perception is scattered among many areas of the cerebral cortex, information access requires a way to bind together separate data. They think the loops from the cortex to the thalamus might do the job. Because planned behavior requires activity within the frontal lobes, access consciousness could come from the fiber tracts running from multiple brain locations to the frontal lobes.

Koch believes there is a physical basis for consciousness that can be explained by existing theories in neurology. He focuses on one aspect of consciousness, perceptual awareness, seeking to discover the *neural correlates of consciousness*, or NCC. He defines NCC as "the minimal set of neuronal events jointly sufficient for a specific conscious phenomenal state." He focuses his inquiry on visual consciousness as the doorway to understanding higher levels of consciousness. Advances in research have helped us understand that the awareness of seeing something involves the complex interaction of many regions of the brain. Say you are driving your automobile, focusing on the cars ahead and evaluating your relative speed and distance, when an object enters your peripheral line of vision. The optic nerve carries an impulse through the thalamus, which directs the sensory input to a cortical processing area. Then the impulses go to the primary visual cortex. At this point, though, you are still not conscious of the object.

In this situation, awareness is the result of competition between a temporary grouping of neurons associated with the as-yet unidentified object and other neural groups associated with the cars, the road, and the traffic signals ahead. Each group activates the thalamus, the primary visual cortex, and other areas within the caudal visual cortex, as well as certain cortical columns in the medial, temporal, and frontal lobes. We are capable of being aware of only one visual perception at a time. Further, awareness is the result of sensory inputs violating our expectations. The neuronal group representing the unidentified object wins out for an instant so that you will consciously identify the object as a threat or as harmless, engage in an appropriate motor maneuver, then switch back to the other neuronal groups.

A person can detect an object when processing only a portion of the visual (or other sensory) input if he or she has a set of neurons, which Koch refers to as nodes, encoded with a representation of the object. The existence of such nodes is a necessary but not a sufficient condition for perceptual awareness. Other necessary conditions include projecting the encoded information to the cortex and feeding back the processed results in a way that meets an intensity and time threshold.

Koch theorizes that this visual awareness has evolved in mammals because of its advantages in hunting, avoiding danger, and, eventually, social activity. While we have subsequently evolved functions involving higher levels of consciousness—such as abstract thought, language, and planning ahead—Koch studies this more primitive form of consciousness because the neuronal mechanisms underlying visual perception are relatively easily studied in animals.

Adopting a different approach, Stanislas Dehaene (2014) has pioneered the use of brain imaging technologies to study consciousness. Although functional magnetic resonance imaging (fMRI) identifies the specific brain areas activated, it permits viewing a static pattern of activation for only a second or two. Other instruments, such as electro- or magnetoencephalography, can record in milliseconds the temporal dynamics of the activation as it progresses through multiple brain sites. Together, these devices have led to significant discoveries. For example, experiments have traced the cortical activation that results from subliminal messages and have shown that a visual stimulus can be processed all the way to the meaning of a word without the subject making any report of consciousness.

This has led to a comparison of brain activity when one is conscious of a word versus when one is not conscious. Two major differences were found. First, in a conscious state there is amplified activation, up to tenfold, in the visual word form area of the brain. Second, other distant brain areas, such as the inferior frontal region and inferior parietal sectors of the prefrontal cortex, activate in a coordinated way. The initial 270 to 300 milliseconds (about a fourth of a second, which is extraordinarily long in brain processing time) of this process were identical between conscious and non-conscious states. However, the divergence between conscious and non-conscious states was marked by measurement of a P3 wave. Small and quickly decaying P3 waves accompany subliminal stimuli. Large, non-linear increases in P3 wave activation occur when stimuli cross the threshold of consciousness.

- *Oscillation*: movement back and forth with a steady, uninterrupted rhythm.
- *Neural oscillation*: rhythmic, repetitive electrical activity within a neuron and in interactions among neurons.
- *P3 waves*: neural event-related potential associated with decision making and measured by electroencephalogram most strongly over the parietal lobe.
- *Hz*: a hertz is a unit of frequency equal to a periodic interval (cycle) of one second; thus, 100 Hz means 100 cycles per second.
- *Gamma waves*: a pattern of human neural oscillation with a frequency range of 25 to 100 Hz.

Along with the large P3 wave, which peaks between 400 and 500 milliseconds, Dehaene has also measured a high level of oscillation in the brain (in the high-gamma band of 50–100 Hz) and a massive synchrony across distant brain regions associated with the conscious state. Prior to consciousness, processing is modular, with several simultaneous activations that are independent and parallel. Access to consciousness is achieved, however, through the synchronicity among multiple brain sites.

As a result of these findings, Dehaene proposes a phenomenological definition of consciousness: *the sharing of information among different brain areas*. For example, the visual processing of an object is shared with the Broca's area of the brain so one can select words to speak; the hippocampus so the object can be stored in memory; the parietal areas so one can decide whether to attend further; and so on. Dehaene hypothesizes that the tightly intertwined long-distance connections in such associative brain areas as the dorsal parietal and prefrontal cortex, or the anterior temporal cortex and the anterior cingulate, send messages among the areas, producing the synchronicity. Thus, consciousness is not created in a single brain site but rather is the product of long distance synchronization among multiple areas.

Andrey Vyshedskiy (2008), adjunct professor at Boston University (chapter 4), proposes that consciousness is the result of a unique human capacity that he calls "mental synthesis." All living creatures have some kind of sense organs, as well as a neurological organ to process and activate a response to stimuli. Creatures that we consider more highly evolved have the additional ability to store the experiences of stimuli in memory to assist in the appraisal of new situations. Vyshedskiy postulates that what makes humans different from other highly evolved creatures is their ability to combine different memories that are encoded in groups of interconnected neurons that he calls "neural ensembles." For example, visualize your living room. Now visualize a kangaroo. Now combine them, resulting in a kangaroo sitting on the couch or chair in your living room. Presumably you are not recalling an actual event, since kangaroos in living rooms are relatively rare. Instead, you are combining two visual percepts stored in your brain by means of the synchronous activity of large groups of cortical neurons.

Imagining kangaroos in your living room is not an apparent advantage for survival. However, the capacity for this kind of mental synthesis underlies a whole host of mental processes like planning, making judgments, adapting, creating, and problem solving. Mental synthesis allows us to ask the "what if?" questions: What if I sharpened a stone and attached it to a long stick? I could more easily kill animals for their meat. What if I make two round wooden objects, call them wheels, and attach them to a basket? I would move food faster and more efficiently. What if I drive through that stop sign? I'll likely crash into another car and be seriously hurt. What if I don't go to work today? I'll be fired. What if a person could travel at speeds approaching that of light? Time would slow down.

> For many winters, my buddies and I have skied five miles up to a camp in a remote area of the Adirondack Mountains to spend a weekend together. When we started this annual adventure, we were in our 20s and 30s, strong and healthy. We would arrive at the cabin overheated from exertion, start a fire in the wood stove when the temperature was as cold as −30° F, and stand

> around for six or more hours until the temperature was tolerable. When a man is relatively young, he labels such an experience an "adventure." As his body ages, he interprets it as "discomfort." Over the years, we have engaged in mental synthesis to imagine how we might make the experience more appealing to our changing interpretations. Insulation, propane heaters, and a snowmobile were the result. Most recently, we mentally created a complex system for instantly heating water from the frozen pond. Implementation is an ongoing, Rube Goldberg–like drama, as well as the source of much entertainment.

In addition to describing mental synthesis as central to human consciousness, Vyshedskiy presents evidence that conscious perception is also associated with the global synchronization of neuronal assemblies in the beta frequency (15–25 Hz). Consciousness is awareness, while conscious experience is any experience of which one is aware. Vyshedskiy thinks that the neurological basis of conscious experience is the synchronous firing of neuronal ensembles in phase and on the upswing of the attention phase. The notion of synchronicity among different brain areas is shared by both Vyshedskiy and Dehaene.

> The notion of synchronicity actually originated with Carl Jung, who sought meaning in coincidences he observed when conducting psychotherapy. Later, scientists discovered what they believed to be a tendency for pendulum clocks mounted on the same base or wall to swing, over time, either in phase, or anti-phase, depending on the research conditions. More recently, phase synchronization between different regions of a person's brain has been identified as playing a key role in the processing of both working and long-term memory.

We can think about consciousness as an illusion, as consisting of multiple psychological processes, or as the product of synchronicity of neuronal activity among multiple brain areas. Each conceptualization requires time and energy to process. To consider all three requires the ability to tolerate ambiguity and cognitive messiness. I trust that any reader who has gotten this far in this book has all these attributes.

The Debate about Conscious Will

I ask that you be *mindful* as you read this next section on conscious will and be conscious of both your thoughts and your emotions as you process the content. In a sense, I am asking that you use your conscious will to monitor your thoughts and emotions as you process the notion that you have no conscious will!

Let's revisit a creature that we might assume has no conscious will—the lowly termite. We look at their elaborate condominium-like nests and wonder how they know how to design such intricate structures. The answers derived from scientific study shed light not only on the habits of the termite but also on human thinking. As described in chapter 4, the mud-ball construction of termites is chemically based. Their building process has been labeled *stirmergic algorithms* and can be observed in the behavior of ants gathering food and geese flying in a V pattern. A scientific interpretation of this behavior would include the notion that there was no predetermined design or plan, that no termite "knows" or is conscious of anything beyond how to instinctively respond to a chemical trace. There is no need for linguistic coding or memory.

But wait! Surely the human brain is more complex than that of a termite and *is* capable of designing and constructing complex structures. This is undoubtedly true. However, the vignette about termites illustrates how the human brain interprets phenomena. Until science discovered the chemical traces that motivated termite behavior, it was assumed that the complex termite construction had to be driven by a design, a leader, and a central plan. This kind of thinking is the basis for philosophy, religion, and even science itself. Further, it shapes our thinking about ourselves as purposeful beings driven by our own internal central leader.

The late Daniel Wegner (2002), professor of psychology at Harvard University, made a distinction between the experience of conscious free will and free will as causation. He referred to the experience of free will as a "feeling." This is not the conventional use of the word "feeling." I understand him to mean that we have a conscious experience of intent and of acting on the intent. This process is different than our subsequent interpretation that we have caused our own behavior.

An immediate problem in studying conscious will is that intent is totally subjective and can only be measured by self-report. In addition, not all action, or behavior, is voluntary. When you pull your hand away from the hot surface of a stove, you experience this action as automatic, not conscious. Taking a walk, driving a car, and playing golf also involve very complex neurological processes, most of which we are not conscious of.

In the 1980s, Benjamin Libet (1982) set out to time both the subjective and objective correlates of simple voluntary movements. On the subjective side, subjects reported the instant they were conscious of willing their arm to move and the instant they were conscious of the movement itself. Objectively, researchers timed the Readiness Potential (RP), a pattern of electrical activity in the brain that precedes voluntary movement, as well as the instant the muscle initiated contraction. The results: Consciousness of willing the arm to move was experienced a half-second *after* the RP. The brain initiates a movement before we are aware of wanting it to happen.

When we see a billiard ball hit another, we don't see the *cause* of the second ball moving. We infer, or interpret, that the force of the first ball caused the second to move. In psychology, as Wegner pointed out, a distinction is made between *empirical will*, which is the causal relationship between thoughts and behaviors as determined by scientific analysis of their covariation, and *phenomenal will*, one's report of the experience of will.

The way we understand causation in the physical world is mechanistic, governed by the laws of physics. We may plead with our sputtering car to will itself home ("Come on, baby, you can do it"), but generally we understand that the vehicle's performance is determined by the proper burning of fuel in an orderly process inside the engine. In psychology, we think of causation differently, emphasizing the role of intent. These two ways of thinking about causation are incompatible, asserted Wegner. Our thinking, feeling, and behaving are the product of incomprehensibly complicated mechanisms functioning as the empirical will. Because we cannot comprehend such complexity, we readily accept a far easier explanation: We did it because we intended to. Of course we are quick to disavow intent when our actions have negative consequences. Nevertheless, the conflict between our innate inability to understand the mechanics of our behavior, on the one hand, and our need to make sense of ourselves and the world around us, on the other, leads to a belief in "the magic of our causal agency" (Wegner, 2002).

It appears that different areas of the brain are involved during voluntary motor actions (frontal lobes) as compared to the experience of conscious will (interaction of multiple brain sites, including those involved with conscious thought, muscle feedback, and visual processing). Further, experiments demonstrate that response to a stimulus is quicker and involves different brain structures than does a conscious response. There is nothing conscious about quick responses to stimuli except our awareness of them after the fact. The illusion of causality arises from two factors: First is Vyshedskiy's notion of mental synthesis, the ability to foresee an outcome before it happens; second is the interpretation of having engaged in a physical or mental effort via feedback from the somatosensory system.

> When salmon fishing on a remote lake in northern Maine, trolling my lure behind the rowboat, I noted my location with respect to a large rock while humming a specific tune. At that moment, my rod was bent over by the strike of a very large fish. After successfully landing it, an experience filled with excitement and a sense of competence, I found myself rowing past the same location while humming the same tune. I paired the visual stimulus of the location with the mental processes of humming and assumed that together they had somehow caused me to catch the big one. Such magical thinking pervades the sport of fishing. As the great fishing philosopher and author John Gierach (1995) put it, "Many of the fine points of fly fishing are lost on the fish."

The interpretation of having exerted conscious will requires three elements: *priority* (the thought must precede the action), *consistency* (the thought must be consistent with the action), and *exclusivity* (the thought must not be accompanied by other potential causes). Where these exist, we interpret the outcome as the product of conscious will. Where these don't exist, we assume the outcome is the result of some outside agent. This is yet another example of duality in thinking.

Compare conscious will to a golf ball. When I say I "have" a golf ball, I conclude this from visual and tactile inputs. I reason that I no longer possess the ball when I process visual stimuli that I interpret as the splash of water where the ball hits the lake. Conscious will, however, is not a physical object. It is a mental construct of a subjective experience. To "have" it, to possess it, is different from "having" a golf ball.

Have you been mindful of your thoughts and emotions as you read the preceding paragraphs? Every reader will interpret them differently. Some might experience anxiety and think that declaring conscious will dead undermines concepts of responsibility. How can you hold someone accountable if he or she does not have conscious will?

Daniel Wegner (2002) used a metaphor, comparing conscious will to a compass. When we sail, the compass does not steer the boat in any physical sense, but it sure is helpful in avoiding disaster and getting us to our destination safely and in the most efficient manner. This is similar to what we label "conscious will": It interprets the relation between our thoughts and behaviors and enhances our functioning and our chances of survival.

Are you thinking about where this line of thinking is going? What emotions accompany your thoughts? We are heading toward one of the most fundamental debates in dualistic thinking: free will versus determinism. The economic stimulus and social benefits created by this dichotomy are unending. It has employed philosophers; been a boon to the paper, ink, and publishing industries; made millionaires of self-absorbed proselytizers; and temporarily distracted hormonally driven college students from further exploration of the limits of self-gratification. Then along came Wegner, putting a Harvard-style damper on all the fun. Employing another metaphor, he declared the debate a false dichotomy: "It is like asking, Shall we dance, or shall we move about the room in time to the music?"

Free will and determinism cannot be compared because they are fundamentally different concepts. Free will is an interpretation of a subjective experience. Determinism is a process that attempts to explain human behavior. You can't *have* free will, but you sure can *experience* free will. Free will is not a psychological mechanism; it is a uniquely human experience.

> The duality of determinism versus free will has been resolved by some with the concept of *compatibilism*, which posits that free will, as required for moral responsibility, is consistent with causal determinism. All the philosophical

> implications of such a position, and the countervailing ones, have been the subject of many a book. Perhaps much of the debate is born of different understandings of the concept of "free will." Wittgenstein's consideration of language seems relevant once again.

Earlier I mentioned that Wegner called conscious will a "feeling." Now we are confronted with another dichotomy—the one between thoughts and feelings—as we struggle with our interpretation of subjective phenomena. As is often the case in what we call higher level thinking, we try to resolve the dichotomy with some new notion, in this case, *cognitive emotions*. Gerald Clore (Clore & Ortony, 1998) identifies the sense of knowing, or the sense of familiarity, as a combinational experience. Wegner classified the experience of willing an action as similar, in that it combines an informative feeling of mind and body through action.

Interpreting our actions as being under our control has survival value because it enhances our psychological and physical health. People who conceive of themselves as powerless are less likely to mobilize their efforts and defenses in service of their survival. Morality is based on the belief in free will—our moral compass. Wegner (2002) concluded that conscious will is useful, even essential to survival, but an illusion, nevertheless. He cited the following metaphor from Albert Einstein:

> If the moon, in the act of completing its eternal way around the earth, were gifted with self-consciousness, it would feel thoroughly convinced that it was traveling its way of its own accord. . . . So would a Being, endowed with higher insights and more perfect intelligence, watching man and his doings, smile about man's illusion that he was acting according to his own free will.

Declaring free will an illusion is engaging in truth-versus-fiction or right-versus-wrong forms of dichotomous thinking. An alternative dichotomy is proposed by John Duncan (2010), assistant director of the MRC Cognition and Brain Sciences Unit in Cambridge, England. Duncan distinguishes between two perspectives on understanding the human mind. One he calls the "inside" view of ourselves as rational creatures who give our own reasons for how we behave, as free agents who do as we choose. This paradigm works well when our decisions are successful, our behaviors meet some definition of expectation, and our reasoning is sound. Our perspective changes, though, when things don't go so well. We intended to run that errand on the way home but forgot. We knew the right answer on the exam but blew it. Now we begin to consider ourselves as biological beings with biological limits. We take an "outside" view, examining the mind to try to understand how it works and how it fails. This outside perspective is the scientific one: the attempt to create order out of chaos by organizing thoughts. Our personal, inside perspective is that we have free will. Our outside-looking-in view recognizes the multiple, complex factors that contribute to those things we call thoughts, feelings, and behaviors.

Duncan views the free will versus biological/psychological (pre-)determinism as a problem of language. He argues that psychology does not deny people their freedom in the sense that people do experience freedom. We know what it means to be free of an unhealthy relationship, of the restrictions of jail, or of worry and fear. But free will? Free of what? We can believe that no one can force us to think or feel in any way we do not choose. Can we also believe we are free of *ourselves*? This doesn't make sense. Rather, these questions reflect different points of view. From the inside, we see ourselves operating as free, independent agents. From the outside, we try to understand how our behavior can be explained in terms of organizing principles. These are not mutually exclusive concepts, just different perspectives, like the differences in perspectives on time that we will explore in chapter 6.

Our Sense of Self

In *Incognito*, David Eagleman (2011) notes the findings of Galileo in the early 1600s that the earth is not the center of the universe and the subsequent outrage and punishment for heresy at the hands of the church. More recent findings in astronomy only serve to create more uncertainty and make our role in the greater scheme of things more minimal. Eagleman argues that advances in neuroscience provoke resistance to the notion that "we are not the center of ourselves," that most of what we do is unconscious, then rationalized in the left hemisphere. He concludes that consciousness, which plays a small but not unimportant role in our survival, has evolved in order to provide us with cognitive flexibility.

Consciousness includes many kinds of awareness born of sensory inputs. Antonio Damasio (2011) notes that the special form of consciousness we label *self* is unique in that it requires a stable reference point to create and maintain continuity over time. He concludes that this reference point is our body. While the body can be thought of as having many parts, an alternative conceptualization is that it has a stable *internal milieu*, biochemical processes that must be maintained within a certain range in order to avoid disease and death. Damasio views this built-in system as the basis for continuity in body and brain, the basis of what we experience as self.

Further, he postulates that the brain stem makes internal maps of the various parts of the body, which connect with each other in a recursive manner. This mapping is based on the primitive emotions that emanate from the brain stem and form the basis for the sense of self. Since other vertebrates have brain stems, he believes they have conscious minds. For him, the difference in humans is that our cerebral cortex is far more developed, producing a richer, more complex consciousness, including aspects that constitute self. He emphasizes that he does not believe that self is the product of the cerebral cortex but originates in the brain stem and is enriched by cortex activity.

Personality is a way to quantify the self. We try to make meaning out of the abundance of data about self by constructing mental categories that share common attributes. As defined in the American Psychiatric Association's (2000) *Diagnostic and Statistical Manual of Mental Disorders* (DSM-IV-TR), personality traits are "enduring patterns of perceiving, relating to, and thinking about the environment and oneself that are exhibited in a wide range of social and personal contexts." Further elaboration of this definition includes behavioral aspects, such as interpersonal functioning and impulse control. Many personality traits have been identified or constructed by psychologists, including introvert/extrovert, contemplative/reactive, trusting/suspicious, and other/inner directed. Our thought processes seek further meaning by combining these constructs into a broad category called personality.

A key building block in this construct is that of "enduring patterns." Thus, there is an assumption that each person is endowed with relatively fixed patterns of thinking, feeling, and behaving. The economy of our cognitive processes reduces each of us to a nice, neat package. Underlying this way of conceptualizing the self is the assumption that there is a unitary self: Each individual perceives, thinks, feels, and behaves in predictable, or patterned, ways. Under this paradigm, the task for science is to identify the biological, neurological, genetic, and social factors and interactions that produce the predictable patterns. This kind of research is generally conducted in laboratory conditions to control for the variables being measured.

Psychotherapists, however, operate in a much more chaotic environment. Some clinicians, including myself, think that the unitary personality concept is limiting, both in our understanding of our patients and our ability to help them. Richard Schwartz, PhD, director of the Center for Self Leadership and an associate professor at both Northwestern University and the University of Illinois–Chicago, has developed a very different way to think about the self. In *Internal Family Systems* (1997), he describes different parts of the person's personality, each serving a different function. He envisions psychotherapy as group/family therapy whose goal is to reduce perceived threats among the parts to bring the core self into its rightful role as leader of the internal system.

Most people will acknowledge that they think, feel, and behave differently at different times. To be sure, fatigue, stress, and hormonal changes are among factors that seem to have significant impact on our psychological functioning. Social context can also affect our cognitive, emotional, and behavioral performance. Most people will be very different in front of a large audience, in the face of hostile questioning in a courtroom, or when performing for large monetary rewards (or punishment). Such differences can be minimal and easily thought of as falling within a personality type. At other times, behaviors in different circumstances may differ enough to cause others to perceive one as a distinctly different person.

Sometimes our most elaborate ways of thinking about phenomena evolve to a point where the whole construct starts to collapse on itself. In quantum theory, for instance, the behavior of light has been thought to be like tiny particles under some paradigms and like waves under others. Atomic scientists continue to struggle with finding a more cognitively satisfying model.

The diagnosis in psychiatry labeled *dissociative identity disorder* (DID) is a similarly disruptive concept. Formerly referred to as multiple personality disorder, it describes a condition in which two or more distinct personalities (alters) exist within the same person and take control at different times. This condition is not the result of substances or medical factors, and it does not include the fantasies and imaginary friends common among children. One way people process such disruptive concepts is simply to reject them. We see this occurring in our daily lives. It is very common for people to construct a simple model of life based on religious and/or political thoughts and beliefs, then reject or modify any ideas that do not fit—thinking known as the *confirmation bias*. Mental health practitioners are subject to the same cognitive bias. Some label people who present as different personalities at different times as hysterical, malingering, or faking. This may be because people generally don't like their paradigms threatened and respond with hostility.

One reason that many clinicians are skeptical about the existence of DID is because they have never directly witnessed the phenomenon. It is estimated that, on average, a person with DID will not develop the trust within therapy to self-reveal until he or she has experienced three years of a consistent therapeutic relationship. Given the increasingly transient nature of our society and the push toward short-term therapy by third-party payers, it is rare now for a patient to see the same therapist for such an extended time frame.

The vast majority of clinicians who have treated people with DID think that each personality represents a partial identity that emerged at different developmental periods to support the survival of the person in the face of enormous, persistent psychological trauma. They have found that one patient's different personalities can have a large diversity of traits, such as age, gender, race, and medical conditions (as actually determined by objective physical findings), as well as distinctive psychological and developmental characteristics, such as language use, cognitive style, and emotional and behavioral expressions. Such striking differences within the same "person" are contrary to the basic assumptions about individual identity and personhood.

> Y, a 56-year-old male, entered therapy to address complaints of chronic depression. He reported a childhood rife with sexual abuse at the hands of a grandfather, an uncle, and a parish priest. After nearly two years of intermittent therapy addressing symptom management, Y allowed his wife to speak with me. She expressed the belief that her spouse was like "two different

people" and described him as being responsible and caring, then shifting to a demanding, childlike demeanor. Thereafter, Y presented to me at different times with very different symptoms. For a time, he complained of an eating disorder and entered an inpatient program. He also had separate episodes of neurological, gastrointestinal, cardiac, and dermatologic symptoms.

After about three years of therapy marked by shifting complaints, Y appeared for a session in an agitated state. Following some relaxation exercises, he fell silent, hung his head for a long period, then looked toward a corner of my office and began speaking in a child's voice. He identified himself as K and said he was seven years old. He explained that it was not until then that he felt enough trust to reveal himself to a male in authority. During subsequent sessions, K described the ritualized, persistent sexual abuse he had experienced.

Over another few years, other identities emerged, at least 10 in all. One was a very young child who spoke with a pronounced lisp, another an angelic figure who mentally transported the children to a safe place when they experienced or remembered the abuse. One particularly challenging alter was a rebellious, hostile adolescent who engaged in persistent verbal attacks toward me. He would describe extreme risk-taking behavior that he allegedly engaged in with a younger, substance-abusing male. Until his wife provided collaboration, I considered this to be a possible delusion, since it was so out of keeping with the moral standards of the host.

After six years of therapy, Y's many personalities had become aware of one another to varying degrees and were beginning to develop a sense of trust and mutual self-interest. Y's behavior modulated, as evidenced by much more stability within the marriage, and his visits to various health specialists were markedly reduced.

Similar clinical reports have been described in many books and articles. *A Fractured Mind* by Robert Oxnam (2005) offers a riveting description of therapy from the patient's perspective. It also is a good example of the importance of the choice of labels to describe such an unusual psychological phenomenon. Professionals in the mental health field often refer to such a condition as "psychopathology." However, clinicians who have had the opportunity to treat such individuals are more likely to see their thinking and their shifting identities as highly creative adaptations to survive persistent life-threatening experiences.

To subject the validity of DID to scientific scrutiny challenges the very cognitive strategies that constitute scientific thought. How do we distinguish between the normal fluctuations in our patterns of thinking, feeling, and behaving and the existence of several distinct personalities within the same body? One conceptualization of the difference is the presence of recurrent memory gaps that are inconsistent with the ordinary memory limitations: The separate identities are often unaware of the existence, behavior, or traumatic histories of other alters.

An alternative to the DID label is to explain the symptoms within the context of another diagnostic entity, commonly either borderline personality disorder or bipolar disorder. However, such relabeling doesn't advance our understanding. How can we come to a more cognitively pleasing way to consider this phenomenon? Perhaps the dilemma can be better be understood as one of *reification*, which is the process of treating an abstraction as if it had a concrete, material existence. The concept of personality is an abstraction we have created cognitively to help us make sense of certain patterns we discern among different peoples' thinking and feeling (abstract concepts) and behaving. We must bear in mind, though, that we cannot scientifically prove the existence of an abstraction. From my perspective as a psychotherapist, the more important issue is to have at our disposal an array of cognitive frameworks that can help patients achieve their goals.

Figures 5.1, 5.2, and 5.3 are drawings done by a child alter of an adult survivor of persistent childhood physical and sexual abuse. These are a visual representation of progress within psychotherapy. The first, in black and white, shows the child's destruction by the perpetrator. The next, done later in therapy, shows the child and other child alters with the therapist inside a protective bubble. Later yet, we see three child alters protected by a large tree, no longer the target of the evil perpetrator. Assimilating the visual representations of child alters into the process of psychotherapy promotes their integration into a more coherent whole.

Conceptualizing DID is but another illustration that the way we think is the product of our sensory experiences, past and present, as processed by multiple areas within our brains.

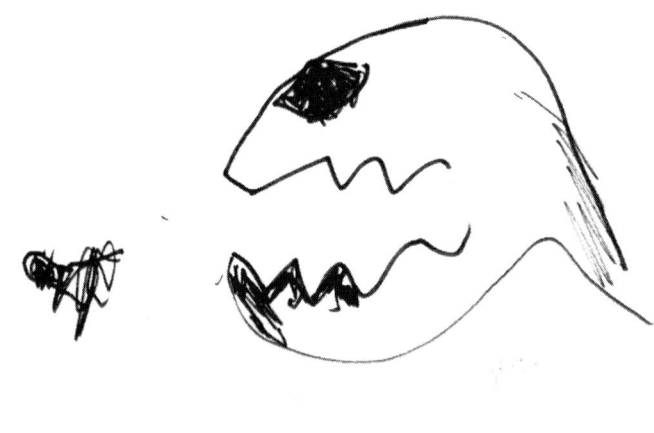

FIGURE 5.1 Drawing by Adult Survivor of Childhood Abuse: Initial Presentation

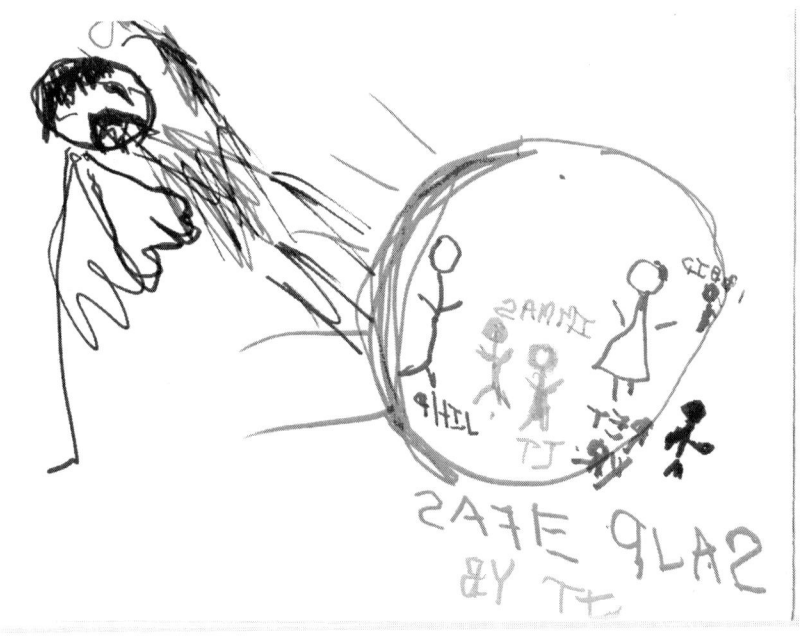

FIGURE 5.2 Drawing by Adult Survivor of Childhood Abuse: Early in Therapy

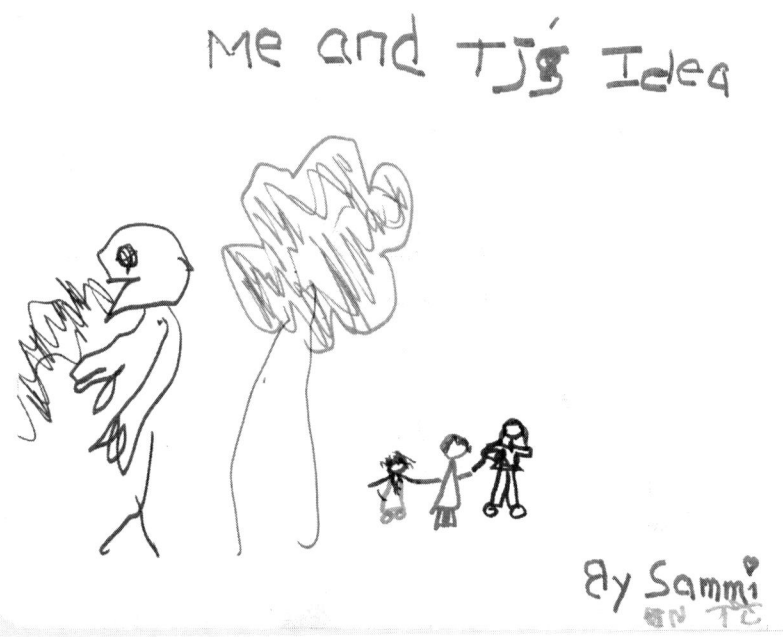

FIGURE 5.3 Drawing by Adult Survivor of Childhood Abuse: After Therapeutic Rapport Is Established

> DID is not the only diagnostic entity that defies our intuitive, day-to-day ways of thinking. Conversion disorder, popularized in the movie *A Dangerous Method*, includes the sudden, unexplained onset of such symptoms as seizures, paralysis, and/or blindness. Referred to as hysteria, it was much more often identified in the patients treated by Sigmund Freud than it is by present-day practitioners. Indeed, the condition seemed to gradually disappear from both psychiatric and neurologic texts starting in the 1940s. More recently, thanks to brain-scanning technologies, conversion disorder has become subject to further investigation. Stress could play a role, causing increased activity between areas of the limbic system and those responsible for controlling motor activity.
>
> When the medical technology available cannot detect any underlying somatic correlate for a symptom, it is easy to assign some amorphous causation such as "it's all in her head." When a correlate is found, it is equally easy (and misleading) to assign causation.

Commonly held assumptions about personality, specifically those traits that we associate with successful outcomes in life, can lead to faulty conclusions. George Vaillant, MD (2012), a professor of psychiatry at Harvard Medical School and director of research at Boston's Brigham and Women's Hospital, was the lead investigator on the Grant Study, which followed the lives of 268 Harvard students beginning in the late 1930s. They were all from privileged families and met the standards of intelligence and achievement required for admission. Subjects were studied every two years using such tools as questionnaires, medical reports, and interviews. Over time, researchers found that early predictions of success were unfounded. Many students possessing exceptional traits associated with future success ended up being labeled mentally ill and/or alcoholic, while those with more mundane traits were ultimately more often considered successful. In a review of Joshua Wolf Shenk's account of the Grant Study entitled "What Makes Us Happy?" (2009), *New York Times* columnist David Brooks observed:

> But it is the baffling variety of their lives that strikes one the most. It is as if we all contain a multitude of characters and patterns of behavior, and these characters and patterns are bidden by cues we don't even hear. They take center stage in consciousness and decision-making in ways we can't even fathom. The man who is careful and meticulous in one stage of life is unrecognizable in another context. . . . There is a complexity to human affairs before which science and analysis simply stands mute.
>
> (Brooks, 2010)

The results of the Grant Study, along with my personal clinical experiences with persons with clear DID, leads me to raise questions about our most basic assumptions in creating categories of people, then making predictions about their future behavior.

Another way to think about how we think about ourselves and others is to examine how we attribute causation to the behavior of others compared to how we think about causation of our own behavior. In studying this, social psychologists have identified the *fundamental error of attribution*, also referred to as the *correspondence bias*. This phenomenon is best illustrated by a simple example:

I am assigned at random to complete a project with Jane, a fellow graduate student. We have never met before. We meet and agree that by next Wednesday we should have each completed selected readings from a bibliography. I have a competing project, plus some personal obligations, that limit my time to read the assigned materials. As a result, I complete just half the readings. When we meet, I hear Jane say that she was also only able to finish half of her assignment. I conclude that she is unreliable and undisciplined. Further, I think that I am unfairly burdened by competing demands and have done well to complete as much as my time would allow.

The fundamental error of attribution suggests that we explain the behavior of others by putting excessive weight on personality traits, while explaining the same behavior in ourselves as the result of situational factors. We have experienced our own situational stressors. In the absence of input about the experience of others, we default to the simplest, most self-serving explanation: I have good reasons; she is a slacker.

A contrasting view of how we view the self as compared to others is offered by Vilayanur S. Ramachandran, director of the Center for Brain and Cognition, University of California at San Diego. He theorizes that a key role in consciousness might be played by *mirror neurons*, a term he uses in this context to describe an awareness of the self through comparison with others. Italian researchers had already discovered in the 1990s that certain neurons in the frontal lobes of monkeys fired both when the monkey reached for an object and when the monkey observed another doing the same task. Using EEG technologies, Ramachandran and others confirmed similar findings in humans, namely the existence of *mu waves* in the motor cortex, whose activity is suppressed by persons observing the motor activity of others. As quoted by John Colapinto in the May 11, 2009, *New Yorker*, Ramachandran explained,

> One of the theories we put forward is that the mirror-neuron system is used for modeling someone else's behavior, putting yourself in another person's shoes, looking at the world from another person's point of view. This is called an allocentric view of the world, as opposed to the egocentric view. So I made the suggestion that at some point in evolution this system turned back and allowed you to create an allocentric view of yourself. This is, I claim, the dawn of self-awareness.

When we observe another person smiling, we experience it through our mirror neurons and express it through our facial muscles and tissues. Mirror neurons likely are implicated also in the contagious effect of a yawn. Such findings are in accord with the embodied model of the mind as involving a dynamic interaction among the brain, the body, and the environment (in this case, other people).

> Reading fiction can be viewed as an exercise in thinking about what other people are thinking. A cognitive approach to literature is an evolving area of study among a group of literary scholars and cognitive psychologists. Lisa Zunshine (2006), a professor of English at the University of Kentucky, is interested in the theory of mind, our ability to interpret another's thinking and feeling, as expressed in fiction. She notes that we can comfortably keep track of three mental states at a time: Barry says that Jennie thinks that Joe has a romantic interest in her. The works of Virginia Woolf challenge our cognitive abilities when they require us to follow up to six distinct mental states, or levels of intentionality. Zunshine plans to conduct a study in which she will use fMRI to examine subjects' brains while they read texts of increasing complexity. Fiction is indeed a format for expressing our thinking and, as such, provides insight into how we think.

Jeanette Norden (2007) at Vanderbilt University looks at those with *agnosia* (loss of knowledge) to create further understanding of the complexities of consciousness. For example, cortical blindness is the result of damage to Brodmann's Area 17. The patient's visual system is intact and he can see; he is just not aware (conscious) that he can see. For the person with this neurological damage, the football game on television does not exist when the sound is turned down. However, for another person in the same room, processing the same visual stimuli, the game might produce a flood of thoughts, awarenesses, and interpretations, resulting in a full range of emotional experiences. What we experience as consciousness is dependent on a dynamic interaction among the sensory stimuli, the body that interacts with them, and the brain that processes them.

The sense of "me" as a unitary, subjective experience created by a brain that is characterized by multiple pathways is called *the binding problem*. Norden postulates that there is no single location in the brain for "me." Rather, "me" is the product of dynamic, synergistic processes.

Complexities of Gender and Sex

Most people can attribute a label of "male" or "female" to themselves and others without much deliberation. For ourselves, we rely on thought processes that are the result of neural pathways formed when we were very young. We heard from others that we are a boy or a girl and internalized that aspect of our consciousness.

We ascribe gender in others mainly from visual cues, some biological (breasts or lack thereof, body shape, characteristics of voice) and others that are socially or culturally inspired (dress, hairstyle).

This economy of thinking serves us perfectly well most of the time in our daily lives. We can almost always address another person with the appropriate gender label or flirt with someone of the gender that we prefer. However, like all economy of thinking, this one masks a more complex reality. Gender is not a simple dualism. In fact, biology and psychology reveal that there are interrelated categories of gender differentiation and that people do not necessarily fall neatly into those labeled "male" or "female." Biology tells us that phenotypic sex is characterized by the presence of internal and external genitalia. When a newborn exhibits visual evidence of a penis and scrotum, it is labeled "boy." A quick glance that identifies labia instead of a penis leads to a label of "girl." Occasionally, this quick visual scan is inconclusive: The visible genitalia are neither clearly "male" nor "female." This situation, referred to as *hermaphrodism*, can lead to agonizing decisions for physicians and parents—decisions that are, at this point in our understanding, as much a crap shoot as a scientific process. These choices involve surgical and hormonal interventions that have life-long consequences for the infant as he or she develops into an adolescent and an adult. The pressure to fit the newborn into one of two gender identities may represent our cultural discomfort with gender ambiguity.

Another way we label by gender is through the biology of genotypic sex, which is the result of inheriting either XX (male) or XY (female) chromosomes. For reasons that are not fully understood, genotypic and phenotypic gender categories are not always the same. However, gender identification is a more subjective interpretation of our sexual sense of self, a construct created by our brain. We can only speculate at this time that such identification is probably the result of the interaction of biological, genetic, and environmental factors. Diagnostic criteria for the clinical label of gender identity disorder require that the patient have normal genitalia.

Brain sex is a more recent development in the field of neuroscience. This gender differentiation is based on actual structural and functional neurological differences between persons labeled "male" and "female." As with most attempts to economize thinking by labeling or categorizing, this one both illuminates and creates shadows. All brains vary. Neuroscientists think that brains regarded as male by some criteria can be differentiated from those labeled female by differences in their size; the number, density, and types of neurons and synapses; and the characteristics of some receptors. Such structural differences are referred to as *sexual dimorphism*.

According to this thinking, the fetal cells that constitute the brain have equal potential to be structurally male or female. In developing males, at a critical time *in vitro*, the brain will be exposed to *estradiol*, an estrogen product of testosterone, resulting in a "male" brain pattern. In contrast, developing females are not exposed to significant levels of estradiol, thus resulting in a "female" brain.

Hence, the structural brain differences are determined fetally, and male or female brain sex can exist in persons who are genotypically and phenotypically either gender and cannot be changed.

There are a number of areas of the brain that are thought to be sexually dimorphic in humans. Within the limbic system, differences have been identified in the amygdala (suggesting differences in emotional response to stimuli), the hypothalamus (where mating and parenting behavior is affected), and the hippocampus (where there are more estrogen receptors in females). Structural differences between hemispheres may explain a higher prevalence of learning dysfunctions such as dyslexia among males. There is no clear difference between males and females with respect to the number of neurons or the subjective concept referred to as "intelligence." However, self-labeled females tend to have better abilities at language and at reading the emotions of others, while self-identified males seem to have better spatial abilities.

Human economy of thinking simplifies our concepts of human differences as conceived by gender, while our culture seems to magnify them. American popular culture is saturated with themes of gender differences, often motivated by appeals to sexual desire. Creators of such themes are aware that, for most of us, sexual behavior is a source of great pleasure, as experienced subjectively via the neurotransmitters in our brain's reward center. These simultaneous needs to both economize our thinking and to magnify our human differences underlie many of our social problems: race relations, differences between rich and poor, international relations, and political discourse.

Psychology has long espoused that mental health is characterized by a multiplicity of ways of thinking, leading to a variety of emotional and behavioral states in response to different stimuli or situations. Conversely, mental illness has been characterized as a rigidity of thinking that results in the same limited emotional and behavioral responses, despite very different stimuli or situations. By this paradigm, the healthiest way to think about yourself is not as simply a male or a female, which grossly simplifies the reality of who we are. Rather, we are best served by a multiplicity of self-concepts, from which we can choose that which best serves us at a given moment. Gender identity should be just one aspect of that complex set of thoughts that constitute our subjective sense of who we are.

Gender refers to a part of our identity. Sex refers to the multi-sensory experience that leads up to behavior that propagates the species. Thinking about sex illustrates the challenges in understanding "self." Research in sexual arousal underscores the distinction between measurable phenomena and their interpretation by the brain. Gender differences further complicate matters. Conventional gender categorizing does not capture its true complexity. Research into gender differences generally uses the male/female model, which contributes to muddled conclusions.

When straight men are exposed to heterosexual and lesbian visual sexual stimuli, their genital response, as measured by a plethysmograph, is in synch with their subjective interpretation of their arousal. Women, however, are different.

Meredith Chivers (Chivers et al., 2004) of Canada's Queen's College reports that straight females have a stronger physiological response (genital blood flow and lubrication) to a well-toned exercising female than to a chiseled man walking nude on a beach. Further, subjective ratings of arousal by females were not consistent with objective measures. When viewing lesbian scenes, straight women reported lower excitement than their vaginas indicated; viewing heterosexual activity, they reported higher excitement than was measured in their bodies. While acknowledging the challenge of separating biological and cultural factors, Chivers cites other findings to support her contention that divergence in women between objective and subjective responses might be innate. Men may rely on physiologic responses to create emotional states, while women may depend on social stimuli. Thus, the discrepancy between women's physiology and their interpretation of stimuli may exist in other areas of functioning in addition to the sexual.

(Note that all these findings have not been replicated and are subject to the interpretations of the investigators. They represent inductive reasoning and are subject to the vagaries of gender labeling and the breadth of individual differences among the categories of male and female. Such hypothesis-creating research requires testing with control groups, then replication.)

The disparity between sexual readiness (lubrication) and lust (thinking/feeling) could be an evolutionary adaptation to surviving unwanted sex or rape. Lubrication is protective against injuries that could lead to infertility and/or death and thus is more likely to be passed on to offspring. Chivers speculates that women may be prone to lubricate at hints of sexual possibilities. Lust, however, falls in the more cognitive domain, where Chivers sees females as more receptive than aggressive, a state that is complementary to that of the lustful male. Lisa Diamond (2009), another contemporary female sexologist, speculates that female sexual desire may be fueled more by intimacy born of social cues than by perceived sexual attributes of a potential mate. For example, she cites more frequent bisexual behavior among females than males as evidence of flexibility that is embedded in female sexual desire. Further, she notes that the oxytocin system, neurotransmitters that facilitate a sense of trust and comfort, relies on estrogen, which has a much higher level within the female brain. The implications for trust and comfort among those labeled male is open to speculation.

Marta Meana (2012) at the University of Nevada–Las Vegas emphasizes the role of being desired, of narcissism as opposed to relational intimacy, in female lust. She cites a study of visual attention in heterosexual men and women that she conducted with Amy Lykins. Sexual researchers often go to extraordinary lengths to take the romance out of sex, like having people perform when hooked up to a *f*MRI. In this study, subjects wore goggles to track eye movement while looking at pictures of heterosexual foreplay. Males stared far more at the female faces and bodies than at those of the males. Females gazed equally at both genders, at the faces of the men and the bodies of the women. Meana also cites research showing that female erotic fantasies center more on receiving pleasure, while men are more likely to fantasize about giving it. She concludes that "women's desire is not relational, it's narcissistic," marked by the desire to be the object of erotic admiration and sexual need.

Psychological research does tend to sanitize the mystery of human experience that gives life its zest. The arts are the opposite: They often honor the unexpected, the unpredictable. The musician Dory Previn unwittingly summed up alternative interpretations of the female sexual experience in her 1971 recording of "Angels and Devils the Following Day" by portraying the power of guilt to negate pleasure (songmeanings.com/songs/view/3530822107858660539/).

Meana is quick to point out the apparent dilemma in what women want, echoing the musings of Freud a century earlier. Then again, perhaps the problem is in our thinking about what women think. One-third to one-half of women subjects report erotic fantasies involving rape. Rape for a woman involves her total lack of control, but fantasy is within the total control of the self. Fantasy strips away the possibility of any and all negative consequences. It is lust without risk, a product of the mid-brain.

Meana's construct of the female sexual response as separate somatic and cognitive systems ignores the role of the somatosensory system in integrating the physiologic responses with her interpretations. I believe the paradox is not in what women want but the result of the ways we choose to think about the little that we understand regarding female sexuality.

Our Inevitable Fate

An essential element of our sense of self is the awareness of our ultimate fate, death. How do we reconcile our interpretations "through the lens of self" with our knowledge that all living things die? Jesse Bering (2012), former director of the Institute of Cognition and Culture at Queen's University in Belfast, Ireland, notes that our fate after death is often characterized as a mystery. His interpretation is that the only mystery is why people think there is any mystery about an afterlife at all. After all, the brain, from which consciousness is created, is an organ of the greater body. When the body is dead, so is the brain/mind.

Bering notes that every culture contains some belief in an afterlife, or at least treats the afterlife as an uncertainty. It would be easy to ascribe such thinking to religious influences, but Bering believes otherwise. It is not our fear of non-existence that drives us to consider immortality, but rather that such "irrational beliefs" are "an inevitable by-product of self-consciousness." Being conscious means never experiencing a lack of consciousness. Sleep or being "knocked out" by drugs or a hard blow to the head do not constitute a "loss of consciousness" despite the common vernacular, since the brain continues to function. Afterward, we may think we have been unconscious. Having never experienced a true lack of consciousness, though, we are incapable of imagining what it would be like to be dead.

A field of social psychology called *terror management* postulates that belief, or at least uncertainty, about an afterlife protects us from the overwhelming anxiety about the non-existence of our ego/consciousness/self. Bering doesn't buy it. He thinks that the evolution of self-consciousness has resulted in cognitive architecture that has been unable to think about our non-existence from the start.

In one of the apparent conundrums that we confront when studying thinking, we find that nothing is something. Those who argue against an afterlife say that what follows life is *nothing*. Yet when we think about *nothing*, we have concrete referents, such as blackness, emptiness, or quiet. Most people are cognitively incapable of conceiving that our minds end in death. Our conscious experiences do not prepare us to conceptualize non-consciousness. Thus, we tend to compare the termination of consciousness with prior conscious experiences, such as sleep.

From an evolutionary perspective, our survival depends on knowing that a threatening creature is no longer threatening when it is dead. Anthropologist H. Clark Barrett (2008) of UCLA notes that being able to conceptualize the termination of our own consciousness has no survival value. However, in yet another of the endless conundrums born of thinking about thinking, perhaps the opposite is true. Maybe not being able to conceive of the end of ourselves actually helps us survive. Barrett suggests that if we could readily conceive of our own demise, we might be less averse to exposing ourselves to risk, or even to purposefully ending our own lives. Our understanding of death in other creatures, including other humans, may have different cognitive and emotional qualities than our comprehension of our personal demise.

Parents who develop healthy emotional attachments with their children will often engage in some variation of a peek-a-boo game. Typically, a mother will hold an object between herself and the young child, thereby blocking the child's visual perception of her. Then she asks, "Where is Mommy?" which maintains an auditory stimulus. Finally, she will peek around the object, reintroducing visual stimulation. With repeated exposure, the young child learns that the object of his attachment is still there despite lack of visual input, thereby reducing anxiety in the near term and preparing the child for the inevitable longer separations from caretakers as he develops. Such *person-permanence* thinking is challenged when the parent figure ultimately dies, unleashing the anxiety that the thinking has held in check. Barrett postulates that this person–permanence thinking is our last cognitive barrier to accepting that death means that all the body's organs are transformed into a soup of organic chemicals.

Philosopher Stephen Cave (2013) identifies four themes of stories we tell ourselves to ameliorate the dread of the inevitable. First is the immortality tale that has existed in nearly every human culture. In times past, it was expressed in myths of the fountain of youth or similar magical elixirs. In modern times, hopes turn to the magical powers of science to somehow cure disease and aging.

The second theme is resurrection, first expressed through scriptures adopted by Jews, Christians, and Muslims, reinvented in modern times by cryonics, the deep freezing of the deceased in hopes that someday science will discover a means to bring life back to the physical body. An alternative approach that circumvents the obstacles posed by the real limits we observe in all physical life, human or otherwise, is the belief in a bifurcated self—one physical, the other spiritual. In religion, hopes of immortality lie in the existence of the soul. In modern, digital times, this notion has been reinvented through the uploading of our minds, our essence, to a computer for eternal storage.

Another means to immortality is through legacy, leaving behind something that perpetuates our previous existence. Having children is such a living legacy. Donating money for named buildings, programs, or professorships, or being honored by others in such ways, are forms of symbolic life extension. As Cave notes, quoting Woody Allen, not everyone equates legacy with immortality: "I don't want to live in the hearts of my countrymen. I want to live in my apartment."

Self and Selflessness

While we struggle with the cognitive challenges of conceptualizing the demise of our consciousness, we seldom think about another state of non-consciousness: the one before we were born. That this cognitive void might be driven by Western culture is suggested by the following Buddhist poem:

My self long
Ago,
In nature
Nonexistent;
Nowhere to go
When dead,
Nothing at all.
    –Ikkyu

The concept of *no-self* is an important tenet of Buddhist philosophy. The Buddha taught that everything was impermanent and that human suffering was the result of attachment to material objects, as well as to thoughts and beliefs. One such belief that leads to suffering is the notion of an individual self, separate from others and the world. Such thinking is false, taught the Buddha, and inevitably leads to pride, narcissism, and craving. The sense of "I" implies an unchanging and autonomous self, craving what is "mine." This attachment to our sense of self underlies our fear of death. In contrast, the Buddha viewed the concept of a separate self as arbitrary. He said that what we call self is part of a greater system made of chemicals and substances, some of which were once part of some other living entity and some of which will be part of a future living thing.

Vilayanur Ramachandran (2009) notes that mu wave experiments show that the brain not only interacts with sensory receptors, but in suppressing their action when observing the motor activity of another is actually interacting with that other person. He states that the only thing separating people is their skin. He dubs mirror neurons "Gandhi neurons" (reflecting his Indian roots) because they dissolve one supposed demarcation between individuals.

Another perspective on the neuroscience of self and selflessness is offered by Zoran Josipovic (2013) at the Center for Neural Science at New York University. He notes that the brain can be thought of as organized into two networks. One is the *extrinsic network*, including those areas of the brain activated when we focus on a task or on external stimuli. The other is the *intrinsic network*, which is active when we reflect on ourselves. These areas are spontaneously fluctuating resting-state networks that are anti-correlated—that is, when one is more active, the other is less. The difference is small, as measured by speeds of > 0.1Hz, but consistent. Josipovic speculates that these antagonistic patterns are adaptive, allowing us to focus on a task without becoming distracted by self-absorption. However, he thinks that the fluctuations between these two networks contribute to excessive fragmentation between the self and others, between the internal and the external. This represents the duality that many contemplative traditions suggest produce human suffering, as described by the Buddha.

Conversely, non-dual awareness, associated with mature spirituality, represents a unity of consciousness, says Josipovic. There is no blocking of the sensory input. A person is fully oriented in time and space, no longer subject to the habit of fragmenting experience into inner and outer, self and others. His preliminary research suggests that focused attention, as in yoga and meditation, can decrease the anti-correlation of the two networks, thereby increasing their functional connectivity. Josipovic suggests the harmony between the inner and outer experience as reported by advanced contemplatives, such as monks or yoga practitioners, is achieved by cognitive control that causes neural plasticity of the two networks. He concludes that "mature spirituality is not a matter of eradicating one's self, but of realizing the natural unity and harmony of existence."

Conceptualizing the self as a separate entity is partly a product of a brain-centered model. Modern brain-imaging techniques create dazzling pictures that appeal to our visual processing mode of creating meaning and elicit emotions of positive valence. "A picture is worth a thousand words." In contrast, understanding the embodied cognition model, as proposed by Andy Clark and others, requires slower cognitive processes. Here, the self does not have a physical location but is the result of a complex interaction that crisscrosses the conventional boundaries of skin and skull. As quoted in the *New York Times* (December 12, 2010), Clark states that "the mind, like bodies, are collections of parts whose deepest unity consists not in contingent matters of undetachability but in the way they (the parts) function together as effective wholes." Here the self is fantastical, dynamic, interactive, and so complex that there could never be two alike. I feel positive emotional valence just thinking about it!

What Makes Us Humans

One method of making meaning of sensory stimuli is to categorize living creatures. Thus, biology has developed a complex classification system, or taxonomy, based on mostly visual sensory stimuli. We start with two groups, which we label living and not living. The living are then broken down into five kingdoms, based on their cellular organization and methods of nutrition. Those deemed animals are divided into 33 phyla, based on similarities of basic body organization. The subphylum that includes humans is the vertebrata, characterized by a complex spinal cord. There are some 58,000 species of vertebrates. These groupings seem relatively easy to derive from visual inputs: Dogs and cats are distinguishable from each other, as are humans and baboons. However, when we consider distinctions lacking in clear visual stimuli, things become less certain—e.g., What, if anything, distinguishes human thinking from that of other primates?

A common answer has been the ability to think abstractly. However, Andrey Vyshedskiy (2008) notes research that identifies the capacity for abstract thinking in a whole host of animals, from pigeons and dolphins to chimpanzees and monkeys. Experiments show the ability of this wide range of creatures to categorize novel stimuli, which is the definition of abstract thinking. Vyshedskiy argues that other characteristics often thought of as unique to humans are, in fact, not: Other creatures have the capacity for speech and communication, can experience emotions, and can utilize memory. As noted previously, what truly distinguishes humans, theorizes Vyshedskiy, is the capacity for mental synthesis.

How does this ability manifest itself in differentiating humans from others? Vyshedskiy cites the example of a dog who can earn a reward, food, by passing through a narrow opening (a picket fence with a vertical board removed) while carrying a stick in its mouth. Only after repeated trial and error does the dog earn the reward accidentally, by tilting his head. Note that the dog will be able to remember the solution the next time it is confronted with the same problem. A human, on the other hand, would be able to quickly solve the problem by visualizing turning his head so the stick would pass through the opening. All creatures with functional eyes are able to form a visual percept with their eyes open. Only humans can form a mental image with their eyes closed, like a kangaroo on the couch.

Vyshedskiy believes that such mental synthesis is uniquely human and is fully developed by ages three or four. The ability to mentally synthesize is essential to acquiring a complex synthesizing language. Chimpanzees teach their children by example: Young chimps see their parents collect termites by putting a stick down a termite mound, then imitate them in trial-and-error fashion with different sizes and shapes of sticks until they get their reward, a tasty mouthful of bugs. Young children also imitate their parents, sometimes in embarrassing ways (repeating swear words, for example). However, as the brain of a child develops, it becomes increasingly capable of imagining alternative solutions to challenges. The unique human ability to engage in mental synthesis supports Noam Chomsky's (1983) theory that the capacity for human language is innate and cannot be taught to animals. Animals can communicate, but they can't develop complex synthesizing language. Their behavior is driven by reflexes and conditioning.

The capacity for mental synthesis evolved in hominids as the product of an improved visual system, theorizes Vyshedskiy. Survival was enhanced with the development of two distinct systems of visual identification: the *holistic system*, which matches visual percepts to complete objects encoded in memory, and the *visual analysis system*, which matches visual cues to an object's parts stored in memory. The holistic system is located in the right hemisphere of the brain, the visual analysis in the left. The latter enhanced survival by allowing the identification of partly obstructed predators and other threats. From the visual analysis system evolved the capacity to voluntarily form a mental template, leading to the ability to manufacture tools that improved the odds of survival. These advances in the visual system laid the foundation for the development of language that could communicate planned activity. Neanderthals could verbally communicate the presence of a threat. The evolution of synthesizing language allowed the development of strategies of escape or attack to respond to a threat, thereby enhancing survival.

The innate human capacity to synthesize language is demonstrated by children isolated from adults who have language. Following the Sandinista revolution in Nicaragua in 1980, the government opened two schools for deaf children. Teachers focused on spoken Spanish and lip reading. The use of sign language was not included. The program failed to teach the children Spanish. However, the children did spontaneously develop their own sign language, complete with syntax, to communicate with one another. Adults thought the signs were a form of mime, but MIT linguist Dr. Judy Kegl was able to determine that the language included verb agreement and other aspects of grammar. This is cited as evidence of a capacity unique to humans and not apparent in any other living creatures (Senghas, 1995).

In 2009 the Public Broadcasting Corporation also explored the question of human uniqueness in a three-part series entitled "The Human Spark." Central to their thesis was that language and tool-making skills evolved at the same time and that both depend on critical processes within the left frontal cortex. It is our mental syntheses and synthesizing language, along with our hand dexterity, that account not only for the survival of hominids but also for our ability to manufacture increasingly complex products, build cities, and develop culture-building fields such as art, music, architecture, and engineering. Consciousness also allows us the opportunity to make changes in what we refer to as "self."

Transforming Ourselves

Religions and cultures are replete with rituals intended to renew or transform us into a more desired state. Buddhists meditate, mindfully focusing on that moment between the past and the future. Muslims engage in *wudu*, a ritualized cleansing, before *salat*, recitations from the Qur'an. Christians might fast, pray, confess, and receive absolution prior to receiving "the body of Christ." These apparently different practices are all intended to alter the internal psychological state, including our sense of self and our sense of our place in the greater world. They affect this subjective change by altering the neural networks that form our sense of self in the same way that other experiences do: by processing sensory stimuli that lead to cognitive, emotional, and somatic/behavioral responses that are transmitted in an interactive manner to the neocortex, creating or modifying a neural network, or memory. Peggy La Cerra, PhD, director of the Center for Evolutionary Neuroscience in Ojai, California, thinks there are six elements to succeeding in intentionally changing the self, whether based on religious, spiritual, or secular principles.

La Cerra (La Cerra & Bingham, 2002) notes that neural networks are rarely changed suddenly and pervasively, and when they are, it is typically in response to an overwhelming traumatic experience. Testimonies that describe sudden conversions in response to a divine encounter are contrary to both our understanding of neuroscience and to the historical experiences of the most revered spiritual and religious figures. Siddhartha engaged in many years of ascetic and meditative practice before "the final veils of ignorance fell," transforming him into the Buddha. Jesus fasted and meditated for 40 days and nights following his baptism by John before finding "the light of God." Muhammad experienced years of religious training and solitude before being "embraced by the angel Gabriel" while meditating in the Cave of Hira. Thus, La Cerra identifies the first element of intentional change as personal transformation.

The second element is frequent practice over time, which changes the neural pathways incrementally and must be done in a manner that maximizes the brain's potential. Neural networks work in an associative manner: An activated network activates other related networks. Our internal representation of self consists of multiple neural networks interacting. To be effective in self-change, according to La Cerra, one must practice reducing the interference from tangential or unrelated networks, a practice known as meditation. Experienced Buddhist monks demonstrate significant changes in their brain functioning while meditating, as measured by both EEGs and *f*MRI. Specifically, monks with 15 to 40 years of meditation practice showed increased, as well as better organized and coordinated, gamma wave activity in the left prefrontal cortex, an area associated with positive thoughts and emotions. Neuroscientist Richard Davidson (Davidson & Begley, 2012), professor of psychology and psychiatry at the University of Wisconsin–Madison and director of the Laboratory for Affective Neuroscience and the Waisman Laboratory for Brain Imaging and Behavior, notes that these results represent long-term changes in brain functioning, which is evidence of neuroplasticity. While scientists used to believe that the brain was fixed in its functioning, now they think differently, transformed by new information in the form of sensory stimuli.

The third element in changing oneself requires a clear conceptualization of the intended outcome. A mental construct is needed as a reference in deciding what thoughts, feelings, and behaviors to embrace and which to reject. This model of self might be based on a religious or spiritual figure or on secular persons or ideals. Trying to be "good" is not enough. Good like whom? Jesus? Gandhi? Mother Theresa? An admired, humble person you know who goes about doing good deeds without recognition? In any case, we can only achieve our goal by clearly defining it.

Fourth, La Cerra says that progress in achieving change must be monitored. Our thoughts, feelings, and behaviors must be judged against our intended outcome. This, too, can be achieved within the meditative process and can be referred to as our witness, our conscience, or our inner coach. Alternatively, our progress can be evaluated externally by a trusted mentor.

Changing ourselves, of course, requires motivation, the fifth element. Motivation does not result from thought alone. As noted previously, a person with intact cognitive functioning is incapable of making a decision without a motivating affective state. Memories are complex interactions among many neural networks involving thoughts and feelings. Awareness of our preferred emotional states and the ability to shift into them motivates us. I get up in the morning to be at the gym by five not because I focus on the sting of the cold morning air or the dull ache in my muscles as I stretch, exert, and lift. Rather, I recall the feeling of strength I experience later in the day or the thrill of being able to hit a golf ball at age 70 as far as I could at 18. Such motivating emotions can also be a response to immediate sensory stimuli: the sights, smells, and sounds related to religious ceremonies or the tactile and gustatory pleasures of an indulgence.

The sixth and final element that La Cerra identifies for intentional change is behavioral. It is not enough to work on transforming subjective experience. This internal change has to be accompanied by overt manifestations. She recommends making a short list of the behavioral equivalents of your desired change. If you want to be more at peace, reduce the number and intensity of emotional conflicts with others. If you want to be more humble, volunteer for jobs that bring no emotional or material recognition. If you want to be more assertive, identify situations where you can stand up for your opinions without being aggressive. If you want to be more charitable, visit a nursing home and find a resident who has no visitors (there are many) and become their relative by proxy.

That we change as we process new experiences is inevitable. La Cerra suggests ways to use our thinking to assert a degree of control over that change, rendering it more intentional than random. Such intention assumes an element of will, a compass to guide us toward our goals.

Human consciousness is an advanced capacity, beyond the sentience of other primates. The ability to debate the existence of conscious will is also uniquely human. Indeed, it is conscious thought that allows us to believe that we can change ourselves, while at the same considering the possibility that we have no conscious will.

6

THINKING ABOUT SCIENCE AND CONTEMPORARY ISSUES

We oppose the teaching of Higher Order Thinking Skills (HOTS) (value clarification), critical thinking skills and similar programs that are simply a relabeling of Outcome-Based Education (OBE) (mastery learning) which focus on behavior modification and have the purpose of challenging the student's fixed beliefs and undermining parental authority.
—from 2012 Texas Republican Party Platform

The dogmas of the quiet past are inadequate to the stormy present. The occasion is piled high with difficulty, and we must rise with the occasion. As our case is new, so must we think anew and act anew.
—Abraham Lincoln

If everyone would agree that their reality is A reality, and that what we essentially share is our capacity for constructing a reality, then perhaps we could all agree on a meta-agreement for computing a reality that would mean survival and dignity for everyone on the planet, rather than each group being sold on a particular way of doing things.
—Francisco Varela,
Global Vision website

On this leg of our trip, we shall apply what we have learned about the way we think to some selected contemporary issues, including the current practice of science and psychotherapy. Perhaps a relevant metaphor is that of the mind as a Model T Ford facing the demands of modern transportation, from the speed and handling requirements of interstate highways to the balance, traction, and power demands of off-road treks. We understand the critical role that emotions play in our interpretations, including our innate bias to interpret sensory input in terms of the survival of the self. We have also begun to consider the limitations of the prefrontal cortex in processing multiple sources of complex data.

In chapter 4, I referenced the knowledge hierarchy, from data to information to knowledge. Technology has allowed us to create an unmanageable amount of data. Jim Gray, the late Microsoft database software pioneer, coined the term "fourth paradigm" to describe the emerging role of computing in science (Hey, Tansley, & Tolle, 2009). The first three paradigms were the experimental, theoretical, and computational sciences. The third paradigm produced an "exaflood" (a surfeit of digital exabytes) of observational data that overwhelmed scientists. While many saw the need for bigger, faster super computers to handle the deluge of data, Gray favored distributed computing, or a world full of personal computers with online access to scientific literature and data. Meanwhile, a new generation of scientific instruments combine sensors and computers that generate and capture even larger floods of data. The result is "computational thinking," with ideas like recursion, parallelism, and abstraction that are expected to redefine science.

As technology advances, new meanings are created for words. The evolution of language reflects the accelerating growth of data. Consider the following:

Recursion was originally defined as the act of running back, or returning. Applied to baking, it was exemplified by the use of starter in making sourdough bread. Placing two mirrors parallel and facing each other created images of infinite recursion. In computer culture, recursion is a programming technique in which one of the steps in a procedure (program) invokes the program itself.

Parallelism referred to similarity or likeness. A newer application refers to computations carried out simultaneously when a problem can be divided into sub-problems that can be solved at the same time.

Abstraction is a concept that retains only attributes relevant to a particular thing. For example, a golf ball is classified as a ball by its shape, even though it differs from other balls in size and surface characteristics. In computer science, abstraction refers to data and programs that capture only details relevant to a particular purpose.

The fourth paradigm is a new generation of scientific computational tools that will manage, visualize, and analyze data. It requires the ability and necessity of sharing data among multiple users, accomplished through the centralization of computing facilities, or "the cloud." Both Microsoft and Google plan to make a range of astronomy data available to anyone who is interested. Similarly, in the neurosciences researchers are developing a shared tool to help us understand the communication among neurons. Imaging the ganglia of leeches has led to the identification of "decision" cells responsible for processing multiple inputs and for creating an action, such as movement. The researchers' hope is to create a three-dimensional display that can overlay a series of inferences about brain behavior that can then be tested. The second level of the knowledge hierarchy is information, which Steven Pinker (1997) defines as the correlation of two or more things, especially data, that result from rule-driven (versus random) processes. As more data is collected, more such correlations are discovered. The company EMC estimates that the world's information is doubling every two years and that by the year 2020 there will be 50 times as much information as in 2011.

English economist Tim Harford (2013) estimates that our hunter-gatherer ancestors were faced with about 300 choices of "products and services." By contrast, a modern Walmart store offers over 100,000 choices, while choices in all of New York City total some 10 billion.

Computer-related technology and modern economies have produced a torrent of data, information, products, and services that have not been well understood, analyzed, or managed. Knowledge, attaining a broader understanding from the data and information, cannot be attained by technology alone. Cognitive scaffolding in the form of technology has far outpaced the capacities of the prefrontal cortex to create knowledge (meaning) from it.

Numerous cognitive errors loom as we try to process the exaflood. One is *data mining*, where the identification of patterns serves as proof of a conclusion rather than the basis for a hypothesis to be tested. Another is *argument from authority*, where a conclusion enjoys the halo of truth based solely on the assertion of an expert or experts. This respect for authority seems to evolve from the survival value of having a trusted leader in group situations. Humans evolved from living in small group and family settings to tribes and nations, which increased the need for leaders. Of course, complete rejection of the views of authorities and experts is another logical fallacy in itself. A related issue is to argue against a position on the basis of the person making it.

Similarly, the *argument from final consequences* has two inherent fallacies. One is that an assertion cannot be true if the consequence is unacceptable. The other is to accept an assertion solely because the anticipated outcome is desired. These fallacies were on display during the debate over the alternatives for reducing the national debt. Those identified as wealthy felt the debt could not be solved by increasing their taxes. Others saw increasing taxes on the wealthy as favorable solely because it reduced the national debt.

Confusing correlation with causation is perhaps the most common logical fallacy. We note an association between phenomenon #1 and phenomenon #2: When #1 happens, #2 follows. Therefore, we assume #1 *caused* #2. Such thinking is fast and economical. It takes time and energy to discern whether the two phenomena were coincidental, were caused by a third variable, or had a causal relationship. Even more time and energy consuming is considering phenomena as the result of emergence.

Special pleading refers to the invention of reasons to explain certain aspects of evidence. Creating theories to explain missing knowledge is a basic scientific approach. Dark matter is theorized to explain missing mass in the universe. This hypothesis is then subjected to testing. The fallacy occurs when the hypothesis is used as a premise or conclusion to argue against incomplete or inconvenient evidence.

There are numerous other logical fallacies, but for now we will limit our consideration to data mining and related fallacies that apply to analysis of large data sets.

Investing and the Economy

In his book *The Quants*, Scott Patterson (2010) describes the catastrophic consequences of failed computer and mathematical models. "Quants" refers to people who conduct evaluations based on the methods of *quantitative analysis* using mathematical models as opposed to *qualitative analysis*, which focuses on more subjective factors such as quality and integrity of management. Morgan Stanley's Process Driven Trading Unit was comprised of brainy traders, financial engineers, and computer whizzes who developed highly sophisticated computer applications that earned huge profits. However, their analysis was not based on traditional data such as a company's performance, management, and competition. Instead, they devised theoretical breakthroughs in the application of mathematics to markets and made bets on which stocks were going up or down. No one outside the unit understood the model, but they did not care as long as it kept generating steady and outsized profits.

Patterson describes how the model went amuck in August of 2007. The stocks that were sold short began to rise while those that were bought in anticipation of their rising fell. It was only later that the bursting of the U.S. housing bubble was identified as the force that had driven a change in market behavior that upended the model and its assumptions. Losses in mortgages propelled banks and hedge funds to sell assets quickly to stem the tide. The easiest assets to sell were the stocks held in similar quant funds. There followed a cascade of selling and losses that revealed the relationship between stock portfolios and housing, a relationship that the brilliant planners had not previously understood. At the time, experts in financial markets were at a loss to explain the dramatic downturn. The most sophisticated quantitative strategies, supported by complex mathematical models and gigantic computing power, had failed. Equally perverse was that the prices of the shorted stocks were rising at the same time that the market was crumbling. Patterson equates the posturing among hedge fund managers to a giant poker game, with each trying to understand who held what, who was bluffing, who was holding out.

The psychology is not complicated. There is a model that has consistently generated profits for many people. The model itself is understood by few, but the rewards are shared by many and have come to be expected. Mathematics and computing power have taken emotion out of the equation: This is a completely objective analysis of patterns based on a complex, if fixed, set of assumptions. The model represents the universal market solution, an investing theory of everything. The positive results were not only financial but also emotional. The reward centers of the participants were stimulated. Thus, while the trading model was strictly objective, its use was sustained by the positive emotions generated by success, or the *illusion of control*. Continuing success in the form of outsized earnings reduced the motivation to continually re-evaluate and modify the underlying assumptions. There was a flood of data and information, but a trickle of knowledge.

In marked contrast, poker player Michael Binger (2008) realizes that success at cards is not simply the product of rational thinking and that poker does not have a universal solution. Rather, it is the balanced interplay between the rational and the emotional that leads to success at cards. The prefrontal cortex is capable of monitoring, and managing, what we experience as emotions. Binger has learned to think about his thinking, including his awareness of his emotions, thereby improving his decision making. This is an apt description of effective, modern psychotherapy.

Following each financial crisis, analysts try to explain how the series of bad decisions occurred. Given the same sensory data about what happened and when it occurred in the markets, and processing it through the experts' existing knowledge and biases, they divide along the usual either/or choice of causation: structure (failure of regulatory processes) or incompetence (lack of understanding).

Author Malcolm Gladwell (2009), however, suggests a third explanation based on the psychology of overconfidence, where emotion overpowers reason. Gladwell, staff writer for the *New Yorker* since 1996, cites a study by psychologist Mark Fenton-O'Creevy in which highly paid professionals were asked to press a series of buttons that might or might not affect the up or down direction of a line across a screen. While the movement of the line was completely random, most of the subjects expressed the belief that they influenced the direction through their actions. This illusion of control permeates much of human psychology and has an adaptive function. Increasing our own assessment of our skill at winning increases our probability of winning, a self-fulfilling prophecy. Over-confidence often breeds increased over-confidence, though, eventually impairing rational thinking in a self-destructive spiral.

In the early 1970s, psychologist Daniel Kahneman was one of the first to question the basic principles on which economic theory evolved: that people were rational, were selfish, and had stable desires. He was astonished that his colleagues in a related field of human behavior (economics being the psychology and sociology of a particular aspect of human functioning) were operating from such a wrong-headed paradigm. Along with his colleague, Amos Tversky, he published "Prospect Theory," a paper that undercut a central premise of economics, *utility theory*—the notion that economic behavior was based on rules of rationality (Kahneman & Tversky, 1979). This planted the seed for a new subspecialty known as behavioral economics. More important, Kahneman exposed cognition as a very imperfect attempt to create meaning from an environment full of random, inexplicable events.

Prospect theory can be best understood by starting with two questions that Kahneman and Tversky posed to their research subjects.

> Question #1: If you had $1,000, which of the following would you choose?
> A. a 50% chance of gaining $1,000, and a 50% chance of gaining $0; or
> B. a 100% chance of gaining $500.

> Question #2: If you had $2,000, which would you choose?
> A. a 50% chance of losing $1,000, and a 50% chance of losing $0, or
> B. a 100% chance of losing $500.

In both questions, the choices are between being risk taking (A) or risk averse (B). From a rational perspective, neither is a superior choice. Rather, the answers reflect a preference, or bias in thinking. The result was that 84% answered "B" to Question #1, while 69% chose "A" for Question #2. How to explain such a discrepancy between risk aversion, on the one hand, and risk taking, on the other?

From an evolutionary perspective, survival is enhanced by adaptation. For example, our visual systems can adjust to different levels of light, from which our cognition can process stimuli from a neutral position, a new reference point. Our interpretations make the same kind of change in processing data. Our calculations depend on how a problem is framed. Kahneman and Tversky (1979) identified a trend among their subjects to settle for a reasonable gain even when faced with a reasonable chance of earning more. Conversely, they found a preference to engage in risk seeking in order to limit losses. Put simply, they found that subjects derived proportionately less joy from gain than pain from loss. Survival is better served by avoiding starvation than achieving satiation.

Figure 6.1 is my attempt to convert these notions from a linguistic format to a visual one with one modification from an economic model. In the financial world, the vertical axis represents value. In my psychological model, that axis represents emotional valence, the emotional state we expect from the increase or decrease in value. Intuitive psychology would suggest a linear relationship between expected loss/gain and the anticipated emotional valence. Prospect theory produces a different visualization, one that not only distorts the emotional value of loss/gain, but does so in a curvilinear fashion: The greater the loss, the more the pain; the greater the gain, the less the pleasure. This explains investors' bias to sell prematurely after small gains but hold on in the face of continuing decline (a loss is not a loss psychologically until the investment is sold).

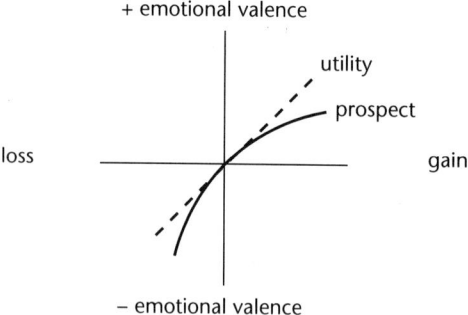

FIGURE 6.1 Utility and Prospect Theories Psychological Model

Peter Whybrow (2005), a neuroscientist at UCLA, presents an evolutionary perspective on the interface between the brain and modern American society. He posits that the brain has evolved over hundreds of thousands of years to survive in an environment characterized by scarcity. Our passions for the essentials for survival are driven by the primitive brain (and rationalized by the neocortex). Our reptilian brain drives us to acquire as much as we can of sex, food, and safety. Faced with the abundances that characterize our modern culture, the brain's primitive reward systems are not easily suppressed. Abundance challenges the capacity for self-regulation. Thus, suggests Whybrow, we create huge amounts of personal and governmental debt, financial bubbles, skyrocketing rates of obesity, McMansions, and addictions to gambling, drugs, alcohol, and sex. How will this end? Not well, he suggests. The trend will end only when we self-destruct or when the environment deprives us of the abundances whose consumption we cannot self-regulate.

> Since the inception of "the dismal science," economists have sought an understanding of why the markets cycle. Their interpretations of economic ups and downs have traditionally focused on data generated from market activity itself: the supply of money, the amount and quality of credit available, the ratios of earnings to investments, rates of interest, and similar quantitative information. More recently, a field of economic theory has evolved that focuses on human behavior: behavioral economics. John Coates (2012), a former derivatives trader who became a neuroscientist, has conducted studies of traders on the London stock exchange. His conclusions: Levels of testosterone and cortisol among the predominantly young male traders produce the wild market booms and busts that destabilize the economy. Heightened testosterone enhances performance in the short-term but after peaking leads to impaired judgment, or the hormonal basis for Gladwell's

> over-confidence, called *the winner effect*. The stress hormone cortisol plays a role in encoding memories, both in the amygdala (for emotional meaning) and the hippocampus (for factual significance). When stress remains high, as on the trading floor where millions of dollars can be earned or lost from a single decision, memory recall is affected: Our survival instincts drive us to recall the most negative outcomes from our past experience. As a result, traders become risk averse, avoid the opportunity to recoup, and thereby magnify the downturn. Coates suggests that market stability can be achieved through hormonal diversity. If trading decisions were made by people of both genders and a range of ages (and hormonal levels), they would be less prone to emotional reactions and more to rational processes. The dilemma: Young males are attracted to the competition and stress, which stimulates their reward systems. Females and older males do not experience trading in the same way and are less motivated to engage in it as a career.

Analogies are powerful but can be misleading. There are both psychological and systemic differences between poker and investing. In card games, there is a continuous and fairly immediate feedback loop. The consequences of mistakes are experienced quickly, and thinking adapts to allow for learning from them. Rules are fixed, as are the numbers and combinations of cards. Poker represents an *ergodic system*, a concept from physics in which nothing is ever added and all elements remain stationary. As explained by Ole Peters (2011), a physicist interested in applying concepts of physics to economic theory, in an ergodic system, ensemble and time averages are the same: An ensemble of people flipping a coin simultaneously will get the same average results as one person flipping a coin sequentially. Financial systems are non-ergodic, yet economic theory has treated them as if they were ergodic. History is replete with individuals who conclude that they have figured out the secret to the markets based on a prolonged period of success. They are certain of their knowledge and abilities and stay with a strategy despite changing conditions that render its assumptions less and less relevant.

Gambling and investing are forms of prediction. There are many others. Philip Tetlock, professor of psychology at the University of Pennsylvania, describes the remarkable failure of well-known political pundits to predict the future. This inability was not significantly correlated to either political biases or thinking style. Tetlock (2006) explains this failure by supposed experts by alluding to the ancient Greek expression, "The fox knows many things, but the hedgehog knows one big thing." Hedgehogs rely on one defensive response: They roll into a ball with their sharp spines protecting them. Foxes, in contrast, employ multiple strategies depending on their interpretation of the situation. Political pundits who think like hedgehogs are certain of their position and often misinterpret evidence to fit their preconceived notions. If emotions originating in the amygdala contradict such a conclusion, these pundits ignore or turn them off. The richness of the brain's processing is thus diluted or negated. However, successful predictors of political trends, like the foxes, are less certain of a single theory, have a higher tolerance for ambiguity, and are able to use diverse brain regions. Like Binger with his success at poker, these pundits are able to think about how they think. Introspection, concludes Tetlock, is the best predictor of good judgment, while certainty limits the capacity of the brain to function optimally.

As in politics and economics, confident thinking based on a singular paradigm constrains successful outcomes in psychotherapy. As we have seen, the human mind is far too complex to be distilled into a single, simplistic theory. It is incumbent on the psychotherapist to assess the cognitive style and beliefs of each patient and approach therapy in an individualized manner.

Comparing betting with investing may offend some finance professionals. Like all analogies and metaphors, this one can either enhance meaning or be misleading. Michael Mauboussin (2009), adjunct professor of finance at Columbia Business School, notes a helpful comparison between betting on horses and investing. In 2008, Big Brown won all five of his first starts, including the first two legs of the Triple Crown. Betters gave him a 77% probability of winning the last leg. He finished last. Mauboussin identifies an analytical error evidenced in both investing and betting on horses. The error is to focus narrowly on specific information that is easily available, what psychologists term the "inside" view. Big Brown won five races. Therefore he would likely win the sixth, a version of the momentum heuristic.

The "outside" view looks for comparable situations that might yield a more solid statistical basis for a betting decision. It turns out that since 1950 just 3 of 20 winners of the first two legs of the Triple Crown have also won the third. Further, compared to the speeds of the most recent Triple Crown contenders, Big Brown was significantly slower. However, this outside view took some time and work. When confronted with complex financial and economic inputs, we tend to default to the inside view, taking immediately available information and processing it through recent experience, generalizing those experiences into patterns, overvaluing dramatic (emotional) examples, and remembering dollars lost more acutely than dollars gained. Moreover, these cognitive and behavioral biases are not limited to novice investors; 80% of mutual funds managed by financial experts underperform the market in any given year.

Finding correlations between seemingly unrelated facts is fodder for conspiracy theorists but can be entertaining in other contexts. For instance, investors have identified a statistically significant correlation between the outcome of the Super Bowl and the subsequent performance of the stock market. When one of the "original" National Football teams wins the big game, the stock market has risen the following year 79% of the time. According to a historical analysis by George W. Kester (2010), a finance professor at Washington and Lee University, published in the *Journal of Investing*, a market-timing investing strategy based on this spurious correlation would have yielded results significantly better than the market averages. (As every serious financial adviser asserts, under governmental pressure, "past performance is no guarantee of future results.") Note that this correlation does meet a scientific standard of statistical significance.

Investment professionals are not the only highly educated, highly compensated members of society who are susceptible to thinking that leads to less than optimal results. Physicians and other health-care providers make similar cognitive errors.

Health Care: Too Much and Too Little

In the 1800s, health care was delivered in our society by overwhelmingly male physicians who apprenticed with older doctors to acquire their limited knowledge and skills to help the body heal itself. As science acquired new knowledge that led to more effective treatments, the health-care system developed hospitals, advanced diagnostic capabilities, a greatly expanded and diversified workforce, and powerful financial incentives that influenced the nature and distribution of medical knowledge. As people processed the sensory inputs associated with these multiple, rapid changes, they had various emotional responses (excitement, wonder, gratitude, confusion, and envy, among others) that contributed to a multitude of thoughts. Further, people experience distinctly different emotional responses to distinctly different sensory inputs. Thus, the ongoing political debate about health-care reform represents a cacophony of emotions rationalized by intricate thinking. Lost in the rhetoric is acknowledgment of the limitations of the health-care system, born of the thinking of researchers, practitioners, and patients.

Following are four examples of contemporary health-care issues: technology and costs associated with complaints of back pain, depression and pharmacology, evidence-based medicine and mammograms, and addictions and abstinence. The way that various parties think about each contributes to inefficient use of resources and less than optimal patient outcomes.

Before the advent of advanced imaging methods, lower back pain was treated with bed rest. This conservative, inexpensive intervention resulted in alleviation of pain in 90% of patients within seven weeks. Doctors had no objective data that might explain the cause, or cure, of the pain. Then magnetic resonance imaging (MRI) provided physicians with numerous detailed visual inputs of the spinal cord. They started to identify all sorts of supposed spinal structural problems in patients complaining of lower back pain. They made correlations between complaints of pain and certain spinal disc "abnormalities," assuming a cause-and-effect relationship. The result was more aggressive, invasive interventions, with associated increases in costs and complications.

The use of epidural injections to anesthetize lower back pain and laminectomies (surgical removal of supposedly damaged discs) was not the result of good science. Lacking was a control group to compare with those patients complaining of lower back pain. A large sample of persons with no back pain underwent imaging along with a sample that did report pain. Doctors, who did not know which patients suffered back pain, identified structural abnormalities in two-thirds of those with no pain (Jensen et al., 1994). In another study (Jarvik et al., 2003), a group of patients with lower back pain were assigned randomly to two groups: One received standard spinal cord X-rays; the other underwent MRIs, which provided far more detailed data on the cord's structure. The second group received more expensive, intrusive interventions, yet the pain relief outcomes between the two groups were identical.

> The failure to use control groups has a long and storied history in psychiatry. Freud and his followers developed elaborate theories about all kinds of people and about supposed "diseases." One example was the pathologizing of homosexuality. Based on a limited sample of avowed homosexuals who sought psychiatric care, Freudian psychiatry concluded that such people suffered from an abnormality caused by overly indulgent mothers and cold, uninvolved fathers. No one seemed concerned that these conclusions were being generalized to a much larger group of people based on observations of a sample that had self-identified as needing professional intervention. In 1954, however, psychologist Evelyn Hooker (1957) did the first blind study of two groups of people who were not seeking care: one of self-identified homosexuals, the other that identified as exclusively heterosexual. She administered a battery of psychological tests to all the subjects, then had three expert evaluators rate the unmarked results. No discernible differences in psychological functioning could be ascertained. Using such control groups and blind processes permit a theory to be disproved, which is a hallmark of scientific thinking.

In the field of medicine, too much information is not only not always better, but it can actually be detrimental by interfering with the prefrontal cortex's limited ability to process it. Our brain has evolved to make meaning out of sensory input and is prone to creating theories about mere coincidences. Even the brains of highly trained scientists are subject to such incorrect conclusions. For example, the awareness of research findings published in the medical journals has had limited impact on the treatment of back pain. Doctors continue to use MRI technology to identify structural causes for back pain despite the lack of validity of such findings, then embark on invasive treatments of questionable value. We develop our initial interpretations as neuronal pathways based on limited sensory input, then reject additional sensory input that does not support our first interpretation. Our confirmation bias is the result of information overload combined with economical processing. Indeed, the way we think is the product of the integration of an enormous number of interpretations of an even more enormous number of stimuli.

Our second consideration of a contemporary health-care issue starts with an examination of how different thinking about depression can lead to different conclusions. We can develop different ways of conceptualizing depression. Implicit in the word "depression," as in all words, is some unifying theme. More than 300 years before the birth of Christ, Hippocrates labeled what we call depression as "melancholia." He thought it was the product of a black substance (melanin) produced by the gallbladder (cholia). The word he constructed was based on the unifying theme of his notion of the etiology of depression. The term "melancholia" continued to be operative into the twentieth century, even as psychoanalytic thinkers reconceptualized the causes of depression in such terms as "unresolved neurotic conflicts" and "anger turned inward."

However, in the mid-1990s neuroscience research began to suspect other underlying causes, and "depression" came into more common use. The unifying theme in this word is profound sadness. The American Psychiatric Association's DSM-IV-TR went into excruciating detail to try to identify different kinds of depression based on symptomatic presentation, context, severity, and presumed etiology, among other things. It is precisely this process of at once seeking commonality, in this case within the concept of depression, while contemporaneously refining differences among our multiple interpretations of the world around us, as in the various presentations and contexts of depressive symptoms, that characterizes human thinking. Mental health professionals who classify symptoms into diagnostic categories effectively multiply the sub-groups of depression by such modifiers as severity, chronicity, and apparent causation. At the same time, those who seek pharmacologic solutions operate within a much narrower paradigm. Some may still be in search of a single explanation, affective science's equivalent to Einstein's theory of everything.

Others, including myself, lean toward a much more complicated model, in which there are many "depressions." I compare depression to the common cold. Both are defined by a list of common symptoms. The common cold is marked by sore throat, inflamed nasal passages, tiredness, diminished appetite, and impaired sleep. Depression is characterized by objective and subjective reports of depressed mood, diminished pleasure, disturbed appetite and sleep, reduced energy, impaired concentration, and negative thinking. Over 200 viruses have been identified to date that cause the symptom complex we call the common cold. Similarly, depression likely has multiple causes, including genetic, physiologic, and environmental contributors. The difference between a cold and depression is that any one virus can cause a cold, while depression is the result of a complex interaction among multiple contributing factors. I use the same paradigm for thinking about the causes of the disorders of anxiety, schizophrenia, and posttraumatic stress, among others.

Literature teaches us the importance of point of view, a visual metaphor that can help us understand the complexities of human depression. We know that the knowledge we acquire from viewing an object depends on the angle, point of reference, and quality of light, all of which influence the input of visual stimuli; likewise for our interpretation of multi-sensory stimuli. Consider the following.

- A person experiencing depression for the first time may think (interpret) that some strange, outside force has taken hold of him.
- A person who experiences persistent or multiple episodes of depression might think either that she will never feel better or, alternatively, that "this, too, shall pass."
- The loved one of a person with depression, impatient in wanting his old partner back, might think the depressed person should just shake it off and return to normal.
- A loving partner who has experienced depression himself might be more tolerant of his partner's slow recovery or might think his partner should follow the recovery regimen that previously had worked so well for him.
- An employer of a person with depression might support her employee's recovery as a means of re-establishing a workplace asset, or she might seek the employee's dismissal on grounds of diminished productivity.

The combinations of these points of view can be multiplied exponentially: employers who have/have not experienced depression, who have/have not had loved ones with depression, who have/have not seen recovery from depression, and so on. Add cultural and moral standards (seeing symptoms of depression as signs of a poor work ethic, failure to do one's fair share, or laziness) and the interpretations get more and more varied. Then mix in the vagaries of the brain processing the stimuli, such as mood and hormonal levels, and we see how each individual can have different interpretations of another's depression at different times.

Point of view also colors the perspectives of the "experts" in the field. There is a tendency among medical and mental health personnel to think that because they have a more scientific education regarding psychology and neurology that they are somehow immune to the ravages of depression (and other human conditions). This is a potentially dangerous delusion. In reality, physicians are among those groups with the highest rates of suicide and chemical addiction (Rubin, 2014), both of which are highly correlated with depression.

While mental health providers and researchers have special knowledge and skills that can translate into very powerful tools for change for patients, their exposure to unique stressors and their common belief that they are rendered invulnerable by their special knowledge make them, in fact, at higher risk of depression and associated psychiatric symptoms.

Moreover, neuroscience researchers are subject to many stimuli that they interpret or misinterpret as they seek to understand and alleviate psychiatric conditions. Certainly their education, experience, and access to top-level research facilities and colleagues are critical factors in honing their knowledge and ability. However, recent revelations of untoward financial influence by drug companies in shaping research findings underscore that the thinking of medical professionals is not immune to the lure of money, status, and recognition.

An article in the *New England Journal of Medicine* (Turner et al., 2008) reviewed drug company studies of unpublished data submitted to the Food and Drug Administration. Of 74 studies showing the efficacy of anti-depressants, 73 were published, whereas most of the drug company studies that found anti-depressants to have negative or questionable results were not published. Erick Turner, a researcher and psychiatrist at the Oregon Health and Research University, states that physicians' lack of access to questionable or negative study results often leads them to make inappropriate decisions when prescribing anti-depressants.

The "chemical imbalance" theory of depression was born of a finding in the 1950s that a drug called Iproniazid seemed to relieve some symptoms of depression in some people. Because Iproniazid increases the levels of the neurotransmitters serotonin and norepinephrine in the brain, a cause-and-effect relationship was assumed. After more than 50 years of research, there is still no explanation for how these neurotransmitters are related to depression. For example, anti-depressant medications (SSRIs) inhibit the re-uptake of serotonin within hours, yet the alleviation of depressive symptoms can take weeks, if it occurs at all. Irving Kirsch (2010), author of *The Emperor's New Drugs: Exploding the Antidepressant Myth*, notes that drugs that both raise and lower serotonin levels have been cited as effective in treating depression. Just how effective? As it turns out, not much better than a placebo.

The placebo effect is a complicated subject, and its power should not be minimized. It has been found to be successful in treating not only depression but also hypertension, pain, Parkinson's disease, psoriasis, rheumatoid arthritis, and ulcers. All of these conditions respond to opiates and dopamine, which are the body's natural biochemicals. Placebos can also trigger their production. The placebo effect on depression has been found to be much more powerful than on the other conditions in which it is effective, statistically accounting for virtually all the clinical improvement of depressive symptoms. On the other hand, other conditions do not show a placebo effect. These conditions include atherosclerosis, cancer, growth-hormone deficiency, elevated cholesterol, infertility, and obsessive-compulsive disorder.

> Depression is not an easy phenomenon to research, since it is an abstract concept applied to a number of subjective experiences (loss of interest, lowered energy, impaired concentration, blunted affect, thoughts of helplessness and hopelessness) that have only some observable equivalents. Peter Kramer, MD (2011), clinical professor of psychiatry at Brown University and

> author of *Listening to Prozac*, notes that recruitment of research subjects can be contaminated by subjects' symptom exaggeration to obtain free care or incentive payments and that given the widespread availability of anti-depressants, subjects who volunteer for an untested drug represent a very small portion of total users and thus might not be typical. In addition, criteria for assessing severity and chronicity of depression are not consistent among studies, leading to contradictory claims about efficacy among mildly, moderately, and severely depressed patients whose symptoms are acute, of moderate duration, or persistent over time.
>
> Dr. Kramer concludes with what he labels a "belief": Psychotherapy is the preferred first step in mild depression. If the response is not satisfactory, he recommends adding an SSRI, often at higher dosages than cited in the professional literature.

Not all psychiatrists are proponents of the "chemical imbalance" paradigm of depression and other psychiatric disorders. David Burns, MD (2006), is among them. In *Feeling Good: The New Mood Therapy*, he makes a compelling case for verbal treatment, cognitive-behavioral therapy, for depression. In *When Panic Attacks: The New, Drug-Free Anxiety Therapy That Can Change Your Life*, he critiques research on anti-depressants that has been supported by drug companies. Ironically, even after the companies exclude the many findings that do not support their products, their "typical" published research still shows anti-depressants to be no more effective than placebos, while their "best" results show that 80% of anti-depressant outcomes are due to placebo effect. He goes on to critique research design and methodology that may lead to findings that are in the best interests of the drug manufacturers.

Let's consider one more twist on the pharmacologic treatment of depression: While one body of research claims that SSRIs are clinically effective in treating depression and another that says that they are no more effective than a placebo, there is a third view, based on anecdotal evidence, that SSRIs cause an increase in suicide and aggression in a small group of patients. So there you have it: The effects of SSRIs are positive, neutral, or negative, depending on the various interpretations of sensory inputs by well-trained researchers.

> Despite limited convincing scientific evidence of efficacy, the use of SSRIs to treat a variety of conditions labeled "depression" has the approval of the Food and Drug Administration. A more concerning practice is the expanded use of medications for off-label purposes, such as the SSRI paroxetine (Paxil) for the treatment of depression in children. With the quiet encouragement of pharmaceutical manufacturers, physicians prescribe medications for

> conditions for which there have been no controlled, double-blind studies. While doing so might seem risky from a medical liability perspective, there is a perverse twist. To be found liable for malpractice, a physician must engage in practices that fail to meet the "prevailing community standards." The moral: It is acceptable to engage in unscientific practices as long as peers are doing likewise. Both drug manufacturers and physicians protect themselves by encouraging widespread practices that are not approved by the FDA.

Why so much time devoted here to depression? First, thinking about depression and ways to alleviate it illustrate the important influence of inputs and how the brain processes them. Medical practitioners are inundated with information and perks from drug companies about their products for treating depression. No such information is readily available regarding psychotherapeutic interventions. No company packages and delivers psychotherapy, and the research findings of its efficacy are rarely published in medical journals.

Second, and just as important, is the effective treatment of depression with cognitive-behavioral therapy, which speaks to the power of thinking to change at least some debilitating psychiatric symptoms. Some research (Butler et al., 2006) has found that CBT exceeds the efficacy of medications in treating anxiety and depression, as measured by outcomes at the end of treatment and the prevention of relapses over time. One explanation might be that medications address only one small chemical factor among the myriad genetic, biological, and environmental influences on mood, while changing the way a patient thinks or interprets himself in relationship to his environment may have a broader healing influence on multiple brain sites, neural pathways, and electro-chemical activities.

> L, a 50-year-old married woman referred to me by her family physician, complained of depression that had persisted for many years. She had been prescribed multiple SSRIs at various doses, to no effect. When her doctor suggested yet another anti-depressant, she asked for a referral for psychotherapy as an alternative. Her history was full of themes of loss: the deaths of both parents, the emancipation of her children, and increasing estrangement from her husband. While L considered other stressors as possible reasons for her depression, she consistently returned to her marriage as the primary concern. She interpreted her husband's expressions of frustration, his irritability, and his withdrawal from her as a failure on her part to meet his needs, a failure to have the kind of relationship she had hoped for once the children left home. She professed love for him but didn't think she was getting any in return.

> Our bias toward personally interpreting our perceptions can have two dimensions, which often co-exist: one as the object of the percept ("He is doing this to me"), the other as cause ("I must be doing something wrong"). The first can trigger anger; the second, depression. Further exploration of her husband's history helped L to a different interpretation: He also had a history of both past and recent losses. His frustration, irritability, and withdrawal were symptoms of his own depression and had nothing to do with her. This perspective changed her emotional response, freeing her from the negative emotions that were impairing her functioning.

With this information about the efficacy of CBT in treating depression, our prefrontal cortex may be tempted to decide that verbal therapy is the solution. There is further confounding data, though. Despite the existence of highly effective cognitive-behavioral techniques, "relatively few psychologists learn or practice these interventions" (Baker, McFall, & Shoham, 2008).

According to Andrew Weil, MD (2011), studies suggest that the rates of depression are much higher in the industrialized world compared with poorer, agrarian societies. He also asserts that rates of depression among Old Order Amish are 10% those of other Americans. He interprets these apparent differences in rates of depression as evidence that the human body, including the brain, did not evolve for living in modern conditions. Specifically, he cites sedentary lifestyles, too much time indoors away from nature, social isolation because of electronic information and communication, and eating of processed foods as major contributors to depression. Weil detects a correlation in this disconnect between our modern lifestyles and the ancient patterns ingrained in our bodies and suggests causation.

An alternative to SSRIs and CBT being researched is transcranial magnetic stimulation (TMS), in which a weak electrical current is applied to targeted brain regions. This is not to be confused with electroconvulsive therapy (ECT), in which stronger currents are applied more diffusely. TMS focuses on specific brain areas responsible for a particular function and either inhibits or stimulates their functioning. Early results show promise in alleviating chronic pain, tinnitus (noise or ringing in the ears), and major depression. Hopefully, further clinical studies of TMS will adhere to strict scientific research protocols. Multiple anecdotes do not constitute scientific proof; each study needs to be evaluated on its own merit.

Modern metaphors tend to rely heavily on science, especially medical and computer sciences. Thus, depression is an "illness," or a malfunction of the hardwiring of the brain. These metaphors represent a *reductive materialism*, a simplifying human experience to biology, complains theologian and psychotherapist Thomas Moore (1992). Psychiatrists dispense pills, focusing on outcomes and thereby ignoring the *meaning* of the symptoms. Psychotherapy, on the other hand, is a quest for meaning on the part of the patient, with the therapist as a knowing and supportive guide. "The unexamined life is not worth living," Socrates famously asserted. Does our society suffer from an over-reliance on scientific solutions at the cost of examining our lives to find meaning in our existence?

Physical pain and depression are subjective, personal experiences. When the cause of pain can be deduced with a degree of certainty, such as correlation with a recently broken bone, repair can alleviate pain in the long-term, while painkillers can provide short-term relief. However, correlating spinal structural "abnormalities" to lower back pain has a lower degree of deductive validity because the pain might be intermittent and no immediate cause can be identified. Other complaints of pain, such as migraine headaches, have no readily identifiable cause and may or may not respond to different interventions. The symptom complex labeled depression may be correlated with an apparent cause (psychological loss, postpartum hormonal changes, or a recurrent mood pattern of mania and depression) or may have no apparent cause. Our culture imbues us with notions of "normal" and "pathological" and values the role of persons, institutions, and products that can restore normality. We become anxious when confronted with the threat of losing our own mood stability or that of a loved one and often seek immediate corrective action to alleviate our anxiety. Our prefrontal cortex cannot process the complexities and uncertainties of the condition and its resolution.

A third contemporary health-care issue that creates widespread anxiety among women and the people who love them is breast cancer. The brouhaha in response to new government guidelines for breast cancer screening illustrates discrepancies between the thought processes of scientists and those of consumers.

With advances in knowledge, medicine has evolved along a continuum from intuition toward a heavier reliance on science. As more—and more expensive—interventions are developed, payers demand a greater evidence of efficacy. Studies have shown wide disparities in the types and costs of care, with no evidence of differences in outcome. Spurred by the Institute of Medicine of the National Academy of Sciences, medicine has been under the strong influence of *evidence-based* thinking: Medical decisions should be as dependent on scientific evidence as possible. Such thinking conflicts with the psychology we employ in our daily lives.

Start with the frequency of breast cancer screening. Our intuition tells us that earlier and more frequent screening will increase the chances of finding a potentially deadly cancer. Applying this intuition, where do we start with breast cancer screening? Monthly screenings of teenagers? This *reductio ad absurdum* helps to illustrate a less intuitive notion: Screening itself introduces a level of risk. These risks include the cumulative effects of radiation and the interventions, both in the form of biopsies and aggressive treatment, for slow-growing but benign tumors. (Tumors, like spinal cord "abnormalities," are not necessarily cause for intervention.)

Next, consider the frequency with which screening identifies a correlate of breast cancer when further examination actually reveals no such cancer. In the case of these *false positives,* a wide gap emerges between scientific and "normal" cognition. The following fictional vignette serves to illustrate this gap. (This is the same scenario introduced in chapter 1. See how you did.)

Suppose a test for a certain enzyme is 95% accurate. That is, if a patient has that enzyme detected in his blood, there is a 95% probability that he has a certain cancer. Further, suppose that among people without the cancer, 1% will have the enzyme in their blood. Finally, assume that 0.5% of all people, or 1 out of 200, have that particular cancer. If you test positive for the enzyme, are you likely to have the cancer? Counter to our "normal" interpretation of sensory input, the answer is "no." The math is fairly simple, but the processing of the mathematical applications differs from the simplistic tendencies of our prefrontal cortex. If you have the cancer, the probability is 95% that you will test positive for the enzyme. However, if you test positive, there is only a 32% probability that you actually have the cancer! Why? Because there will be significantly more false positives among the positive test results. Suppose this screening is done on 100,000 subjects. Of those, only 0.5%, or 500, will have cancer, and 95% of the 500, or 475, will test positive. Yet 1% of the 99,500 who do not have cancer, or 995, will also test positive. Most of the positive test results, 995 of 1,479 (995+475), will be false positives. The identification of false positives often leads to further tests and treatment of those patients, raising the likelihood of harmful outcomes.

Now let's move from fiction to reality and consider an example of mammograms and the incidence of breast cancer (McGrayne, 2011). Mammograms are a reasonably accurate screening test: They identify about 80% of 40-year-old women with breast cancer, with a false positive rate of 10%. A 40-year-old woman with neither symptoms nor a family history of breast cancer undergoes a mammogram as part of her routine medical care. She tests positive and is advised to get additional testing. What is the probability of her actually having the disease?

Bayesian statistics take into account disease rates, and breast cancer is relatively rare. Further, it considers that the probability of breast cancer is higher in a woman with a lump in her breast as compared to one without. Finally, it factors in false positives. As noted in chapter 2, Bayes' rule states that the probability of a cause, given an event, is proportional to the probability of an event, given a cause. Applied to our example, this yields the following equation:

$$\begin{pmatrix} \text{Probability of} \\ \text{cancer given} \\ \text{a positive} \\ \text{mammogram} \end{pmatrix} = \begin{pmatrix} \text{Probability of} \\ \text{a positive mammo-} \\ \text{gram among} \\ \text{cancer patients} \end{pmatrix} \times \frac{(\text{Probability of having breast cancer})}{(\text{Probability of a positive mammogram})}$$

To solve the equation, we need three facts: 1) the probability of breast cancer for a 40-year-old woman having a mammogram = 4/10 of 1%, or 40 in

10,000; 2) the probability of a woman with breast cancer getting a positive test result = 80%, or 32 of the 40; and 3) the probability of getting a positive mammogram = 1,028 (32 positive tests plus 996, or 10%, false positives).

The probability of cancer given a positive mammogram is then calculated as:

$$P = \frac{\frac{40}{10,000} \times \frac{32}{40}}{\frac{1,029}{10,000}}$$

Calculation yields a 3% probability, or 97 chances out of 100 of being cancer free. Conclusion: Routine screening absent symptoms and family history creates needless worry, leads to further testing that has its own added risks, and diverts resources that could be used to improve screening while reducing false positives (McGrayne, 2011, pp. 259–261).

Early medical screening results in another cognitive distortion. We calculate survival rates from the time a condition is detected. If more frequent and earlier screening identifies more positive test results, including false positives, survival rates improve, even without any intervention. For example, assume that both Mary and Jane have the onset of an identical cancer at age 50. Mary has her first testing and diagnosis at age 55, while Jane's occurs at age 60. Both die at age 65. Mary's length of survival is double Jane's, irrespective of any interventions. Apply this anecdotal information to groups of patients, and an irrational case for early screening results.

According to John Allen Paulos (2009), professor of mathematics at Temple University, two additional cognitive biases are at play as people consider the frequency of breast cancer screening. One is the anchoring effect identified in chapter 4. People have become anchored to the notion of annual screenings and are resistant to change, despite the evidence. A second is the *availability heuristic*, the tendency to interpret frequency based on the quickest correlation our mind makes. When we consider cancer, we quickly experience the visual and emotional memories of a dying friend or relative, as opposed to picturing the suffering of an anonymous person from unnecessary treatment.

A related medical/psychological conundrum involves the *omission bias*. Here, scientists note that patients tend to worry more about the low risk of harm from an active intervention (taking a medication, receiving a vaccine) versus the higher risk of harm that results from doing nothing. Resistance to taking tamoxifen to prevent the occurrence or recurrence of breast cancer is cited as an example, as is parental refusal of vaccinations to prevent whooping cough in their children. Prospect theory suggests that people are more concerned with losing something by taking action than they are about gaining something by taking that action.

This latter conclusion, generalizing to all people, is where scientific thinking can get overextended. The prefrontal cortexes of researchers are probably more adept at handling multiple, complex data than the average Joe, but they still tend to winnow information down to that which is consistent with their own established neuronal pathways. Mistaking correlations with causation and struggling with loosely defined conditions are constant challenges for those seeking a better understanding of what we process cognitively. Understanding how people process probabilities and the influence of the availability heuristic, the anchoring effect, and the omission bias are all important insights into how we create meaning. Processing all this requires more advanced prefrontal cortex structures than most of us now possess. In the meantime, we will all benefit from optimal use of the cognitive faculties we do possess. Careful consideration of the risks and benefits of medical screening is hard cognitive work, beyond the capacities of many. We must hope that our physicians can advise us based on their having completed that work in a thorough and objective manner.

Our fourth and final contemporary health-care issue begins with common misinterpretations of scientific psychology research, caused at least in part by selective attention and memory and the promotion of unsubstantiated conclusions for personal gain. In *50 Great Myths of Popular Psychology*, Scott Lilienfeld and colleagues (2010) expose some of the most egregious examples. One is the belief that the direct expression of aggression tends to diminish aggression. Why do we continue to believe that we need to "let it out"? We see a correlation between the expression of the anger and its diminution, and therefore we assume a cause-and-effect relationship. Research, however, shows that anger will probably subside on its own, independent of whether it is expressed outwardly.

Regarding health care specifically, another popular myth has sustained an extensive addictions treatment system and in the process has limited psychological access to substance abuse services. The myth is that once a person is an alcoholic, he is always an alcoholic, that a person who has abused alcohol can never again consume in moderation. Indeed, total abstinence *seems* to be the only course for those with severe alcohol dependence and associated physical and psychological complications. Alcoholics Anonymous and treatment programs operating on abstinence models are seen as the only effective interventions for such folks. However, these models have their limitations: Some two-thirds of drinkers drop out of AA within three months, and AA helps just 20% of participants abstain completely. Nearly all alcohol abuse treatment programs mandate abstinence as a condition of successful completion, despite the proven success of controlled-drinking interventions for persons with less severe conditions. Such persons might be more likely to seek help if they knew that total abstinence was not the only acceptable outcome. Interventions with a goal of controlling the amount of alcohol consumed address, among other things, a cognitive distortion known as *restraint bias*, by which our success at habit control leads to an inflated sense of control, over-exposure to temptation, and giving in to it.

P, a 39-year-old married father of one, referred himself for psychotherapy as a condition of his probation, to which he was sentenced for a second driving-while-intoxicated offense. He had completed two previous out-patient alcohol rehabilitation programs, both of which had required total abstinence as the goal. Sensing that the alcohol abuse was symptomatic of unaddressed psychological issues, his probation officer had suggested he consider psychotherapy as an alternative to another course of alcohol rehabilitation alone.

It is common for persons with alcohol abuse problems to report a family history of alcoholism and associated chaos and abuse, and P was no exception. He described surviving his childhood by vowing to himself that he would ultimately defeat his overpowering, sadistic father by being a successful adult. Indeed, he had achieved that goal: He held a well-paid job as a construction supervisor, had a satisfying marriage and family, and had literally built a home from the ground up.

Confirmed by his probation officer, P reported long periods of total abstinence, followed by episodes of increasing anxiety that ended with a short period of binge drinking and legal consequences. The focus of our therapy was not on the drinking behavior but what preceded it. What were the circumstances, and his interpretation of them, that led to his anxiety and then the drinking?

Freudian psychoanalysis focused on internal conflicts between the *id*, instinctual impulses, and the *superego*, the learned sense of right and wrong, resulting in neurotic anxiety. While the concepts of id and superego have lost their prominence among most contemporary practitioners, the notion of internal psychological conflicts has not. Such conflicts are conceptualized in different ways by different schools of thought, such as those involving approach–avoidance, or two strong motives, or two or more parts of the psyche. By definition, a conflict involves an increase in anxiety if one choice is favored over the other. In addition, conflicts can involve unconscious elements.

As P explored his chaotic childhood, he was able to develop an awareness of a previously unconscious motive. Despite the abuse, he maintained that apparently instinctual desire to win his father's approval. The more success he experienced, the more he experienced conflict between success and dad's approval. His pattern was to eventually self-medicate the anxiety with alcohol.

Within the confines of a safe therapeutic environment, P was able to become aware of his unconscious desire to please his dad and his increasing levels of anxiety and alcohol abuse since his father's death. When gently transformed from the shadows of the unconscious to the light of conscious awareness, the desire lost its potency, and the conflict resolved. P has been able to consume an occasional beer at family and neighborhood gatherings without any desire to drink more. His ability to liberate himself from unwelcome desires and anxiety has become a source of ongoing self-affirmation.

Thinking about these four contemporary health-care issues illustrates how disparate fields of medicine can be the victims of cognitive distortions or biases, leading to overuse of intrusive surgical and screening methodologies, dependence on questionable research findings, and generalized assumptions about outcomes necessary for recovery. The wise health-care provider is one who can do the hard, slow cognitive work to discern and transcend the assumptions, biases, and routine practices that are the consequence of our usual thinking and interpretation.

Consumerism and Persuasion

Making decisions about items to purchase, and the price to pay for them, illustrates further aspects of human thinking. In *Priceless*, William Poundstone (2009) notes that the prices we are offered are not calculated in a highly scientific way but are determined by "coherent arbitrariness." Consumers don't know the "right" price for an item. Indeed, there is no right price. We decide based on relative prices and price increases.

Manufacturers are well aware of consumer psychology, so they hide a price increase by reducing the size of the product while maintaining its price. This strategy is particularly effective with frequently purchased items where the price is easily remembered. When this strategy of price inflation has run its course, a new, improved package and price will confound customers' attempts to compare price.

The anchoring effect is powerful in determining the value we ascribe to a potential purchase. Poundstone cites a study of two groups of licensed real estate agents who were shown the same house. One group was told the list price was $30,000 more than the price the other group was told. When asked to predict the eventual purchase price, the first group estimated $16,000 higher, on average, than the second. Like the intelligent graduate students in chapter 4, the agents were influenced by the reference point, even though they knew it was irrelevant.

Daniel Kahneman's previously referenced prospect theory describes the role of risk, and risk aversion, in decision making. According to Kahneman (Kahneman & Tversky, 1979), consumers over-value certainty and have a high aversion to loss. The popular TV show *Deal or No Deal* has become a kind of laboratory for behavioral economists to prove the power of risk aversion over strategies to maximize returns. In the July 2009 *International Review of Finance*, Robert Brooks et al. (2009) presented their exhaustive analysis of data from the Australian version of the show, concluding that risk aversion increases with the stakes, that younger age and male gender are significant determinants of risk taking (surprise, surprise), and that reframing the choice from gains to possible losses increases risk aversion. Applying these findings to everyday economic decision making, however, has been criticized on the grounds that there is no real risk involved to the contestant, since they are not risking anything that they possessed prior to the game show.

Running for political office involves the ultimate study of consumerism. Research psychologist Kevin Dutton (2010) of the University of Oxford has elucidated the basic psychological principles of persuasion. Let us see how they apply to contemporary political life.

The first such principle is simplicity. While most people can acknowledge the complexity of issues our country and the world face (climate change, immigration, the economy, and health-care delivery, to name a few), we are most persuaded by positions presented in three simple parts. While we tend to think in dichotomies, just two points of persuasion run the risk of seeming simplistic. A third can add confirmation, a sense of completion. More than three, and you begin to lose your audience. Caesar famously summed up his ruling philosophy with *Veni, vidi, vici* ("I came, I saw, I conquered"). Ask a friend to explain her position on a complex issue, and you will likely get a three-part answer, thinking that is a variant of the decoy effect.

Further, simplicity applies not only to content but also to presentation. Psychologists Hyunjin Song and Norbert Schwarz (2008) at the University of Michigan found that subjects estimated the time to prepare a recipe to be significantly longer if it was presented in a fancier typeface than in a simple font. Subjects cognitively confused the complexity of visually processing the information with the estimated effort needed to implement it.

A second principle of persuasion is to frame the information being presented in a way that is easily interpreted as being in the listener's self-interest. Buy a particular breakfast cereal for your kids because it will make them healthy and happy, thereby making you a good parent. (How accurately do those happy family breakfast ads for cereal and Pop-Tarts reflect the morning experience in your household?) Effective politicians don't ask us to support them for their benefit but because the outcome will be good for us. Even on those rare occasions when a politico asks for constituent sacrifice, he will frame it in terms of the ultimate benefit to the voter.

Dutton refers to his third principle of persuasion as confidence, although I interpret his point with nuance. He cites research demonstrating that subjects will rate a wine said to cost $90 as tasting better than one said to cost $10, even though both bottles contain the same wine. Taking the research further, subjects were examined by a functional MRI scan. The allegedly expensive wine generated more activity in the brain's pleasure center, the medial orbitofrontal cortex, than did the supposedly cheaper one. Indeed, it did taste better! The same results have been replicated when the subjects were wine experts. It is a matter of interpretation, though, whether these findings speak to the role of confidence or that of expectation (the placebo effect).

Empathy is the fourth principle Dutton cites in analyzing persuasion. As mentioned in chapter 2, patients will recover more quickly from the common cold if they interpret their physician's demeanor as empathetic. Similarly, we will be more persuaded to vote for a candidate whom we think shares our interests and concerns. Scott Brown's upset in a special 2010 election for Ted Kennedy's vacated Senate seat in Massachusetts was likely a product of his campaigning in jeans while driving his battered pickup, compared to his opponent's perceived indifference to the common voter.

Finally, according to Dutton, we are perhaps most influenced by incongruity. The neurology of incongruity involves the processing of the unexpected, shown by increased activity in both the amygdala and the temporoparietal junction. This activity suggests not only that the unexpected gets our attention but that it also interrupts our normal cognitive functioning. In hypnosis, confusional techniques are employed to temporarily disable the usual thought processes, opening the way to reframing the subject's thinking. Incongruity is also the essence of humor. Laughter is our response to unexpected (and unthreatening) auditory and visual stimuli. In politics, self-effacing humor is the most unexpected. Barack Obama's effective use of the gentle personal put-down, including regarding subjects for which some element of the electorate might have felt discomfort (read race), may have contributed to persuading some voters to be more open to his candidacy.

> Milton Erickson, MD, was an early leader in clinical hypnosis. His effective use of confusional techniques was legend. Following multiple failures to lose weight, a woman professed an unwavering belief in her inability to change. Under hypnosis, Erickson instructed her to gain three pounds in the next week. The perplexed subject appeared a week later, having complied with her doctor's suggestion. During the second trance, the good doctor suggested she lose one pound. A week later, she had succeeded again. While she was in a subsequent trance, Erickson was able to disabuse her of the "no-control" cognition. She reportedly went on to attain her weight-loss goals (Havens, 2005).

These principles of persuasion are not limited to consumer, political, or clinical situations. They are equally applicable to occupational, social, and relational matters. Our emotional reactions to such applications will shape our thoughts about them.

What Are the Chances?

Consider this: In advertisements for his 2007 campaign for the Republican nomination for president, Rudy Giuliani was quoted as follows: "I had prostate cancer, five, six years ago. My chances of surviving prostate cancer—and thank God,

I was cured of it—in the United States? Eighty-two percent. My chances of surviving prostate cancer in England? Only 44% under socialized medicine" (Gigerenzer et al., 2009). Statistics are a relatively new way of accumulating and analyzing one burgeoning source of new information, mathematical data. Scientific thinking requires more than intelligence and can be sidetracked by dysrationality, as was the case with candidate Giuliani. Statistical illiteracy renders us vulnerable to commercial and political manipulation and can cause us to make misguided decisions. The practice of medicine in our culture is rife with statistical confusion and obfuscation.

Let's go back to the second example of dysrationalia posed in chapter 1: Do these results of a test of a new medical procedure prove its efficacy?

	# Patients Improved	# Patients/No Improvement
Treatment	200	75
No treatment	50	15

The common cognitive error is to focus on the largest number, 200, and conclude the treatment works. The statistical improvement rate of those receiving treatment is 72.7% (200/275) while that of those not receiving treatment is 76.9% (50/65). Treatment is no better than no treatment.

Gigerenzer and colleagues identify aspects of modern medical practice that enable such misapplication of statistical methods. They posit that medicine has an historical ambivalence toward statistics, a tension between the practitioner as scientist and as artist. In turn, patients tend to trust their doctors rather than take the time and cognitive energy to analyze the data themselves; thus, they seek the illusion of certainty, which is at odds with statistical orthodoxy. Returning for a minute to the issue of screening for breast cancer, the authors say that both doctors and patients overestimate the benefits and underestimate the harm of mammography. In fact, mammography reduces the risk of a woman dying of cancer in the following 13 years from about 5 to 4 in 1,000, while patient surveys find belief in a reduced risk rate up to 80 times as high. Similar concerns are expressed about the perceived benefits of prostate-specific antigen (PSA) testing for prostate cancer in men.

As a result of modern technology, both doctors and patients face a vast array of decisions. One area of statistics in which Gigerenzer et al. (2009) argue for a better understanding is the difference between absolute and relative risk. They cite the 1995 warning by a governmental safety committee that a particular oral contraceptive increased the chance of a life-threatening blood clot by 100%. The result was a media blitz, a significant reduction in the use of the contraceptive, and thousands of additional pregnancies and abortions (both of which correlate with a higher risk of blood clots than the contraceptive). The increased risk of a blood clot with the contraceptive was from 1 to 2 in every 7,000 women. The *relative risk* increased by 100%, but the *absolute risk* increased from .014% to .028%.

> The mixing of absolute and relative risks in medical literature and advertising is common. Materials intended to educate patients can be totally misleading. A brochure for hormone replacement therapy stated that HRT increased protection from colorectal cancer "by up to more than 50%" while possibly increasing the risk of breast cancer 0.6% (6 in 10,000). The choice for the patient is obvious. Or is it? The 50% protection increase was less than 6 in 10,000. HRT causes more cases of cancer than it prevents.
>
> Medical advertisements are fertile ground for statistical misrepresentation. Consider this advertised claim: Lipitor reduces the risk of stroke by nearly one-half in patients with Type 2 diabetes and at least one other risk factor. In absolute terms, the reduction is 1.3%: After four years, 2.8% of such patients taking sugar pills had a stroke, versus 1.5% of those taking Lipitor (Gigerenzer et al., 2007).

Even physicians have difficulty processing statistics accurately. Gigerenzer and colleagues (2009) queried 160 gynecologists about a scenario similar to the one presented earlier.

- The probability that a woman has breast cancer (prevalence) is 1%.
- If a woman has breast cancer, the probability that she tests positive (sensitivity) is 90%.
- If a woman does not have breast cancer, the probability that she nonetheless tests positive (false-positive rate) is 9%.

A woman who has just tested positive asks, "What are the chances I have cancer?" Which is the best answer?

- 81%.
- Out of 10 women with a positive test, about 9 have breast cancer.
- Out of 10 women with a positive test, about 1 has breast cancer.
- The probability she has breast cancer is about 1%.

Prior to further statistical training, 60% of the gynecologists grossly overestimated the probability of cancer (81% and 90%), while only 21% chose the best answer, 10%. Gigerenzer argues that both practitioners and patients would be better served by presenting data as natural frequencies. Thus,

- 10 of 1,000 women have breast cancer.
- Of those 10, 9 test positive.
- Of the 990 without cancer, about 89 test positive.

This format is easier for the neocortex to process, increasing the likelihood that both doctors and patients will make informed decisions.

Gigerenzer and colleagues (2009) cites Giuliani's use of data contrasting British deaths from prostate cancer with survival rates in the United States, suggesting that American males are nearly twice as likely to survive as their British brothers, which he attributes to differences in medical care. This all sounds logical enough until we add some additional stimuli to the cognitive mix. The PSA test is widely used in the United States but not in Britain. Thus, five-year survival rates are going to differ dramatically because men will be diagnosed earlier here than in Britain and therefore will live longer after the initial diagnosis. The more important statistic, however, is the *mortality rate*. Here the difference is insignificant: 26 prostate cancer deaths per 100,000 American men, versus 27 in Britain. As with the matter of mammography and breast cancer, these statistics do not take into account the added costs of testing and unnecessary treatment, which can often result in impotence and incontinence.

> Simpson's paradox is another statistical anomaly, this one resulting from the averaging of different sizes of sub-groups. There are many examples in the medical and economic literature, but both professions have suffered enough under my scrutiny at this point. So I will turn to a more benign area of study, baseball statistics. In both 1995 and 1996, Derek Jeter (New York Yankees) had a lower batting average than David Justice (Atlanta Braves). For the two seasons combined, Mr. Jeter had a higher average.
>
> | Player | 1995 at-bats | 1995 percentage | 1996 at-bats | 1996 percentage |
> |---------|--------------|-----------------|--------------|-----------------|
> | Jeter | 48 | 250 | 582 | 314 |
> | Justice | 411 | 253 | 140 | 321 |
>
> The explanation: Combining the two years, Jeter batted .310, Justice .279. Averaging the sum of averages of different-sized groups produces a wrong answer.

Another misinterpretation of statistics is the common conclusion derived from the fact that humans share 98% to 99% of their DNA with chimpanzees is that humans and chimps are therefore almost identical. Wrong! Geneticists understand that small differences in genes can produce dramatic differences in living creatures. DNA is, in fact, a discrete combinatorial code, so there is no correlation between the percentage of DNA difference and the percentage of functional difference. A 1% difference in the content of a genetic code can translate into a 10%, 20%, 50%, even 100% difference in living beings, depending on how the difference is combined in code construction.

Social sciences and medicine have relied on significance testing as the standard for measuring a meaningful correlation between two factors. By this approach, a correlation is significant if the probability of it occurring by chance is less than 5%.

(The 5% test of significance was invented in 1922 by English mathematician Ronald Fischer. The number is arbitrary, based on the ease of statistical calculations made by slide rule or pencil.) Stated another way, the probability of it not being by chance is 95%. Sounds pretty conclusive. As it turns out, the smaller the effect being measured, the higher the over-estimation of the effect. Statistician Paul Speckman and psychologist Jeff Rounder, both from the University of Missouri, provide the following example: A flipped coin comes up heads 527 times out of 1,000. Classical statistics concludes that the chances of this occurring are less than 1 in 20. It is therefore statistically significant, and this significance could be used to support the conclusion that the coin is weighted. However, a different interpretation is that the 1 in 20 probability refers to the odds of getting any number of heads in flips above 526. To understand if the coin is weighted, researchers would need to calculate the probability of getting 527 heads with a weighted coin and compare it to the probability of getting 527 heads with a fair coin. They report that this calculated probability as no higher than 4 to 1, not strong evidence of a meaningful relationship. This latter approach reflects the thinking of Thomas Bayes and his Bayesian school of statistical analysis (Rounder, 2013). A fundamental principle of this form of analysis is to compare the probability of a finding with another known probability.

A related notion is the *null hypothesis*, the probability that no relationship exists. Here, researchers try to disprove. Researchers who neglect the null hypothesis risk adverse outcomes. Consider the following example:.

Hypothesis: Sweet corn will grow at a higher rate when planted in organic compost rather than in soil enhanced with chemical fertilizer.

Null hypothesis: Sweet corn will not grow at a higher rate when planted in organic compost rather than in soil enhanced with chemical fertilizer.

Differences in growth rates will support one hypothesis or the other. However, a poorly conceived null hypothesis invalidates the whole experiment. Consider:

Poor null hypothesis: Sweet corn shows no differences in growth rates when planted in organic compost rather than in soil enhanced with chemical fertilizers.

The flaw is that if the corn grows more slowly in compost both the hypothesis and the null are disproved since there is a difference in growth rates and the experiment has no valid results.

Researchers often succumb to the binary notions of "success" and "failure" when evaluating experimental outcomes and equate success with proving a hypothesis. Instead, accepting or rejecting any hypothesis or null hypothesis is a positive result, advancing understanding. The concept of experimental failures applies only to errors in design or execution.

Scientists are human and, as such, subject to the seductive power of recognition for their discoveries. However, there is no recognition for proving an insignificant relationship among factors being studied. This publication bias is not limited to drug therapies. As early as 1959, statistician Theodore Sterling surveyed published psychological studies and found that 97% of those with statistically significant data confirmed the hypothesis they were testing. We like to be right and hate to be wrong.

A foundation of scientific thinking is *replicability*. The results of an experiment have to be confirmed by other researchers using identical methods under identical circumstances before they can be accepted as "truth," which means that a finding can be generalized to all identical circumstances. Since there are always a multitude of variables at work in any research endeavor, though, there can never be certainty that one study fully replicates another.

Neuroscientist John Crabbe (2004) at the Oregon Health and Science University demonstrated the challenges of replication by conducting an experiment on mouse behavior at three different labs located in the United States and Canada. He tried to standardize every conceivable variable. The same strains of mice were shipped on the same day from the same supplier. They had been raised in the same kind of enclosure with the same sawdust bedding and incandescent lighting, were living with the same number of litter mates, and were fed identical diets. Researchers handled them with the same surgical gloves, and they were tested on identical equipment at the same time of day. The results were anything but consistent. The behaviors being measured varied from site to site and strain to strain. The results that were outliers, where one lab had significantly different results from the other two, could be the product of invisible variables that we don't comprehend.

Replication produces another confounding phenomenon, *the decline effect*: Statistically significant findings decline in subsequent trials. One explanation is mathematical: Replication cancels out outliers, a phenomenon known as *regression to the mean*. Another is inherent to the scientific method: Observation leads to a hypothesis, which is then tested on a small sample. Replication expands the study to a broader, more diverse sample, resulting in the *dilution effect*. A more skeptical interpretation cites experimental designs that skew outcomes in the desired direction and the lack of incentives to publish countervailing findings. A fourth view considers the nature of that which is studied. Psychology is one academic discipline that tries to apply scientific inquiry to abstract concepts within non-ergodic systems. The resulting findings can be important, but must be carefully evaluated.

> A telling example of regression to the mean and the decline effect was illustrated by Duke University's J. B. Rhine. He set out to test the existence of extrasensory perception (ESP). On one side of a deck of cards he devised, one of five different symbols was printed. Subjects looked at the blank side and guessed which of the five symbols was on the reverse. As expected,

> nearly every subject guessed correctly 20% of the time. There was one exception, a subject who correctly identified the hidden symbol 50% of the time, including nine in a row. The statistical odds of the latter are around one in two million. Over the course of thousands of more guesses, however, the apparent ESP of the subject showed a steady decline and finally was not significantly better than the others (*Skeptic's Dictionary*, 2014).

Why do scientific notions continue to persist in education and practice, despite ambiguous, declining, and conflicting effect sizes? A conspiracy theory explanation would immediately conclude that fraud was at play. Our slower thought processes, though, would consider the cognitive influences at play: confirmation bias, perceptual heuristics, and our need to make sense of our environment, including the results of our experiments. Too many of us are uncomfortable and experience negative emotional valence when confronted with ambiguity. Any explanation is better than none. Thus, we confront perhaps the most fundamental cognitive bias of all: *the meaning bias*. We need for the world around us to make sense, to have meaning. We create meaning whether it exists or not.

The fundamental result of our emotional-cognitive interface underscores the importance to us of making meaning. The patriotic cry "My country, right or wrong" mimics the cognitive imperative "My beliefs, right or wrong."

> Science can be contaminated by common methodological flaws: failure to use control groups, inaccurate use of randomization, ignoring regression to the mean, and publication bias. Then there is plain old fraud, masked in fancy diagrams and charts, referencing studies with no attribution, and "scientists" with vague or misleading credentials. Take British TV nutritionist Gillian McKeith, whose website reports her PhD in holistic nutrition from the American Holistic College of Nutrition and her "certified professional" membership in the American Association of Nutritional Consultants. British physician and author Ben Goldacre (2007), in his "Bad Science" column in the *Guardian*, reveals that the college was not accredited and offered a correspondence course PhD for $6,400. Dr. Goldacre was able to obtain the requisite association certification for his dead cat at a cost of $60. The college closed in 2010. The appearance of "scientificness" appeals to our fast thinking, triggered by emotions of positive valence. Critical analysis is slower and often less rewarding. Self-deception can be more satisfying than reality.

In the 2003 book *Moneyball*, Michael Lewis wrote of the success that Oakland As' general manager Billy Beane had in assembling a winning baseball team despite a limited payroll. Lewis cited the availability heuristic that underlay the thinking of baseball "experts," which was based on the simple fact of repetition. As a result of this bias, baseball had created an entire culture of language and beliefs to explain the chance happenings on the diamond from which a value for individual players was derived. Beane was able to go beyond such conventional explanations, finding valued players among those rated lower by others.

After receiving an undergraduate degree in psychology, Daniel Kahneman (Kahneman 2011a) was assigned to the psychology branch of the Israeli Army, where he was part of a team that studied the performance of soldiers in order to select the best candidates to enter officers' training. The team observed the candidates as they participated in a series of group activities and graded each on leadership abilities, consolidating their individual impressions into a rating predictive of each soldier's suitability to succeed as an officer. Kahneman noted two lessons from this experience: First was the confidence that the team had in its predictions. Second was that the predictions turned out to be meaningless. Candidates identified as possessing leadership qualities ultimately succeeded at a rate no better than those not identified as officer material. Faced with these results, however, the team operated undeterred, continuing to use the same means of assessing leadership potential as if its earlier predictions had been valid. Kahneman labeled this cognitive fallacy the *illusion of validity*. Later, he studied the performance of 25 anonymous wealth investment advisers for eight years. He concluded that over time their results were identical. Yet the culture of these advisors was built on the illusion of skill. As in most areas of human endeavor, "people come up with coherent stories and confident predictions even when they know little or nothing."

Evolutionary biologist Stephen Jay Gould (1996) sums up our response to statistics beautifully: "The old Platonic strategy of abstracting the full house as a single figure (average) . . . and then tracing the pathway of this single figure through time, usually leads to error and confusion." Because our cognitive processes "have a strong desire to identify trends," they often lead us "to detect a directionality that doesn't exist" (Kahneman, 2011a).

Deep Thoughts

Finally, let us consider the limitations of our cognitive abilities to interpret the findings of modern science regarding the origins and nature of the totality of everything outside of ourselves, what we call the universe (or, based on recent findings, the multiverse, since there is considerable evidence that what we previously thought was "everything" is just a small part of something bigger).

I noted in chapter 1 that we perceive the external world as analog, while our brains interpret it as digital—e.g., the interpretation of light waves of certain frequencies as a specific color. A fundamental question raised by quantum physics relates to the exact nature of reality. A tool to understanding the physical world is mathematics, which expresses reality as integers. Might we be confusing the tool with the reality? David Tong (2012), professor of theoretical physics at the University of Cambridge, states, "God did not make the integers. He made continuous numbers." Discreteness is arbitrary, a function of our definition of terms. Tong gives as an example the number of planets that circle the sun. The traditional answer, 9, was superseded when scientists declassified Pluto. Still, Pluto is but 1 of 6 "dwarf planets." So, depending on an arbitrary standard, there are 8, 9, 14, or 15 planets. Integers are not an input to theories; rather they are outputs, an emergent quantity molded from underlying continuity.

Our thinking, as expressed by our language, has evolved to interpret the sensory stimuli around us in order to enhance our survival. As Steven Pinker (2007) has noted, there is an innate notion of physics in our language that aids us in our pursuit of our everyday objectives. Yet our interpretations are not always consistent with the reality that has been discovered by science. Consider the following fundamental concepts of physics as treated by language and as elucidated by Pinker:

Space is expressed in prepositions and has multiple aspects. *Location* is binary in our ordinary language, such as high and low, or over and under. This digitizing is our brain's way of making meaning of an analog, the continuous world around us. *Scale* is a relative concept, so we use the same prepositions, whether a distance is small ("baby Thomas crawled across the floor") or large ("the plane flew across the ocean"). Pinker continues: Concepts of *shape* ignore certain dimensions, thereby simplifying them into a useful geometry. We live in an apparent three-dimensional world, yet our language often uses one- and two-dimensional descriptions. Thus, we think of a stretched rope as a line, although it is a cylinder in reality. Likewise, we think of a paved parking lot as a two-dimensional surface, ignoring the depth not seen by the eye. *Boundaries* are transformed linguistically into objects: the edge of a knife, the end of a rope. When we dive into a lake, we think of ourselves as underwater, because we are under the surface of the water. In reality, we are surrounded by water. These ways of thinking about space are helpful in understanding our everyday lives by establishing relationships among objects.

Pinker notes the same utility in our language for other basic concepts of physics. Our concepts of *substance*, as expressed in nouns, are a messy taxonomy at best but provide a means for understanding the nature of the stuff itself. Language considers the difference between the matter something is made of ("water droplets," discrete objects) from the entity itself ("puddle," an amorphous mass). Pinker uses apples to illustrate four kinds of matter. First, we have a countable object (one apple) and collections (a dozen apples). Also, there are masses (apple sauce) that can be conceptualized as countable (a jar of apple sauce) and as collections (five jars of apple sauce). These different concepts of matter help us label and measure the material world we perceive.

Next, Pinker notes, the way we conceive of *time* is expressed in verb tenses and is transformed from an analog to a digitized format. Unlike space, though, a point in time is conceived as being among three locations: The *present* might be a split second or an era, the *past* extends indefinitely backward in time, while the *future* is an eternity. Einstein referred to this tripartite notion of time as a "stubbornly persistent illusion" creating an intellectual straightjacket, yet another example of path dependence. Events within time are conceived like shapes: They begin, proceed, and end. Linguists refer to these as *aspects*. Language makes rough distinctions among events that begin and end ambiguously ("Phil missed the putt"), those that are instantaneous ("The ball hit the bottom of the cup"), and those that have vague beginnings but a clear ending, as characterized by goal achievement ("He shot a 75").

Language packages time and space and can make an amorphous concept ("ice cream") into an entity ("an ice cream"). An event can also be divided into parts (a play, a concert). Finally, Pinker notes that verb tense represents more than a simple representation of order; it has deeper meanings: The present tense refers to our awareness of the moment before it becomes memory; the past refers to what we *believe* to be known and fixed; the future, intrinsically an unknown, and the extent to which we think we can influence it are subject to endless philosophical pondering.

Inherent in verbs is a theory of *causality*. Language expresses the degree to which we interpret an actor as having influenced an outcome. Pinker cites psychologist Philip Wolff, who showed subjects two scenarios with the same result. In the first, an actress uses her hands to open a door. In the second, she opens a window, and a breeze blows the door open. When asked "Did she cause the door to open?" subjects answered yes to both scenarios. When asked "Did she open the door?" subjects answered yes to the first but no to the second. When causation is conceived as direct, predictable, and intended, we assign responsibility. When it is muddled by intervening variables, our assignment of responsibility becomes less clear.

Wray Herbert (2010a) suggests the momentum heuristic as another basis for our intuitive physics. Also called the "propensity effect," it is the product of our innate sense that speed, motion, and direction are powerful forces that are not easily altered. In both sports and politics, the language of momentum is frequently employed to predict outcomes. Herbert also cites the "hindsight bias," or the I-knew-it-all-along syndrome, in which we delude ourselves by altering our memories of our predictions. Our sense of self has trouble tolerating our imperfections and mistakes.

These concepts of physics have evolved into a useful way for humans to go about fulfilling their needs and wants. They were utilized by classical physics to develop theories to explain phenomena such as motion, energy, gravity, space, and light. Underlying this science is an assumption, a belief, that there is a world external to us that is objective and measurable. Philosophers call this realism. We refer to what is external to us with words such as "reality" and the supposed rules that govern it as the "truth." We create meaning by developing elaborate models that we label as science, or religion, or spiritualism, or some other -ism. The science of psychology is a model in which our sensory systems process stimuli external to us to create meaning in order to enhance our survival. Theoretical physics has sought the ultimate simplification of meaning: a unifying theory of everything. Beginning in the 1970s, hope for the ultimate explanation of the physical world around us rested in string theory.

The "laws" of classical science were confounded when they were inadequate to explain quantum phenomena, the behavior of the tiniest particles of matter. The nature and behavior of light cannot be explained as a single phenomenon. The light by which we interpret our environment through vision consists of electrons and photons that we do not perceive directly. These basic components of light cannot be explained by classical physics, but they can be by quantum theory.

Quantum theory challenges the most basic assumptions embedded in our cognitive processes. Take substance and location. In the subatomic world, particles have no definite position or velocity until measured by an observer. Even the existence of individual objects is not clear. And time? Our everyday understanding of time as having boundaries, beginnings, and endings is confounded by modern science. The analogy of time with matter is problematic.

> Lera Boroditsky (2011) studies how people think about time. Apparently all people visualize the passage of time spatially, but their visualizations vary. The experiment was simple: Subjects were given four pictures of a person at clearly different ages and were asked to place them in chronological order. Most English speakers would put the youngest on the left and place the others chronologically, with the oldest on the right. Israelis tend to order the pictures from right to left. In both cases, the direction of the flow of time is the same as the direction of the written language. Mandarin Chinese visualize the past as "up" and the future as "down" and order the photographs accordingly. Finally, members of a remote Australian tribe, the Pomoraawan, have no system of spatial relations that uses their bodies as the basis. Rather, they use geographic directions. They think about time the same way, arranging the four pictures from east to west: If facing south, the pictures are arranged left to right; if facing east, they are arranged in sequence toward the body, and so on. They spontaneously know and use spatial orientation to represent time.

We experience time as the interpretation of changes in properties. I know my wife is getting older because her hair is getting gray and her face wrinkled. (Having acquired a degree of wisdom during 48 years of marriage, I have learned to interpret gray hair and wrinkles as being sexy, a cognitive restructuring from my younger days.) Dividing the linear model of time into past, present, and future assumes an objective means of ordering all events independent of the observer. Likewise, the duration of time in our everyday usage must be observer independent. When my wife and I go our separate ways at 9 in the morning and meet up as scheduled at 11, the same amount of time must have elapsed for both of us.

Einstein's special theory of relativity challenged the absolute nature of time by showing that it depended on how fast you are traveling relative to another observer. Events do not happen at a point in space at an exact time. Instead, an event happens within the union of space and time: spacetime. Two observers moving in different directions at different speeds will disagree on when and where an event occurs but can agree on its spacetime. Einstein muddled our thinking about time further with his general theory of relativity, which extended the concepts of special relativity to include the force of gravity. Gravity distorts time, so there is no single, absolute measure of time. It becomes impossible to determine if one event precedes or follows another. Causality, however, requires time. Thus, Einstein theories shatter our classical, intuitive model for making meaning.

David Kirsch and Paul Maglio (1994) have suggested that cognitive science will similarly need to replace the independent notions of physical space and information-processing space with a unified physico-informational space. They cite their study of the real-time, interactive video game *Tetris*, in which certain perceptual and cognitive problems are best solved by performing actions in the world rather than by mental computations. They distinguish between pragmatic actions, performed to bring one physically closer to a goal, and epistemic actions, performed to uncover information that is hidden or hard to compute mentally. Such a combination of physical and information-processing space is the inevitable product of an embedded, embodied paradigm of cognition.

What we know of the world around us is a construct created by our interpretive faculties from various sensory inputs. It is not possible to remove the observer from the equation. And yet, the observer has structural limitations, both perceptual and interpretive, within the observing apparatuses. Think about the origin of the universe. Was it created by God in seven days? Was there a Big Bang? Is it just the creation of our imaginations? Whatever explanation one chooses, it is based on a model of thinking that assumes beginnings and endings. The same model governs not just time but space. Where does the universe end? What is its shape? Does it curve back onto itself?

> The 2011 Nobel Prize in Physics was awarded to Saul Perlmutter, University of California–Berkeley; Brian Schmidt, Australian National University; and Adam Riess, Johns Hopkins University. They provided evidence that the expansion of the universe was not slowing, as would be inferred from

> classical physics. Instead they found something counterintuitive: The expansion of the universe is speeding up! Any explanation for this phenomenon is speculative at this point. Physicists do think that we can only account for approximately 5% of the matter that makes up the universe. The remainder is thought to consist of dark matter and dark energy. The former is the subject of searches by particle detectors. The latter is a complete mystery but seems to be what accounts for the expansion of the universe.
>
> We know very little about the universe. Our cognitive capacities, aided by technological cognitive scaffolding, will need to expand in order for us to understand the expansion of the universe. Meanwhile, keep paying off the mortgage and the credit card. The world is not likely to end soon.

Davis Deutsch and Artur Ekert (2012), both at Oxford University, posit that the adoption of "bad philosophy" by physicists such as Erwin Schrodinger produced resistance to new understandings derived from quantum theory. They cite logical positivism (requiring verification by experiment), instrumentalism (focus on predictive strength rather than explanation), and relativism (culturally rather than objectively determined truth or falsehood) as philosophies that deny reality. To them, the philosophy of reality is the simple notion that there is a physical world and it can be understood through scientific means. This common sense reasoning produces the not-so-common idea that physical entities can have concurrent multiple values. Deutsch and Ekert view such understandings as liberating philosophy from the constraints of "the supposed limits of knowledge."

In *Philosophical Problems of Quantum Physics*, Werner Heisenberg suggests that a common motivator among scientists who study elementary particles is "the centuries-old desire for a unified understanding of the world" (1979, p. 95). Physicists Steven Hawking and Leonard Mlodinow (2010) suggest that there can be no single, theory-independent concept of reality, only a model that connects to interpretations. Such model-dependent realism applies to the conscious and subconscious mental models each of us creates to make of our lives. They further assert that the quest for a unified theory of everything is untenable. The hope that string theory would somehow provide a unified understanding of the forces of nature has faded. There are now five different string theories, each giving good results under specific circumstances. Hawking and Mlodinow conclude that there is likely a network of interconnected string theories, each useful in different situations. The dream of a unified theory may be the ultimate expression of the brain's operating principles of economy and simplification.

> Psychotherapy is a process whereby the patient expresses her interpretation of her experience, the therapist shares his interpretation, and ideally the patient is able to modify her thinking in a way that leads to the relief of

distress. However, this simplistic model doesn't always work to explain the complex, dynamic process. Indeed, there are instances when the therapist is unable to create meaning of the patient, the problem, or the therapy, although the outcome is deemed a success.

Take the following example: V is a 12-year-old female referred by her distraught parents after she began leaving them notes describing intense and persistent homicidal thoughts. The notes started appearing when V began to menstruate. The parents described a normal, healthy development up until then, reporting that V had always been creative and happy in her play, had high grades in school, and had been active in multiple sports. Further assessment, though, revealed significant depression and the appearance of a cluster of new behaviors concurrent with the notes: V's ordering of athletic gear accompanied by a belief that her performance would suffer if certain gear were to come in contact with other gear, excessive hand washing, ritualized eating, and vague references to homosexual concerns. Her grades dropped significantly, and she acknowledged impaired focusing in class because of intrusive, disturbing thoughts.

Diagnostic impression was the emergence of depressive and obsessive-compulsive symptoms concurrent with puberty. V exhibited no resistance to coming to therapy sessions but appeared guarded when asked about her thoughts and feelings. When I tried to discuss the homosexual or homicidal references in the notes, she would acknowledge them but provide no elaboration. After a few sessions, she stopped leaving the notes, explaining that she didn't want to upset her parents. I tried to implement a structured cognitive-behavioral treatment. She would listen passively as I described the homework assignments I wanted her to try, but she would never follow through on them. She was unresponsive to psychological teaching but would become animated in describing her athletic endeavors and interests. Both she and her parents were strongly opposed to the use of antidepressants, citing the unknown long-term consequences and the concerns expressed in some professional literature that SSRIs can increase the suicidal risk in adolescents.

V expressed an interest in going to college to study engineering (a not uncommon choice for persons with obsessive-compulsive tendencies). Given her apparent resistance to the cognitive-behavioral approach, I tried to appeal to her engineering interest by introducing a crude system of graphing her level of emotional distress through the school day. Her distress peaked when she had visual contact with another girl her age, either passing her in the hall or sharing a class. V's response to the visual stimulus of this peer seemed phobic, or like a panic attack. She refused to talk about any past experiences with this girl, but the parents noted that they had been friends and playmates when younger. Concurrent with the graphing of her distress levels, I introduced a board game, Othello, that involves complex visual/

> spatial processing and the manipulation of black and white discs. V took to the game immediately. My interpretation was that the game provided her with relief from psychological inquiry and an opportunity to satisfy her competitive needs. Our conversation during the many games we played focused on two shared observations: the advantage of one player or the other could shift dramatically with one key move, and an overall strategy to assure victory eluded us both. V began reporting significant reductions in her distress levels. My initial reaction was skeptical. I wondered if she was reporting less distress in order to play the game. However, the parents noted a dramatic lifting of her depression and elimination of the obsessive-compulsive rituals at home. She improved her academic performance back to the honor roll level. I commented to her that the disappearance of her serious, debilitating symptoms was a mystery, just like the strategy for winning at Othello. She responded with a big smile. We agreed that we enjoyed winning, even if we didn't understand how we did it.
>
> There are a number of alternative explanations for this positive outcome, including the possibility that it had nothing to do with therapy, that her symptoms were some kind of transient and extreme response to puberty that would remit on their own. The more experience I have as a therapist, the less need I have to explain, or rationalize, the outcome. An element of mystery tweaks my reward center, or so I like to think.

In his *Tractatus Logico-Philosophicus* (1921), Ludwig Wittgenstein considered the limits of thinking, or at least of the expression of thinking. Contradictions, paradoxes, and conundrums represent the limits of both language and thinking. In *Philosophical Investigations* (published posthumously in 1953), Wittgenstein asserted that words have no single, essential core. Just as objects cannot be precisely located in space, the meaning of words is not fixed and there are no fixed boundaries. We cannot measure the distance between different uses of the same word or concept. Wittgenstein used the metaphor of traveling with the word or concept through "a complicated network of similarities, overlapping and criss-crossing."

> A young psychiatrist once complained to me that his patient only wanted to talk about philosophy. His interpretation was that the patient was using philosophical discourse to deflect attention from the "real" issues. The psychiatrist was clearly frustrated. While sympathetic to his complaints, I did gently suggest that the real issue in this case might be his own frustration. Further, I mused that philosophy could play a meaningful role in effective psychotherapy. (Psychiatric training today has moved away from intensive immersion in

the intricacies of psychotherapy, emphasizing instead psychopharmacologic interventions.) He was open to my suggestion and subsequently reported successful use of philosophy as a medium to promote psychological healing and growth.

Much philosophy was born of logic, which is binary: Statements are either true or false. The language of logic attempts to digitize an analog world. Wittgenstein rejected the pursuit of logic, or any other generalizations. Philosophers are seduced by the temptation to generalize in order to unify. The real task of philosophy, he concluded, is to make us aware of the temptation to simplify and generalize and to show us ways to overcome it. Thus, he sees philosophy as a new way of looking at language and, as such, as a kind of psychotherapy. Unlike the young psychiatrist who complained that his patient was wasting time by engaging in philosophy, Wittgenstein makes no distinction between therapy and philosophy. They are the same, or at least share "a complicated network of similarities."

Current computer technology depends on transistors to store information based on a binary, on–off, format. The next generation of super-fast computers could be based on *qubits*, which store information in the form of electrons, sub-atomic particles. This quantum computing utilizes *superposition*, so a qubit can represent both a 1 and a 0 simultaneously, making it possible to perform a mathematical operation in both states at once. Thus, unlike a conventional computer, the amount of information in a quantum computer doubles with the addition of each qubit: a two-qubit system might compute 4 values at once, a three-qubit system, 8, a four-qubit system, 16, and so on. A 20-qubit quantum computer requires more than a million numbers to describe it. This phenomenon represents yet another example of basic notions in our everyday lives being turned on their heads in the atomic world—binary and unitary at once. The act of observing a qubit changes it, potentially stripping it of its potential to compute. Scientists hope to use quantum entanglement, linking particles so that observing and measuring a property in one reveals information about the other, to solve this challenge. As the miniaturization of computer technology approaches atomic levels, basic concepts and patterns of thinking continue to evolve.

A theological parallel of the contemporaneous on–off status of the qubit is the Christian notion of Christ as both fully human and fully divine. Much intellectual energy has been devoted to both sides of the binary distinction, the either/or paradigm. At least in the sub-atomic world, there are special cases where both are both.

Wittgenstein seems to advocate a mode of thinking that eschews simplifying and generalizing, that is contrary to our current understanding of cognition. Regardless, a fundamental aspect of survival is the ability to adapt to change. The rate of change of the sensory stimuli around us, and of our interpretations (which become stimuli in their own right), increase exponentially. Julian Jaynes (2000) suggested that even consciousness is a relatively recent psycho-neurologic development. Inherent in an evolutionary model of cognition is the expectation that thinking will, of necessity, adapt to changing survival needs. The alternative is to not survive.

In summary, then, our ability to make meaning is limited by the digital nature of language. In psychotherapy, utilizing our visual capacities can be a powerful tool to get beyond apparent contradictions or dead ends. The meaning we achieve via visualization cannot always be clearly expressed through language, but it can have significant and measurable effects on our emotions and behavior.

A, a 40-ish male, was referred by his employer because of outbursts of frustration in the workplace that were endangering his continued employment. He was a valued employee who had just recently begun to demonstrate these difficulties, and the employer hoped A could address whatever was underlying these episodes and return to his prior level of productivity.

The history and clinical presentation were suggestive of a combination of attention-deficit and anxiety symptoms (which are not always easy to distinguish from each other). His current situation involved increased financial, familial, and marital stress. He noted that as his levels of stress rose, he increasingly obsessed about their causes.

Obsessions are intrusive, repetitive thoughts over which the patient interprets himself as having an increasing lack of control. In an insidious cognitive twist, the patient starts to believe that clinging to the thoughts and worries is the only way he can maintain his sanity and prevent overwhelming anxiety and meltdown. No amount of logic can break down this irrational belief, but interventions that bypass logic can be highly effective.

I explained to A that there is a part of our brain that thinks not only in words but also in visualizations, as evidenced by our dreams. I asked him to create a visual image of the concept of "letting go." At first he seemed confused. (As noted previously, confusion can be seen as a good prognostic indicator, a sign of openness to different ways of thinking.) I provided him with an example of slowly releasing strings from his hand that are attached to helium-filled balloons.

After a long silence, his demeanor brightened as he described the sensation of releasing a brook trout: holding it gently in both hands, feeling the coolness and flow of the stream on his hands, and the wiggle as the fish returns to its natural habitat. He smiled broadly at the recollection that he associated with many pleasant fishing trips he had had since childhood.

At the next session, he declared loudly, "I've released a lot of trout this week!" He went on to explain how he had applied the visualization to his daily stressors. Without any direct instruction, he had learned to substitute a positive memory when confronted with potential stress. He was able to return to work and resume his role as a valued, productive employee.

Insight is not the only way to overcome psychological distress. For some patients, arming them with tools such as visualization can change their cognitive, emotional, and behavioral experience.

Thinking Better

Given our current understanding of thinking, what practical steps can we take to maximize our cognition in order to enhance our survival as individuals, as groups, and as a species? The first is to take the best possible care of the systems that create thinking. This includes the entire body and the environment with which it interacts. Aerobic exercise, a balanced diet, good hydration, and stress management are a good beginning. Avoidance of toxic sensory and material intakes is next. Exposing oneself to experiences that stimulate the creation of new neural pathways and evoke emotions of positive valence is yet another.

As for improving the content of our thinking, we turn once again to Steven Pinker. As reported by David Brooks (2011a), Pinker asked 164 experts this question: "What scientific concept would improve everybody's cognitive toolkit?" James McWhorter, a linguist as Columbia University, answered that we should be more aware of path dependence (referenced in chapter 1). Our cognitive concepts, like our customs and tools, began with choices that were perfectly sensible at the time they originated "but (have) survived despite the eclipse of the justification for that choice." When first invented, typewriters would jam when people typed too fast, so designers developed keyboards that would slow typists. Electronics sped up the typing process, but the arrangement of the individual keys on the keyboard remained the same. The distinction between thought and emotion was helpful in developing a beginning understanding of human psychology, but in light of findings in modern neuroscience, these mental categories have less utility in advancing understanding.

Another suggestion for improving cognition came from Evgeny Morozov, author of *The Net Delusion*. He cites the "Einstellung Effect," our tendency to try to solve problems based on solutions that have worked previously rather than by evaluating each situation on its own merits. This tendency to lean toward economy of analysis represents fast thinking, as compared to the energy- and time-consuming slower process. It is especially evident in politics, foreign affairs, and economic matters. Ascertaining the most pertinent information from our past as it relates to the present is hard cognitive work. Nowhere is this more evident than in our modern political discourse. Slower, deliberative thinking does not create positive emotional valence in the vast majority of the electorate. Imagine a candidate in a multi-person debate responding to a question about immigration, the economy, or health care with a long, nuanced analysis of the myriad of factors related to the topic at hand. The debate format does not allow for it, and most listeners would not choose to follow the argument. Our proclivity to fast thinking has been reinforced by modern communication technology, which creates the expectation of quick, simple answers. How this will play out in the context of our survival as a society, and a species, is a matter of complex conjecture.

The *focusing illusion* is cited by Daniel Kahneman: "Nothing in life is as important as you think it is while you are thinking about it" (Brooks, 2011a). He uses the espoused value of a formal education as an example. Our society has become obsessed with the notion that education is the most important determinant of income and the easy route to improved income equality. Public education and institutions of higher learning have milked this idea to seek ever-increasing levels of both public and private support. More recently, proprietary colleges and universities have jumped on the bandwagon to advance their profits, while creating degrees and graduates of undetermined quality. Slower, more analytic thinking, however, leads to a far different conclusion. Says Kahneman, "If everyone had the same education, the inequality of income would be reduced by less than 10%. When you focus on education, you neglect the myriad of other factors that determine income. The differences of income among people who have the same education are huge" (Brooks, 2011a).

Applying cognitive psychology to an understanding of fiction and literature represents one aspect of the concept of *supervenience*, as cited by Harvard philosopher and neuroscientist Joshua Green (Brooks, 2011a). Supervenience posits that the mind is wholly determined by the physical nature of its components. New discoveries about the way the brain works do not diminish the products the mind creates. The screen saver on my computer screen can be interpreted on a gross level as the image of my beloved grandson and at a micro-level as an arrangement of colored pixels. The first interpretation supervenes, and is dependent on, the second, which does not reduce the wonderment of the birth and development of a young child any more than a psychological insight into the relationship between cleanliness and evolution renders *Macbeth* any less a literary creation.

Supervenience is closely related to the concept of emergence, cited by many of the responders to Steven Pinker's query about how to improve cognitive functioning. Too often we try to understand a phenomenon by taking it apart and studying its individual parts. As illustrated by the elaborate structures created by termites, this approach can result in misleading conclusions. Similarly, consciousness can be thought of as an emergent property of the dynamic interaction among body, brain, and environment.

Modern marriage is an emergent system. Less than half the adults in our society are married. Effective marital and relationship counseling and therapy are often the result of identifying understandings that go beyond the characteristics of the two partners.

S sought therapy because he discovered suggestive telephone messages from a male friend on his wife's cell phone. (There seems to be a significant increase in referrals for marital and relationship help as the result of a vast new source of incriminating evidence: cell phones, e-mail, and Internet communications.) S was angry and depressed. The foundation of his sense of security, his friend's loyalty and his spouse's fidelity, was suddenly shattered. His wife and the friend admitted to harmless flirtation but denied any wrongdoing. She refused to participate in therapy, telling S that his concerns were foolish. He described obsessive thoughts about what his wife and friend might have done in the past and was suspicions that they were together whenever she was not in his presence.

A common intuitive strategy for dealing with stress is to try to suppress the thoughts that are associated with emotional distress. S used both alcohol and cannabis in an attempt to disrupt the worry and tried to distract himself with more positive experiences. Despite his best efforts, his worry and associated distress persisted.

S met the clinical criteria for a major depressive episode: depressed mood, diminished interest, significant weight loss, poor sleep, general slowing of his motor activity, loss of energy, impaired concentration. The symptoms persisted for two years and impaired his performance at work and his role as a father and husband. His family physician initiated two different antidepressant medications, neither of which resulted in any symptomatic relief. In addition, S underwent a course of psychotherapy, which terminated after he and the therapist agreed that they were stuck. He sought a consultation about alternative approaches to his persistent distress.

This phenomenon we call depression can be conceptualized as a disorder caused by a chemical imbalance in the brain or as faulty thinking associated with past experiences. Neither conceptualization had led to a positive outcome for S. As an alternative, I suggested that his depression might not be a disorder at all but rather an adaptation to enhance his survival. Further, I suggested that he reframe his depression as a normal reaction to an obvious, but unaddressed dilemma—namely, whether to commit to the marriage or seek to terminate it.

He agreed to a two-pronged approach: first, to re-engage in the regular aerobic regimen he had before the revelation that immediately triggered the depression, and second, to ruminate not on what had happened or might happen between his wife and (former) friend but on weighing, on a cost/benefit basis, the options of renewed commitment versus divorce.

> After four weekly sessions, during which we reviewed the results, his symptoms remitted. He decided to remain in the marriage. My chance encounter with his wife (something therapists in small communities experience frequently) more than a year later revealed that the union remained stable and mutually satisfying.

Many of the significant social, political, economic, and governmental issues with which we struggle are also the product of emergent systems, consisting of the interaction of multiple elements that produce outcomes that are greater than the sum of the parts. Take the economy. Readers of the media and investors are inundated with data and analysis from multiple perspectives, often reaching contradicting conclusions. As Philip Tetlock (2006) has shown, experts are typically less accurate in their predictions than folks with less detailed data. I am reminded of the nephrologist who proclaimed that the heart existed merely to support the kidneys. That specialist knew a lot about a particular organ but had little appreciation of that emergent quality we call life. Likewise, value investors, technical analysts, and commodity traders have very narrow vantage points from which to create meaning of our complex economic system.

The ability of experts to make predictions was examined in detail by Paul Meehl (1954), a statistically sophisticated psychologist at the University of Minnesota. He compared the accuracy of expert predictions to those arrived at via simple algorithms and found that the latter performed consistently equal to or better than the experts. One example is the Apgar scale, used to assess the overall health of a newborn. A score of 0, 1, or 2 is assigned to five observable variables (heart rate, respiration, reflex, muscle tone, and color) and provide an immediate guideline to identify infants needing intervention. The Apgar rating system is used in virtually every delivery room, can be administered by staff after minimal training, and has been credited with significantly reducing infant mortality. By contrast, the experts rely on intuition, a form of pattern recognition as delineated by Herbert Simon (2002): "The situation has provided a cue; this cue has given the expert access to information stored in memory, and the information provides the answer. Intuition is nothing more and nothing less than recognition."

A single experience can become an indelible memory when accompanied by emotion and in extreme cases can be traumatic. Being an expert in complex tasks involves a different learning process. For example, expertise in chess, golf, and psychotherapy is acquired in a slow, methodical manner; each consists of a collection of mini-skills dependent on the quality, consistency, and speed of feedback. Chess masters acquire their understanding of complex positions at a glance only after many thousands of hours of disciplined practice. Professional golfers master putting after prolonged training on the practice green and with immediate feedback to refine their abilities. Psychotherapists observe both the overt and subtle reactions of their patients, leading to the development of intuitive skills to respond in verbal and non-verbal ways that shape emotions, focus attention, and create the opportunity for more functional interpretations. These clinical skills are different than the ability to predict long-term outcomes.

WYSIATI, an acronym coined by Daniel Kahneman (2011a), stands for What You See Is All There Is, which refers to the simple fact that we can process only those stimuli of which we are cognizant. An expert psychotherapist is constantly reminding himself that he is dealing with only a minimum of the variables that go into the complex and dynamic process that results in human thoughts, feelings, and behavior. He offers alternative meanings in a manner that the patient can evaluate in the frontal cortex with minimal interference from the biases originating in the more primitive brain regions.

Economist Tim Harford (2011b) coined the term "God complex" in reference to our overwhelming belief in our ability to make meaning, no matter how complicated the problem. If we can't personally or organizationally find a solution, we call in an expert, a consultant, a "God." Harford cites the case of Unilever's efforts to improve the production of powder laundry detergent, made by forcing liquid detergent through a nozzle that mixes the liquid with air, producing flakes. The challenge from the corporate perspective is to design the most effective and efficient nozzle in order to maximize profits. Following typical protocol, Unilever hired the foremost nozzle experts. Despite their best efforts, they were unable to understand the principles underlying the best nozzle operation. The solution, according to Harford, was the same system that underlies evolution: trial and error. Engineers identified the best of 10 nozzles, tweaked its design into 10 variations, tweaked the best again, and continued the process until they eventually came up with the best nozzle of all, absent an understanding of the underlying reasons. Harford extrapolates this thinking to explain the success of the American economy: The United States has the highest rate of business failures (10%) of all the world economies. This doesn't mean 10% of Americans fail. Rather, these failures are a critical component in the evolution of a surviving, growing capitalism. Failure breeds success.

As Daniel Kahneman (2011b) concluded from his studies of cognitive fallacies, human psychology interprets the world as more regular and predictable than it is. The rules that govern our memory systems make a story that is as coherent as possible, as determined by the ease with which it is processed, resulting in an emotion with positive valence. Our thinking is not perfect, but it has been sufficient to sustain our survival. Whether it will continue to do so in the changing world we face remains to be seen.

We have explored the limits of our sensory input and processing, the unreliability of memory, the flaws of our cognitive functions, the interference of our emotional needs and biases, and our inclination to make decisions for unconscious reasons and then rationalize them. How then might we apply the principles of scientific thought to improve our interpretations and decisions?

Critical thinking refers to a systematic application of scientific principles to compensate for our multiple cognitive limitations. A starting point is the recognition that the greatest self-deception of all is that we are rational creatures. To apply *scientific skepticism* to our own cognition requires a great deal of humility and a corresponding dearth of confidence. Professor Steven Novella (2012) of the Yale School of Medicine offers the following insights into improving our critical thinking skills:

- While we cannot change our basic evolved emotional needs and reactions, we can change our responses to them (a fundamental premise of psychotherapy).
- Such change involves neural pathways in our frontal lobes that have been formed by learning, and modifying them requires effort (slow thinking) and repetition.
- We should avoid over-investing in theories and beliefs, as there is no absolute right or wrong, just degrees of confidence.
- Comfort with ambiguity and uncertainty is essential.
- Be aware that when our valued beliefs are challenged, we tend to cling to them more strongly.
- To counter this reaction, we need to engage our higher cortical functions to filter and limit our primitive brain parts.
- Our society, as reflected by our educational systems, values authoritative answers over critical thinking process.
- The awareness of updating prior knowledge with new information is important and a hallmark of Bayesian thinking.
- New information can lead to cognitive dissonance, which can either make our prior beliefs more rigid or empower us to engage in metacognition, with the attendant reward of expanded awareness.

While metacognition requires slow thinking and increased investment of time and energy, it leads to thinking that has a higher probability of being a product of facts and logic rather than biases and emotion.

As illustrated by the first quotation at the beginning of this chapter, the notions of critical thinking and observer dependence evoke strong negative emotional reactions among those who interpret them as having the potential for, among other things, "challenging . . . fixed beliefs and undermining parental authority." Others will respond to these ideas, not as a threat, but with excitement and heightened intellectual curiosity.

It's all in the interpretation.

7
RE-THINKING PSYCHOTHERAPY

Neurosis is the inability to tolerate ambiguity.

—Sigmund Freud

When your mind is more clear, you see the true way the world is made.
When you see the true way the world is made,
you feel at peace inside.
You see how you make your own world,
so then you can make it different if you want.

—Roland Marullo,
Breakfast with Buddha

Psychologists who undertake to set themselves up as judges
in the field of truth and knowledge are shipwrecked
by the laughter of the Gods.

—Albert Einstein

Congratulations on your persistence! Assuming you have read most of what precedes, you have tolerated a lot of ambiguity, an achievement that Freud would applaud. This last leg of our journey will either enlighten or confuse and runs the risk of evoking the laughter of the Gods. My hope is that we, and I include myself, can pursue an understanding of psychotherapy that incorporates advances in both scientific research and thinking. To begin, let's consider how we got to our existing models of psychotherapy.

Psychotherapy and Science

First, a brief look at psychotherapy and its relationship to science. The ancient Greeks were the first to classify disorders of thinking, feeling, and behaving as medical/scientific in nature, though some of their notions seem bizarre today (hysteria in women was the result of a wandering uterus, psychosis was best treated by bloodletting). The Middle Ages witnessed a return to earlier conceptualizations of supernatural causation, including demonic possession requiring torture or worse. While talk, encouragement, and support were acknowledged as helpful for those in distress, it wasn't until 1853 that an English psychiatrist, Walter Cooper Dendy, introduced the term *psycho-therapeia*. The turn of the century saw Sigmund Freud begin the application of a scientific approach to the developing field of psychotherapy: observation of the content of patient's thinking as expressed through talking, identification and classification of different kinds of disorders, and the development of theories that focused on unconscious processes. He focused by necessity on verbal expression as the only means to access cognition at the time. It would be close to a century before imaging and other technologies could begin to uncover the biological underpinnings of mental processes. While Freud's formulations were crude by today's standards, they were consistent with the science of medicine in his era.

Unfortunately, the practice of psychoanalysis remained largely stagnant during the first half of the twentieth century, while the rest of medicine made dramatic advances through the synergy of applied science and emerging technologies. Psychoanalysis did not employ empirical research methods such as hypothesis testing, use of control groups, double blind studies, or adoption of objective outcome measures. Rather, psychoanalytic journals consisted of anecdotal reports on a single patient or a small number of patients, with no measurable way to assess outcomes. Eric Kandel describes psychiatry in the 1950s as "strangely unconcerned with empirical evidence or with the brain as the organ of mental activity" (2006, p. 364) as compared to medicine's evolution into a therapeutic science.

Psychotherapy's avoidance of more rigorous scientific inquiry began to change with the advent of behavioral theory and its emphasis on observable, and therefore measurable, outputs. While early behaviorists were unconcerned with thinking, it was inevitable that psychological theorists would explore the connections/associations between thinking and behavior. Psychiatrist Aaron Beck (Beck & Beck, 2011) was an early proponent of cognitive therapy, with its focus on conscious, not unconscious, thinking. Theorizing that disorders of emotion and behavior have their roots in distortions of thinking, cognitive-behavioral therapy embraced scrutiny by scientific methods. Thus, researchers developed behavior rating scales that operationalized such concepts as depression, anxiety, and attention-deficit, allowing for pre- and post-intervention ratings applied to randomly selected treatment and control groups.

Concurrent with this embracing of science by psychotherapy was the development of an ever-growing number of psychotherapeutic medications, all of which had to support their claims of treatment efficacy to the Food and Drug Administration before they could be marketed. This rush to science in the mental health field in the last half of the twentieth century, which continues today, also involved a major shift in professional roles. Under psychoanalysis, psychotherapy was the almost exclusive role of the psychiatrist, while psychologists and clinical social workers assumed support functions. In the last 50 years, psychiatric training has shifted its focus to treatment with medications, while psychotherapy has become the responsibility of psychologists, social workers, and other professionals. Both psychotropic medications and psychotherapy are based on scientific inquiry and assessment. The lack of consistent research outcomes reflects the limitations of scientific approaches, failure to utilize appropriate methodologies, and such phenomena as regression to the mean.

One obvious difference between research utilizing a specific pharmaceutical agent, as opposed to a psychotherapy, is that the former can be controlled for consistency (the subject is always getting the identical dose of an identical chemical agent), while no two psychotherapeutic interventions can be exactly the same (reminiscent of Leibnitz and his indiscernability of identicals). Thought of this way, one is tempted to conclude that pharmaceutical research will produce more meaningful and practical results. Such a conclusion rests on an unstated assumption—namely, that all the subjects are identical and that their bodies process the chemical(s) in exactly the same way. Of course, we know that cannot be true. Thus, a lack of consistent outcomes among subjects.

Unlike psychotropic drugs, psychotherapy can individualize the intervention via the dynamic interaction between the therapist and the patient. The therapist receives a massive amount of immediate feedback to her verbal and non-verbal expressions, and, to the extent that she can process it, she can modify her behavior to achieve more therapeutic outcomes. Outcomes in psychotherapy are an example of emergence, a result of the dynamic interactions among the brain, body, and environment that constantly stimulate and modify the process. Psychotherapy has the potential to be self-correcting. Thought of this way, psychotherapy's apparent lack of consistency is transformed into its greatest strength, an individualized intervention.

The following critique is not unique to psychotherapy and can be applied to a broad swath of human endeavors, including health care, investing and economics, manufacturing, government, politics, and the practice of science itself. Thus considered, it reflects the limits of human cognition, not the idiosyncrasies of any particular process or undertaking.

Our current model of psychotherapy is the product of an evolutionary process that began with the intuition that many of the wide variety of problems that humans face can be solved or ameliorated by the synergistic interaction of two or more minds. Adaptations of this process have been constrained by all the usual cognitive suspects:

- the meaning bias, our cognitive/emotional need to create coherent meaning from the persistent stimulation of our environment interacting with our

prior stored experiences and meanings, even when such meaning may be misleading;
- the confirmation bias, our selecting stimuli and making meanings that create cognitive harmony and positive emotional valence;
- the illusion of validity, our persistent use of concepts and practices that have not been subject to empirical testing but provide emotional rewards;
- mental constructs as concrete realities (examples in science include integers and wave function, examples in psychology include intelligence and personality);
- reality as singular and fixed, rather than observer dependent;
- path dependence, in which the evolution of ideas in small adaptations retains concepts that actually constrain advancements in understanding;
- causation as central and linear, rather than continuous and reciprocal.

The resulting model of psychotherapy is based on the following practices and beliefs:

- Thinking is largely or solely brain based and can be exclusively altered by the linguistic exchange between a therapist and a patient.
- The brain can solve human problems solely through epistemic processes alone, ignoring the pragmatic.
- A singular, coherent theory of human cognition, emotion, and behavior is both possible and preferable.
- Such a singular and coherent theory can explain human psychology in general, as well as that of a specific individual.
- The cognitive/emotional/behavioral process we call "psychotherapy" can be broken into its constituent bits, from which understanding of it can be reconstructed.
- The practice of psychotherapy reflects a rational and comprehensive integration of current scientific thinking and practice.

Finally, I hope to re-think that abstraction labeled psychotherapy in a way that reflects our current science by:

- being consistent with scientific knowledge and principles;
- applying theories that honor the individuality of each patient;
- favoring the interactive model of emergence over central causation;
- utilizing the full range of cognitive resources;
- recognizing its non-ergodic nature.

An ergodic system is closed or contained, one in which no new elements can enter or existing elements leave. A simple example is the teakettle on the stove. The water is contained in the kettle. Heat is applied. The kettle, water, and heat constitute the entire, closed system. The results can be measured accurately with a thermometer. The experiment is replicable and can be repeated as many times as desired, with the same result (except in the highly improbable, but theoretically possible case of the water freezing). This represents a *deterministic model* in which there are (virtually) no probabilities since all conditions are known. Adding more variables to a closed system, such as alcohol to the water or altitude to the setting, yields further measurable results, as long as all variables are known. The method of scientific inquiry is *nomothetic*: Large numbers of experiments lead to general laws.

In contrast, cognition is highly complex, involving an unknown number of variables. It is non-ergodic, or open, comparable to other living systems that survive by a continuous interaction with their environment. An organic system constantly builds up and breaks down its components. In cognition, this process includes the organic components, the body and the brain, as well as those abstract components referred to as thoughts, emotions, intelligence, personality, and beliefs. Psychology subjects these abstractions to statistical analysis, but they shouldn't be confused with concrete entities. They are statistical descriptions of abstract system components, the whole of which is too complex to be considered deterministic, at least at our current level of technology and comprehension. Much of psychology research, and virtually all of psychotherapy research, is *idiographic* in nature: It generalizes from individual cases.

What are the implications of ergodicity for the practice of psychotherapy? First, therapists must recognize that in their attempt to find meaning in their patient's presentation, they may seek and ascribe a constancy to the patient's thoughts and emotions where none exists. We create abstractions to make meaning of the information we process regarding the patient, then treat the abstract as if it were concrete and fixed.

Second, therapists need to appreciate that both they and their patients are not the same from session to session. Everyone undergoes a multitude of experiences every day, both endogenous and exogenous, that modify their cognition and emotion. In therapy, patients often seek a more solidified and satisfying sense of self. A gentle and supportive awareness of our ever-changing natures can provide relief and new meaning.

As a non-ergodic system, psychotherapy itself represents an abstraction. It is the dynamic interaction of two cognitive systems, that of the therapist and that of the patient, and can be best described by probability since all variables are not known or understood. Enough variables are known so that, as in all medical and other science-based practices, it is far from random.

Non-ergodic systems are not subject to the same modes of scientific inquiry as are ergodic ones. There are far too many variables, both known and unknown, for which to account. It could be argued that science can measure the relative effectiveness of an individual therapist more accurately than it can any particular therapeutic system, since the therapist might be construed as more constant than the application of the therapeutic approach. Attempts to demonstrate the efficacy of a particular type of therapy are fraught with difficulties.

A Science-Based Model of Psychotherapy

Nevertheless, scientific thinking can contribute to improved psychotherapy, both through its methods of inquiry and the application of its research findings. These potential contributions are significant. However, as stated by Steve Andreas (2013), "Therapy is not brain science. . . . A danger in this fascination with the brain is that therapists will use neuroscience to convince themselves that they know more than they really do, and thus must be practicing effective therapy." The caution expressed by Andreas is deserved. However, I am suggesting that we apply both the principles of scientific thinking and a broader scientific understanding of cognition, broader than just neuroscience.

Psychotherapy remains an art that is increasingly informed by science, as is true of most medical practice. Indeed, it is the dynamic and creative nature of the process that yields such potential for change. Language expresses our cognitive efforts to create meaning via categorization. Science and art are digitized abstractions that convey meaning about two different ways of thinking.

To explore the potential synergies of melding these two seemingly disparate approaches in order to improve understanding, let's return once again to the seemingly paradoxical world of quantum mechanics—more specifically, how we think about quantum mechanics. This brings us back to a question raised in the opening chapter: Can thinking be the tool for investigating itself? Hang on! Quantum theory, unlike evolution, does not apply itself to our general understanding of the world we experience on a daily basis. That we can't locate objects in space and that time is relative, making cause-and-effect meaningless, seem just plain weird and irrelevant based on our day-to-day experiences.

Since an apparently unique human cognitive capacity is the ability to ask "what if?" questions, consider this: What if we applied a different model of thinking to quantum theory? And what if that model included the probability theory that originated 200 hundred years ago by our friend, Presbyterian minister Thomas Bayes? Just such a "what if?" was posed in 2002 by three quantum information theorists, Carlton Caves, Christopher Fuchs, and Ruediger Schack (2002).

Up until then, the conventional notion was that an electron was represented by its wave function, a mathematical depiction of its qualities. The result was a calculation of the probability that an electron would have a particular quality, such as location in space. This probability was based on the frequentist model of how the electron's wave function evolves in time. Applying Bayesian probability instead changed the whole paradigm. Under it, the wave function is not real but rather an abstraction, a computational tool created by the mind. As described earlier, Bayesian probability is subjective, based on belief that changes as new information is added.

This combining of quantum theory and Bayesian probability theory, referred to as *Qbism*, negates the reality of the wave function but not the reality of the phenomenon. The interpretation of the wave function is transformed from a reality to a belief that can be calculated and modified with new data derived from experience. Thus, its very nature is analog. The apparent paradoxes no longer exist. They were the product of our cognitive processes. They were all in our minds. A famous paradox posed by quantum theory was that of Schrodinger's cat. Using the standard interpretation of wave function implies that the cat is at once both alive and dead. The Qbism approach refers only to the mental state of the observer. The cat itself is either dead or alive.

Language digitizes our interpretations of the sensory stimuli we receive from our environment. Further, the words we create are conceived as a concrete reality rather than an abstraction. How might we apply these insights to the theory and practice of an analog, human interaction whose unique features we digitize with the word "psychotherapy"?

Like economics, psychotherapy has been mistakenly conceived as an ergodic system, one in which nothing is added, where all elements remain stationary. A more helpful conceptualization is that psychotherapy is the complex, dynamic interaction between two highly complex, fallible, inherently limited cognitive systems, shaped by the continuous reciprocal causation of evolutionary adaptation. (Evolution here refers to both the long-term process of cognitive development of our species and the short-term adaptations within psychotherapy.) Nothing remains stationary: perception, memory, mood, and interpretation are all fluid. Indeed, it is this very fluidity that underlies the therapeutic process. Without it, we could never change.

When practitioners began to question the theories and practices of psychoanalysis, there was an inevitable outcome, one predicted and feared by opponents of critical thinking: the undermining of the authority Freudian doctrine had achieved. Into this theoretical vacuum rushed a multitude of alternative explanations of human emotional and behavior difficulties, each with an attendant set of methods to ameliorate or resolve them. As many as 400 distinct schools of psychotherapy were eventually identified, the vast majority of which did not meet the standards of science.

> A similar phenomenon occurred when the authority of the Roman church over Christian beliefs and practices was undercut by the Reformation in the Western world. There was unleashed a torrent of new conceptualizations of Christianity, each represented by its own denomination. This process continues today, including the creation of non-affiliated community churches that are free to pick and choose from among the variety of beliefs and practices available and even to create their own.

In order to meet the criteria for inclusion as a scientific process, psychotherapy needs to be systematic, rule governed, and replicable. At the same time, its effectiveness rests on its unique ability to be flexible, dynamic, and individualized.

Barbara Held, PhD (1995), of Bowdoin College has addressed these apparently contradictory requirements in her book *Back to Reality* by proposing an ideal generic model of psychotherapy. Held's model digitizes psychotherapy into three components. She argues that any model that lacks any one of the three fails to meet the minimal criteria as a scientific undertaking.

Held asserts that the first essential component of scientific psychotherapy is a *theory of problem causation*, from which the focus of treatment flows. Problem causation is reduced to a single, or at least primary, source. Examples include biological (neurotransmitter imbalance), psychoanalytic (intrapsychic conflicts), interpersonal (family/systems factors), cognitive (distortions of thinking), and sociopolitical (poverty, discrimination) conditions. This component rests on a central planning paradigm, assuming a simple cause-and-effect relationship as opposed to the more dynamic continual reciprocal causation of the embodiment model. Historically, causation has been predetermined by the therapist, based on her cognitive style, beliefs, and biases, all shaped by her own prior life experiences, including professional training.

Held's second identified component is a *theory of problem resolution*, again defined by the therapist. Problem resolution is predicated on a centralized cause that is identified and modified. Resolution, or at least management, of the problem is achieved by addressing its content by a process: A biological intervention might involve SSRIs; a psychoanalytic intervention might use free association and other techniques to evoke and identify unconscious thoughts; an interpersonal intervention, family therapy; a cognitive intervention, corrective thinking; and a sociopolitical intervention, empowerment via social action.

Third is the specification of *patient/problem categories*, or digitizing the seemingly infinite array of human problems into a series of meaningful and manageable groupings. These might include broad categories (psychosis, depression, family dysfunction), subcategories (schizophrenia, major depression, sexual abuse), and further specifications (paranoid type, postpartum, incest). To each can be added qualifiers of the problem (severity, chronicity, and contributing stressors) and the patient (chronological and developmental age, gender, and ethnicity or race). Further complicating this delineation of patient/problem categories is that problem categories are not discrete. The same patient can have problems with cognition, emotional modulation, self-limiting behavior, and social functioning. Labeling the patient's problem involves a complex cognitive process by the therapist, based on sensory inputs shaped by prior learning stored in memory and evoked emotions.

Setting aside these complications in this idealized generic model, let's turn to the apparent tension between the need for systematizing and individualizing. Some therapeutic approaches try to systematize through a strict, manualized approach, not unlike some approaches to education. The therapy is designed to address a specific patient/problem (Held's third component), such as an adult survivor of trauma. The theory of causation (first component) is that the trauma has caused one or more distortions of thinking (interpreting stimuli immediately preceding the trauma as threatening in the present, or interpreting one's actions or inactions as causative or contributory to the trauma). Finally, the theory of resolution (second component) is to challenge the faulty cognitions/beliefs and replace them with more reality-based and functional ones.

The systematic process of problem resolution is achieved through a structured intervention: Therapy is of a predetermined length, say 12 sessions, each of which has presentations and exercises that are completed in either an individual or group format. A pre-test of thoughts, emotions, and/or behaviors establishes a baseline from which a post-test can measure change, hopefully in a positive direction. Such an intervention meets the criteria for being systematic, rule driven, and replicable, just as do drug studies. What it lacks is individualization. There is no allowance for the therapist–patient relationship, a positive one being a powerful predictor of outcome. Nor is there flexibility to adapt to the patient's cognitive functioning, including learning style, education, intelligence, and existing level of knowledge.

At the other pole of the dichotomy is therapy that has been labeled *post modern* or *narrative*. In its extreme form, it asserts that every patient is so different that no theory of causation and problem resolution can be applied. There is no cause-and-effect relationship to be uncovered. Rather, each patient has constructed his own story, and it is this story alone that the therapist has to mold to improved functionality. Like the wave function in quantum mechanics, the patient's narrative *is thought of* as the reality from which meaning is calculated. Language is the tool to modify that presumed reality. This approach to psychotherapy is completely individualized but lacks a system, rules, or replicability.

Once more, we seem to be confronting a conundrum: Effective psychotherapy seemingly cannot be both scientific and individualized. Perhaps it is time for some additional "what if?" questions. What if we apply the principles of critical thinking to the way we think about psychotherapy? What if we minimize path dependence and instead conceptualize psychotherapy within the context of current understandings of cognition? What if we abandon the simplistic cause-and-effect paradigm of human thinking, feeling, and behaving and substitute a model based on the principles of emergence? What if we expand our tools of intervention to include more than the vicissitudes of language and instead capitalize on the full range of cognitive resources? What if we acknowledged the relativity, the observer dependence, of truth (note Einstein's warning in the quote that begins this chapter) and, like Bayes, accepted the scientific powers of probability and belief to bring us closer to meaning that is more functional? What might psychotherapy look like then?

In order to communicate my vision of systematic and individualized psychotherapy, I need to digitize it, break it into a small collection of meaningful bits. To do this, I will modify slightly Held's three components. My three components are a *problem conceptualization model* that is systematic, rule governed, replicable, yet individualized; a *hypothesis of causation and resolution* based on all relevant scientific findings; and *psychotherapeutic intervention*, or hypothesis testing, that maximizes potential effectiveness, is highly individualized, utilizes the full spectrum of cognitive resources available, and includes a dynamic system of multiple feedback loops that constantly guide and modify a process of evolutionary adaptation.

First, a word of caution. This is a way of thinking about psychotherapy. It is not by any measure a "how to practice" psychotherapy. The latter involves an array of skills acquired under expert supervision and repeated practice over many years, as well as that highest level of cognitive function—wisdom. Nevertheless, this model of conceptualizing psychotherapy can provide a framework for effective practice.

Re-Thinking Problem Conceptualization

Clearly defining the problem(s) to be addressed by psychotherapy provides the foundation for intervention. Problem definition begins with the patient: his current interpretation of what brings him to therapy, as well as his cognitive style and his expectations. From this, the therapist begins to construct a hypothesis, utilizing the vast amount of scientific knowledge and theory available. Beware of therapists who use the confirmation bias to fit the patient to a pre-existing theory. Like in another complex non-ergodic system, quantum mechanics, there can be no one theory that explains everything. Excellent therapists construct individualized theories that value continuous reciprocal causation.

In line with Daniel Kahneman's (2011b) notions of fast and slow thinking, we might be tempted to conclude that slow thinking is the only route to optimal outcomes. Sole reliance on our higher order thinking to achieve therapeutic outcomes represents path dependence originating in psychoanalysis, conceptualizing psychotherapy as a lengthy, deliberative process. Not all patients seeking help with psychological issues benefit from that approach. My case vignettes have included two examples of single-session interventions—the patient seeking a quick fix to an airplane phobia and the man with chronic obesity who had little hope of success. When a patient responds to "How might I help you?" with "I don't know," I interpret the response as an opportunity to be creative, unconstrained by the patient's pre-existing expectations. In the first case, the patient was highly motivated but had no idea what to expect from our single meeting. In the latter case I made the intuitive (fast thinking) judgment that a confusional technique might (a probability) circumvent the cognitive processes that were blocking his weight loss. Both interventions were based on many years of accumulated psychotherapy experience and are not generally part of the standard psychotherapy training program.

Many of my vignettes illustrate relatively short-term interventions, most fewer than 10 sessions. In part, this reflects the culture of the rural area in which

I practice, where practical problem solution is valued over protracted rumination. Thus, patient expectation determines the amount of data to be collected and the complexity of the therapeutic process. At the other end of the continuum (analog) is long-term psychotherapy, which involves the conceptualization of a much more detailed and complex psychological system, requiring a thorough collection of relevant data.

Psychiatric diagnosis serves the purpose of providing generally observable criteria that justify intervention and some minimal guidance for initiating an intervention. There are limitations of this attempt to classify disorders of thinking, feeling, and behaving. The diagnostic categories are not discrete. Rarely does a practitioner in the real world encounter a patient who fits neatly into a single diagnosis. Further, diagnosis can be misconstrued as a real entity and become the focus of treatment, seen as a product of central causation rather than interpreted as the product of the emergence process. Cognitive efficiency tops slow thinking, at the expense of a richer, more nuanced understanding. (To be fair, the cognitive hyper-efficiency of some practitioners is reinforced by the economic interests of third-party payers who seek the seemingly cheapest, short-term intervention and mental health employers who demand increased productivity in the face of fixed reimbursements and rising costs. The long-term costs of such short-term fixes cannot be computed by standard actuarial models but might be subject to Bayesian analysis.)

Conceptualizing the patient's problem(s) was historically the responsibility of the therapist. This model underscored the hierarchical power relationship between the therapist/expert and the patient. It also subjected the process to the biases and cognitive idiosyncrasies of the therapist and compromised the probability of a good patient-therapist "fit," or positive therapeutic relationship.

With the exception of intuitive quick fixes, my proposed model of problem conceptualization begins with patient education about basic concepts/words used in psychology in order to enhance communication by making word usage more public (per Wittgenstein). This education focuses on the four pillars of psychology (perception, cognition, emotion, behavior) and their interaction and multiple feedback loops. During this beginning phase, the patient is an active participant, providing examples of basic psychological principles from his own life. Not only does this education provide a basis for more effective patient–therapist communication, but it also begins to frame the presenting problem(s) within the context of normal, as opposed to pathological, psychological processes, thereby reducing the common initial anxiety that a patient experiences. (I use a similar but simplified approach with children, describing examples of problems of thinking, feeling, and behaving, then asking the youngster if he thinks he is having any of those kind of problems.) Only after this introduction, which might take a session or two, do I begin collecting relevant data.

Because it is not my intent to provide a "how to" for psychotherapy, I will not detail the specifics of a comprehensive database. Suffice it to say that it should include as much as possible the data that has been scientifically shown to be associated with psychological development and functioning: family history, including psychiatric and medical details; trauma history; physical and mental health history and current treatments; current levels of functioning within the physical, social, and cognitive arenas; and self-help strategies known scientifically to be correlated with improved cognitive functioning, including aerobic exercise, sleep, nutrition, and meditative/spiritual practice. For children, there should be a thorough developmental and sensory processing history and assessment of current functioning.

Next comes the patient's narrative, which is a rich source of information, yet it must be recognized as the patient's interpretation and therefore subject to all the perceptual and cognitive biases and shortcomings previously considered. When appropriate, reports from other sources (subject to their own biases and limitations) enrich the assessment process. For children, this can include parent, teacher, and caretaker input; for adults, feedback from spouses, family, and significant others. Records of prior medical, educational, and psychological assessments and interventions enhance the process. The rules of patient consent and confidentiality guide this part of the assessment.

Historically, psychotherapists have self-identified with a particular theoretical orientation: psychoanalytic, behavioral, cognitive, to name a few of the more common ones. Such labels guide the therapist's search for meaning regarding the patient's problem(s) and their remediation. The choice of what data to collect involves underlying theoretical assumptions about problem definition and causation, as well as about appropriate interventions. Data collection can be complicit in confirmation bias: Like both Marx's economic theories and Freud's psychoanalytic school of thought, confirmation can be found everywhere.

Rather than gathering data with a predetermined theoretical paradigm, a scientific approach calls for accumulating a database of all information that has an empirical basis, then constructing an individualized theory/hypothesis based on the most logical and relevant information.

> The process of selecting what is judged to be most pertinent to a particular situation is called *eclecticism*. In *Back to Reality*, Barbara Held (1995) digitizes eclecticism into three types: *pluralistic* (the coexistence of different schools of thought, each with a degree of validity and success); *synthetic* (the melding of the essence of different theories into a metatheory); and *technical/systematic*, in which different conceptualizations have been empirically demonstrated to be effective with specific patient or problem categories. I label myself a *pragmatist*, focused on therapeutic outcomes, not theoretical purity. Like string theory, there cannot be one psychotherapy theory that explains everything.

Organizing data in a way that increases the probability of a positive therapeutic outcome requires a process that is systematic and rule driven, while cognizant and respectful of the observer dependence of the therapist and patient interpretations. This involves the adaptation of scientific principles to the realities of both medical and psychotherapeutic practices, a challenge elucidated by Lawrence Weed, MD (Weed & Weed, 2011):

> Whereas the good scientist focuses on a single or very limited number of problems, pursuing each until he finds a solution, the physician is asked to accept the obligation of multiple problems in a given clinical situation and yet to give each the single-minded attention that is fundamental to developing and mobilizing his enthusiasm and skill. The university education a physician receives suggests that his attitude should be scientific in focus, but the multiplicity of tasks that confront him during his clinical training often defeats the goal. He can *act* [emphasis added] as a scientist, however, if he is able to organize the problems of each patient in a way that enables him to deal with them systematically.

In other words, how we think about, and therefore systematically organize, the sensory inputs we process from and about the patient is a fundamental application of the scientific approach. An initial problem list is jointly developed by the therapist and patient, based in the interpretation of both relevant subjective and objective information. Inclusion of the patient in defining the problem(s) is critical, given the role of observer dependence in seeking the abstraction we call reality or truth. This list is dynamic and revised as additional sensory data, memories, and interpretations evolve via multiple feedback loops.

The Problem-Oriented Medical Record developed by Weed (1972) and associates in the 1960s and 1970s mimics the scientific approach. The following demonstrates the parallel nature of the methods.

Scientific Method	**Problem-Oriented Medical Record**
Data gathering/observation	Subjective, objective data
Theory/hypothesis construction	Assessment
Theory/hypothesis testing	Plan/treatment/intervention
Outcome measurement	Outcome measurement
Hypothesis confirmation or revision	Assessment confirmation/revision
Hypothesis retest	Treatment modification
Hypothesis confirmation or revision	Treatment success or re-assessment

The problem list/medical record becomes a scaffold for making meaning out of a variety of data collected from multiple sources. It also serves as a conduit to receive additional information via dynamic feedback loops.

To find a metaphor for this process of refining the problem/theory, we need to go back to Thomas Bayes. Some psychotherapy seeks explanations for current difficulties in past experiences, an exercise in inverse probability, or trying to discern a past probability from the present effect. Other approaches seek corrective actions in current functioning. A combination of the two can be the most effective. Bayes, like many great scientists, devised a thought experiment (McGrayne, 2011), which I modified slightly by changing his generic table to a billiard table that provides containment on the sides. (As a Presbyterian of his era, Bayes could not have endorsed such a sinful activity as billiards.) Imagine that you have your back to a billiard table. A colleague tosses the cue ball at random onto the table, and you assume it could stop anywhere with equal probability. You have a paper on which you have drawn a grid representing the tabletop. Your colleague then tosses a second ball randomly and reports if it lands either left or right of the cue ball. If right, you conclude that the cue ball is more likely toward the left side. This process continues with another ball. If told it is to the left of the cue ball, you conclude that the cue ball cannot be on the far left side. The more balls that are tossed, the more you can narrow the probable range within which the cue ball is located, although you can never know its precise location. This thought experiment represents Bayes's insight into how observations about the present can lead to an increasingly probable and meaningful understanding of it. In a similar way, constant feedback from psychotherapeutic interventions can increase the probability of a more accurate and effective understanding of a psychological problem, its network of probable interactive contributing factors, and, most important, its remediation.

> Seven-year-old D was referred by her pediatrician with a puzzling mixture of symptoms. A year prior, she had been identified as having significant problems with focusing, sitting still, and controlling her impulses in the classroom. She was prescribed stimulant medication, which seemed to have some positive impact. She continued to appear anxious, express multiple worries, and isolate herself (playing video games in her room at home and avoiding interactions with peers at school). The school psychologist reported her IQ was in the superior range (121 to 146). Referral to a specialty clinic had yielded an additional diagnosis of pervasive developmental disorder, not otherwise specified, based on structured observations that identified "odd" behaviors and a lack of emotional reciprocity. Based on the presenting information, a beginning problem list might include attention-deficit symptoms, anxiety, autism spectrum symptoms.
>
> My initial evaluation included an extended interview with both parents, which uncovered a significant dynamic not previously noted: About the time that the teacher was expressing concern about D's classroom difficulties, the parents were experiencing increasing marital conflicts that ultimately led to a separation. (This revelation represented a number of billiard balls in Bayes's thought experiment.)
>
> Seven-year-olds have limited capacities to express themselves through language. Rather than focusing on their verbal expressions, child therapists

> interpret the child's play, including drawings, as expressions of underlying cognitions. D's drawing of a house lacked ground and included a dark, menacing cloud above it. When asked to draw a picture of her family, she excluded her father, and the remaining members appeared small, constricted, and unhappy. Later, when given the opportunity to draw whatever she wanted, she drew her family again, this time including her father, each member facing the front, much larger in size, with a smile on each face. When seen with both parents, D's mood would shift rapidly from laughter to tears and back, seemingly unrelated to anything that was happening at the time (more billiard balls). During these affective shifts, she would cry and say, "I'm so sad, and I don't know why."

The initial, simplified Problem-Oriented Medical Record for patient D would look something like this:

Problem: Complex of behavioral and emotional symptoms
Subjective: Behavioral and emotional instability appeared a year ago. Clinical interview and drawings reveal significant worry and anxiety about the family status and her role in it.
Objective: Both parental- and teacher-structured behavioral rating scales are significant for lack of focus, inability to sit still, and disorganization. Psychological assessment shows high intelligence and autism-spectrum characteristics. Parents agree that their conflicts manifested about a year ago. Patient says she is sad and exhibits tearfulness.

Next, the therapist arrives at a problem assessment in a systematic manner, combining multiple information sources, recognizing observer dependence, following rules of rationality, assuming emergence over linear cause and effect, and posing as a probability subject to further testing.

At this point, I need to interject a cautionary note about the notions of subjective and objective as they relate to the assessment of psychological problems. A physician can order a complete blood count and obtain an accurate measure of such values as white blood leukocytes and differential, red blood count, and hemoglobin and their relationship to a range that has been agreed upon as "normal." The practitioner then incorporates that information into a larger database from which she develops a hypothesis. In this case, "objective" refers to a measure of an actual physical reality.

In the practice of scientific psychology, tests and assessment tools have been developed to operationalize (create objective measures of) abstract concepts that have been subjected to the scientific standards of reliability and validity. Thus, IQ tests provide a number, based on answers to questions, that can be compared to large groups of numbers from other tests to infer relative intelligence. Behavior rating scales consist of a series of items in which patients and observers can rate the frequency of specific behaviors at a given moment/time period. ("I feel sad or depressed" or "Appears fidgety or squirmy"). These items are categorized and scored to derive measures of such abstract concepts as depression and hyperactivity. Science tries to digitize our understanding of our experiences into objective and subjective, which, like all categorization, has aided our understanding of a whole range of phenomena. However, in keeping with scientific principles, we need to be cognizant of the dangers of confusing objective measures of physical realities with objective measures of abstract concepts.

A patient's initial problem is subject to observer dependence, his cognitive style, his cognitive biases (starting with personalization), and an assumption of central causation. A basic maxim of psychotherapy is "Start where the patient is." Thus, it is common for a patient to start therapy by interpreting the problem as external: a nagging spouse, a recalcitrant teenager, an unfair boss, limited finances, an unresponsive medical system, the loss of a loved one, or a traumatic experience. While any or all of these circumstances can be contributory, they narrow the cognitive focus of intervention. Before I delve into interpreting the patient's problem, I like to ask the following: "If coming to see me is successful, what will be different *for you*?" The focus shifts from external causation to internal states, usually affective. Patients want to feel better, less depressed. They want to experience a broader range of positive emotions and feel less anxious, less angry, more content and in control, affirmed and valued.

Re-Thinking Causation and Resolution

Eric Kandel (2006) explored the biological processes underlying learning and memory in organisms with simple neurological systems and was able to track the response to a stimulus applied to a single neuron in the sea snail, *Aplysia*. From this early understanding came an appreciation of the complex biological processes that produce human memory. Human cognition, combining stimulus processing with memory, is far too complex to reduce to a single cause and far too imperfect to understand itself. Perfection, however, is not necessary. We are capable of astonishing intellectual accomplishments despite our individual and collective limitations.

Defining a psychological or medical (or other) problem requires the collection of all scientifically relevant data, a rational sorting and weighing of possible contributing factors, and the construction of a theory/hypothesis based on the probable weight of these factors. Due consideration must be given to the possible synergistic effects between/among some factors and an appreciation that problems may be symptoms of the process of emergence.

One consequence of specialization in health care is the influence of the confirmation bias, the tendency to find what one is looking for. A pediatrician sees or hears of unfocused, unsettled behavior and concludes ADHD; an autism clinician sees or hears of isolation and emotional withdrawal and concludes autistic spectrum. (Think of trying to discern the location of the cue ball after just a few trials, a low-probability endeavor.)

In D's case, to test the theory/treat the problem, my experiment/treatment was a series of family therapy sessions focusing on D's unspoken worries. The hypothesis was that this intervention would result in improved classroom behavior and social performance.

> **Assessment:** Anxiety and depression reactive to parental conflict/separation combined with attentional and autistic tendencies, resulting in a functional tipping point
> **Plan:** A series of family therapy sessions focusing on D's thoughts and beliefs about the past, present, and future of the family
> **Goal 1:** Reduction in symptoms of depression
> > **Obj. 1a:** Child-administered depression inventory within the normal range
> > **Obj. 1b:** Depression scales on both teacher and parent behavior inventories within normal range
> > **Obj. 1c:** D observed to not cry in three consecutive therapy sessions
> **Goal 2:** Improved concentration in classroom
> > **Obj. 2a:** Academic performance on quarterly report card average up by at least 10%
> > **Obj. 2b:** Focusing/concentration measures on teacher-administered behavior rating scales within the normal range
> **Goal 3:** Reduction in social isolation
> > **Obj. 3a:** Playground observation by school counselor records interaction with at least five peers during 15 minutes
> > **Obj. 3b:** Parents report D plays with a peer outside of school at least twice a week

The goals refer to abstract concepts of functioning: depression, concentration, and social interaction. Objectives are measurable and are based on expected improvement over pre-intervention metrics.

There are manuals available that provide pages of purported behavioral objectives for every conceivable problem for which patients might present. Such manuals came into existence to ease the cognitive and paperwork load on therapists who face heavy demands, often in public settings. While addressing the needs of therapists, administrators, third-party payers, and regulatory agencies, these manuals provide no benefit to the patient and impair a truly individualized therapeutic experience.

Re-Thinking the Therapeutic Process

Like all thinking, digitizing the psychotherapy process into three phases I label as problem conceptualization, hypothesis of causation/resolution, and psychotherapeutic intervention both enhances and limits meaning. I need to reiterate the dynamic process of multiple feedback loops among these abstractions. They are not independently functioning entities.

Psychotherapy is sometimes referred to as *verbal therapy*, or *talk therapy*. Both labels do a serious injustice to the process by limiting its scope and potential influence. The term *cognitive therapy* is more comprehensive, encompassing the full range of the embodied cognitive experience. Not that language and all its nuances are not important and potentially powerful. Take, for example, the influence of the metaphor "thinking outside the box" and its influence on creative thinking. Test subjects who were allowed free movement scored higher on creative thinking than did subjects whose physical motion was constrained. During a therapy session I will stand, walk about the office, and change seats and encourage the patient to do likewise.

Psychotherapy is a highly creative process, a search for new meanings regarding the self and its relationship with the non-self. Its effectiveness is heavily influenced by the physical environment in which it occurs. Consider the following unsolicited feedback I have received regarding my (not typical) office:

- My fireplace conveys warmth and security during the cold season.
- The thick brick walls and shading of large trees provide coolness, comfort, and relief on hot summer days.
- The location in a home in a residential area promotes relaxation.
- The color of the walls, which my wife labels aquamarine, is soothing.
- The presence of a small sand tray with tools (toy brush and rake) and children's toys promotes a playful ambience.

Metaphors can be conveyed both through language and via the body. The expression "harboring anger" is linguistic but its visual correlates in the right hemisphere of the brain might be accessed in pursuit of a more functional way to express, release, or transform anger. For example, visualizing a sailboat being pushed gently by a breeze—complete with accompanying sights, sounds, smells, and tactile details—then pairing that with an early somatic correlate of anger such as muscle tightness, can, with repetition, transform triggers of irrational rage into triggers of calmness.

Hand gestures likewise can communicate important metaphorical information about the patient's thoughts and emotions. Pressing the hands inwardly together or waving them wildly might convey unarticulated emotions. Similarly, the tight wrapping of the arms around the torso when describing a feeling of hopelessness might be interpreted as the patient feeling "shackled." Asking the patient to describe the situation again with the arms open wide can result in new associations. Giving a homework assignment of a breathing meditation with open arms while in the physical proximity of the distressing situation can have similarly positive effects. These interventions are examples of the emotionally focused therapy (EFT) and sensorimotor approach cited in chapter 3. Because interpretation of such gestures is subject to the biases and prior life experiences of the therapist, it is best to ask the patient about ways in which he might interpret his own gestures.

Our narrative about our self is our construction of meaning from our past experiences, our memories. Daniel Kahneman is an eminent psychologist but not a psychotherapist. He can have something of an outside view as a non-practitioner, as when he states, "I'm not an expert on therapy, but much of what therapists seem to do is help people re-imagine the situations in their life and acquire new mental habits.... So insights in therapy, to the extent that they lead you to a different labeling of situations, can change people's emotional response" (Kahneman, 2013). He describes our fast thinking, System 1, as immediate and associative. By contrast, System 2, slow thinking, is contemplative and requires an increased consumption of energy to fuel attention and cognitive work.

Kahneman also describes how our fast thinking maintains an ongoing, automatic, associative narrative about ourselves, one that is simpler and more coherent than the complex interactive feedback loops that constitute the actual process of the mental interactions between our self and our non-self. We construct explanatory causes by connecting events, principles, or concepts in the most energy-efficient manner.

To make further meaning of our cognitive functioning, Kahneman distinguishes between two concepts of self, the Experiencing Self and the Remembering Self, and illustrates the difference. Asking a person to remember his vacation does not necessarily elicit the actual experience. The end of an experience, be it positive or negative, colors the memory. To underscore the importance of memory on our decision making, Kahneman suggests a thought experiment in which you imagine that following a vacation you will be given a drug that causes total amnesia of the vacation experience. Would you choose to go on the vacation anyway? Perhaps some would not. Our decisions are motivated not only by the anticipation of positive emotional experiences. They are predicated on remembering them as well (Kahneman, 2013).

Memory is the framework from which we interpret the present. Current experience has no meaning in a vacuum. Yet memory is notoriously unreliable, subject to a variety of errors of commission and omission. It is an abstraction, stored bits or gists, not a replication of reality. The exploration of memories in therapy must include education of the patient to the vicissitudes of memory in a way that does not challenge credulity. Techniques for doing so, and for considering possible errors of memory, are best acquired through expert clinical supervision.

Our creation of meaning through pattern discernment is also subject to errors. As noted by Einstein, it is not the role of the psychotherapist to judge the "truth." Rather, the therapist makes suggestions regarding ways in which the patient's pattern discernment might be contributing to cognitive and emotional dysfunction. Our fast thinking infers cause and effect and assigns agency. In science, pattern discernment is the basis for hypothesis creation and testing, via slow thinking. Introspective psychotherapy reframes the patient's pattern discernment from confirmation into a hypothesis subject to further testing.

Our cognitive biases are legion. The most common one is personalization. An endless amount of stress and depression originates in our primitive, self-centered interpretation that everything that happens involves us. We view ourselves as more competent and more influential over ourselves and our environment than could be possible. Such an exaggerated view of self has had evolutionary survival value and likely serves us today as a self-fulfilling prophesy and a defense against the existential dread of our own insignificance. A related bias is the fundamental error of attribution: our tendency to see our own failures as situational, while those of others represent an inherent character flaw. It is clearly not the role of psychotherapy to strip patients of their inflated belief in their own importance. (Nor, indeed, is it my role to strip therapists of their self-worth as professionals.) However, helping to reframe patients' roles in particularly distressing situations is an effective strategy to reduce symptoms.

Addressing irrational thinking is yet another psychotherapeutic technique that requires considerable time and energy. For patients with the requisite time, energy, cognitive capacity, and discipline, the results can be generalized from specific situations to their interpretation of their whole life experience. Patients like this do not constitute the majority of most therapists' caseloads. Their cognitive fallacy is to draw conclusions, then seek evidence everywhere to support it. The corrective cognitive experience is to start with premises and engage in logical thought processes from which to draw conclusions that are consistent with all the objective evidence.

Andy Clark (1998) views language as the ultimate, man-created scaffold, a reverse adaptation, for creating meaning of our experience. Language has limitations, as elaborated by Wittgenstein. Non-linguistic expressions of our thinking and feeling are also available to aid the therapy process. Visual metaphors can be a powerful tool where language itself is inadequate, as in asking adults to express a visual image of a problem when they are stuck, then crafting their own creative visual solution. Depression may look like a dark cloud; visualize a breeze slowly pushing it aside. Stress might be conceived as electrical impulses coming from above; picture a dome covering you that deflects them. Anger is often seen as fire; contain it in a furnace that shrinks in size. A persistent, recalcitrant issue or worry might appear as a brick wall; float over it in a balloon. Letting go of anxiety and worry might involve converting it to a light gas, blowing it into balloons, and watching the balloons float away. The metaphors do not solve the problem, but they do establish the cognitive conditions for creativity, for making new associations that can alter the nature of the problem and its resolution.

Cognition involves continuous reciprocal causation among the brain, the body, and the environment. Altering cognition can begin in any of the three. My office ambience has been complimented as aiding the therapeutic process; patients may want to consider alterations in their home or work settings, or in places where they spend their leisure time. If they are unable to identify something to change, I suggest they make a random change, assume the role of observer, and note any effect on their thinking and feeling (thereby creating an observation subject to hypothesis testing).

In addition, changing the somatic experience can alter cognition and associated affect. If patients are curled up when remembering a stress-provoking incident, I will gently suggest that they stand and open their arms while staying with the memory. Changing the somatic experience helps to separate the past from the present, altering the current emotional connections to the memory. Movement therapies, such as dance, can alter cognition by addressing the somatic component of the continuous reciprocal process.

Another somatic intervention involves patient education about physical health. We cannot assume that patients understand what constitutes good diet and nutrition. Regular aerobic exercise and moderation of personal habits are essential to good cognitive functioning. Addressing medical needs with a trusted primary care provider will help ensure that the body is an optimal functioning component of the cognition process.

Many of these notions of psychotherapy are in direct conflict with the earlier models espoused by Freud and Rogers, in which the therapist would passively reflect on the patient's verbal expressions, interjecting occasional interpretations. This older model reflected the understanding of its time, and the process of path dependence has sustained it. Advances in scientific understanding of cognition suggest that a more active process will increase the probability of more successful outcomes.

Family therapy was one source of interventions that went beyond language. Virginia Satir (1983) used sculpting, in which family members would enact their visualization of the family dynamics by placing members in physical positions and proximities that reflected their interpretation. For example, a dominating member might be placed standing on a chair, with others taking appropriate submissive poses. Similarly, Cloe Madanes (2014) advocates the use of physical activity combined with the unexpected and incongruous. She cites a case in which a woman experienced panic attacks every morning that lasted throughout the day and had persisted despite years of psychotherapy. The patient's husband described his daily ritual of reassuring her before leaving for work. The therapist suggested a radical change in the morning routine. Instead of the usual support, the husband was advised, in the wife's presence, to communicate a paradoxical message before he left in the morning: telling her he didn't love her, that she should "drop dead," and if she did, he would remarry. The theory behind this seemingly drastic approach was that a minor change in the context in which the symptom appears can set in motion other, often unexpected changes. In this case, the changes provoked by the disruption of the usual symptom context appeared in unknown, unresolved issues within the extended family.

Let's return to seven-year-old D to see how these ideas about the therapeutic process guided the work with her and her parents. Family therapy with such a young child must be oriented to her developmental cognitive level. All four of us sat on the floor at the beginning of our sessions. I gave all of us verbal permission to move about the room as appropriate. (I needed to calm the mother's anxiety, which she expressed by repeatedly telling D to sit still.)

We engaged in three types of play. In one, each of us did picture stories to create in our minds a specific, assigned affective theme (worry, joy, anger, success). Each story had a beginning, a middle, an end, and a moral. Next we drew a picture illustrating the essence of the story. Finally, we shared our pictures and stories and responded with our thoughts and feelings to each other's. This activity was a medium for D and her parents to express their interpretations of the family situation in a safe setting and provided D with alternative meanings of her personalizations. As therapist, I used my participation to demonstrate how one can construct different interpretations of the same phenomenon.

In a second activity each of us used sets of family dolls to enact a family dynamic such as conflict, separation, problem solving, and safety. Multiple sensory experiences were encouraged—having the dolls talk about what they saw, heard, smelled, tasted, and touched; moving about the room; assuming multiple family roles; and demonstrating diverse interpretations.

Third, we played the board game Ungame, using cards for young children and general purpose cards. As I explained to D, the game has no end and no winners and losers. It is played for the experience of sharing in a non-competitive environment. In addition to specific questions posed on cards—some serious, others just plain silly—there are opportunities for question or comment, which provide open-ended openings for interpretation, support, and modeling by the therapist.

D engaged quickly in the therapy process, taking advantage of the opportunity to interact with both parents in a safe, supportive environment. She was able to express her fears that she had somehow caused (personalization) the family breakup and resulting financial stressors. Uncovering her unconscious and/or unexpressed worries evoked parental assurances to the contrary, alleviating her anxiety and sense of loss.

Family therapy uncovered somatic issues that could be contributing to D's problem. Since the parental separation, her nutrition had not been consistently supervised as she moved back and forth between homes. Her sleep patterns were interrupted. She spent an inordinate amount of time alone, playing video games at the expense of aerobic exercise. The stress that each parent was experiencing had interfered with their attention to these important child-care responsibilities.

Young children interpret their world with a heavy dose of fast thinking and personalization. Even though D's executive functioning in her frontal cortex is not fully developed, she can be freed of the burden of personalizing circumstances over which she has no control by processing positive, assuring messages from adults. These messages must be repeated over time to effectively change her habits of thinking.

Family therapy sessions were held bi-weekly. Both parents and D participated actively. Parents reported that nutritional, sleep, and exercise habits were altered. After a trial without stimulant medication during a school vacation, during which D exhibited no behavioral problems, she returned to school drug free. Behavior rating scales by both the parents and the teacher identified no further focusing or behavioral issues and social interactions within the normal range. In addition, her drawings no longer included symbols often associated with depression.

Many of my case vignettes might be interpreted as suggesting that dramatic changes of thinking, feeling, and behaving can be produced by a single, sudden insight. While these summaries are intended to illustrate a point and are intentionally simplistic, the reality is that much effective psychotherapy requires a great deal of repetition to change mental habits. For example, treatment to improve anger management succeeds not by identifying a single common trigger but rather by a process of repeated review of real-life experiences. Change is a process of slow evolutionary adaptation.

Research findings are contaminated by the publication bias. Researchers publish successful hypothesis testing far more regularly than failures. The case of D, and many of those preceding, represent my intentional publishing bias in order to illustrate a therapeutic technique or approach. In actual therapy, hypothesis testing is almost always continuous. From a macro-therapy perspective, the hypothesis is amended as outcomes meet or fail to meet expectations. From a micro-therapy perspective, the therapist is constantly adapting his interpretations and behaviors based on the multiple sources of feedback available from the patient.

There is a wide range of interventions and experiences that can lead to personal growth and change: psychoactive substances, meditation, spiritual practice, education, and exposure to a variety of cultures and values, to name a few. Psychotherapy that incorporates the latest science has the potential (high probability) to be the most powerful method of promoting individualized desired changes in thinking, feeling, and behaving. Its effectiveness depends on the application of the full range of science-based knowledge regarding cognition.

Finally, invoking a visual and geometric metaphor, I come full circle to the first dictum of any therapeutic intervention. David Eagleman (2011, p. 223) notes that people who have been blind from birth do not know what is missing. Likewise, our current understanding of cognition is based on what we know: "We do not experience a gaping hole of blackness where we are lacking information—instead, we do not appreciate that anything is missing." Based on our current knowledge, cognition cannot be reduced to material causation. Making sense of our thinking requires such non-reductionistic notions as belief, gist, probability, desire, and intuition. I believe there will be discoveries that will require a whole new paradigm for conceptualizing cognition. I envy the young people who will be taking the next portion of the journey.

And thus, dear reader, our voyage together has reached its end. As your guide, I have been rendered more humble than when we set out. I take Stephen Jay Gould's (1996) warning to heart. Out of my need to make sense of things, especially that thing called "thinking," I may have detected multiple "directionalities" that do not exist. This notion does not discourage me, however. Daniel Kahneman (2013) describes wisdom as the interaction between our slow and fast thinking in order to increase our awareness of automatic errors that result from the biases that are inherent in our cognitive operations. Invoking a need to include probability in order to understand highly complex systems, I would add that wisdom increases the likelihood of increased self-awareness. Given all that we know about human cognition, and especially all that we don't know, I find that idea hopeful. I have been energized by the trip. At least, that's my interpretation.

BIBLIOGRAPHY

Ainsworth, Mary D. S., Blehar, Mary C., Waters, E., and Wall, Sally. (2014) *Patterns of Attachment: A Psychological Study of the Strange Situation.* New York, NY: Psychology Press.
ALS Association. (2011, August) "Astrocytes Toxic to Motor Neurons." *ALS Association Newsletter.*
American Psychiatric Association. (2000) *Diagnostic and Statistical Manual of Mental Disorders* (4th ed., Text Revision). Washington, DC: American Psychiatric Publishing.
American Psychiatric Association. (2013) *Diagnostic and Statistical Manual of Mental Disorders* (5th ed.). Arlington, VA: American Psychiatric Publishing.
Amsten, Amy, Mazure, Carolyn, and Sinha, Rajita. (2012, April) "Your Brain on Stress." *Scientific American.*
Anderson, Adam K. (2005, May) "Affective Influences on the Attentional Dynamics Supporting Awareness." *Journal of Experimental Psychology.*
Anderson, Lorin, Krathwohl, David, and Bloom, Benjamin. (2001) *A Taxonomy for Learning, Teaching and Assessing.* New York, NY: Longman.
Andreas, Steve. (2013, July/August) "Therapy Isn't Brain Science." *Psychotherapy Networker.*
Baker, Timothy B., McFall, Richard M., and Shoham, Varda. (2008, November) "Current Status and Future Prospects of Clinical Psychology: Toward a Scientifically Principled Approach to Mental and Behavioral Health Care." *Psychological Science in the Public Interest.*
Barrett, H. Clark. (2008, October 22) "Never Say Die: Why We Can't Imagine Death." *Scientific American Mind.*
Beck, Judith J., and Beck, Aaron T. (2011) *Cognitive Behavior Therapy* (2nd ed.). New York, NY: Guilford Press.
Bering, Jesse. (2012) *The Belief Instinct: The Psychology of Souls, Destiny, and the Meaning of Life.* New York, NY: W. W. Norton.
Bernstein, Carol A. (2011, March 4) "Meta-Structure in DSM-5 Process." *Psychiatric News.*
Bilalic, Merim, and McLeod, Peter. (2014, March) "Why Good Thoughts Block Better Ones." *Scientific American.*
Binger, Michael. (2008, February) "Winning the Meta-Game with Yourself." *Bluff Magazine.*

Blackmore, Susan. (2011, April 13) "The Curious Illusion of Consciousness." IONS Society, www.noetic.org/library.
Bor, Daniel. (2012) *The Ravenous Brain*. New York, NY: Basic Books.
Boroditsky, Lera. (2011, February) "How Language Shapes Thought." *Scientific American*.
Branan, Nicole. (2010, March) "Chimps Talk with Their Hands." *Scientific American Mind*.
Brat, Ian. (2010, February 17) "The Emotional Quotient of Soup Shopping." *Wall Street Journal*.
Brewin, Chris R., Gregory, James D., Lipton, Michelle, and Burgess, Neil. (2010, January) "Intrusive Images in Psychological Disorders: Characteristics, Neural Mechanisms, and Treatment Implications." *Psychological Review*.
Brooks, David. (2010, December 12) "They Had It Made." *New York Times*.
Brooks, David. (2011a, March 28) "Tools of Thinking." *New York Times*.
Brooks, David. (2011b, October 28) "The Life Report." *New York Times*.
Brooks, Robert, Faff, Robert, Mulino, Daniel, and Scheelings, Richard. (2009, March–June) "Deal or No Deal, That Is the Question: The Impact of Framing Effects on Decision-Making under Risk." *International Review of Finance*.
Brooks, Rodney A. (1991, January) "Intelligence Without Representation." *Artificial Intelligence*.
Burns, David. (2006) *When Panic Attacks: The New Drug-Free Anxiety Therapy*. New York, NY: Morgan Road Books.
Burns, David. (2008) *Feeling Good: The New Mood Therapy*. New York, NY: Barnes and Noble.
Butler, Andrew C., Chapman, Jason E., Forman, Evan M., and Beck, Aaron T. (2006, January) "The Empirical Status of Cognitive-Behavioral Therapy: A Review of Meta-Analysis." *Clinical Psychology Review*.
Callender, Craig. (2010, June) "Is Time an Illusion?" *Scientific American*.
Carey, Benedict. (2010, December 6) "Tracing the Spark of Creative Problem-Solving." *New York Times*.
Carmel, David, Nasrallah, Maha, and Lavie, Nilli. (2009, October) "Murder, She Wrote: Enhanced Sensitivity to Negative Word Valence." *Emotion*.
Carpenter, Siri. (2011, January/February) "Body of Thought." *Scientific American Mind*.
Carr, Thomas H., Posner, Michael I., Pollatsek, Alexander, and Snyder, Charles R. (1979, December) "Orthography and Familiarity Effects in Word Processing." *Journal of Experimental Psychology: General*.
Castellanos, Francisco. X., et al. (1998, September) "Lack of an Association between a Dopamine-4 Receptor Polymorphism and Attention-Deficit/Hyperactivity Disorder: Genetic and Brain Morphometric Analyses." *Molecular Psychiatry*.
Cave, Stephen. (2013, July) "Four Stories We Tell Ourselves about Death." TED Talk. www.ted.com/talks/stephen_cave_the_4_stories_we_tell_ourselves_about_death
Caves, Carlton M., Fuchs, Christopher A., and Schack, Ruediger. (2002, February) "Quantum Probabilities as Bayesian Probabilities." *Physical Review A*.
Chang, Ruth. (2014, May) "How to Make Hard Decisions." TED Talk, www.ted.com/talks/ruth_chang_how_to_make_hard_choices
Changizi, Mark. (2011) *Harnessed: How Language and Music Mimicked Nature and Transformed Ape to Man*. Dallas, TX: BenBella Books.
Chivers, Meredith L., et al. (2004, November) "A Sex Difference in the Specificity of Sexual Arousal." *Psychological Science*.
Chomsky, Noam. (1983) "The Psychology of Language and Thought." In *Dialogues on the Psychology of Language and Thought*, Robert W. Reiber (Ed.). New York, NY: Plenum.

Clark, Andy. (1998) *Being There.* Cambridge, MA: MIT Press.
Clark, Andy. (2010, December 12) "Out of Our Brains." *New York Times.*
Clore, Gerald L., and Ortony, Andrew. (1998) "Appraisal Theories: How Cognition Shapes Affect and Emotion." In *Handbook of Emotions* (3rd ed.), Michael Lewis, Jeannette M. Haviland-Jones, and Lisa Feldman Barrett (Eds.). New York, NY: Guilford Press.
Coates, John. (2012) *The Hour Between Dog and Wolf: Risk Taking, Gut Feelings and the Biology of Boom and Bust.* New York, NY: Penguin Press.
Cohen, Patricia. (2008, March 1) "The Art of the Save, for Goalie and Investor." *New York Times.*
Colapinto, John. (2009, May 11) "Brain Games: The Marco Polo of Neuroscience." *New Yorker.*
Colcombe, Stanley, and Kramer, Arthur. (2003, March) "Fitness Effects on the Cognitive Function of Older Adults: A Meta-Analysis." *Psychological Science.*
Crabbe, John. (2004) *The Development of Science-based Guidelines for Laboratory Animal Care: Proceedings of the November 2003 International Workshop.* National Research Council (US) Institute for Laboratory Animal Research. Washington, DC: National Academies Press.
Crick, Francis, and Koch, Christof. (2003, February) "A Framework for Consciousness." *Nature Neuroscience.*
Cunningham, Aimee. (2011, August) "Painkillers Thwart Prozac." *Scientific American.*
Damasio, Antonio. (1994) *Descartes' Error.* New York, NY: Harper Collins.
Damasio, Antonio. (2011, March) "The Quest to Understand Consciousness." TED Talk. www.ted.com/talks/antonio_damasio_the_quest_to_understand_consciousness
Davidson, Richard and Begley, Sharon. (2012) *The Emotional Life of Your Brain.* New York, NY: Hudson Street Press.
Dehaene, Stanislas. (2009) *Reading in the Brain.* New York, NY: Viking Penguin.
Dehaene, Stanislas. (2014) *Consciousness and the Brain: How the Brain Codes Our Thoughts.* New York, NY: Viking Penguin.
DeRubeis, Robert, Gelfand, Lois, Tang, Tony, and Simons, Anne. (1999, July) "Medication versus Cognitive Behavioral Therapy for Severely Depressed Outpatients: Mega-Analysis of Four Randomized Comparisons." *American Journal of Psychiatry.*
Deutsch, David, and Ekert, Artur. (2012, August) "Beyond the Quantum Horizon." *Scientific American: Extreme Physics.*
Diamond, Lisa M. *Sexual Fluidity: Understanding Women's Love and Desire.* (2009) Cambridge, MA: Harvard University Press.
Diemand-Yauman, Connor, Oppenheimer, Daniel, and Vaughan, Erikka. (2011, January) "Fortune Favors the Bold (and the Italicized): Effects of Disfluency on Educational Outcomes." *Cognition.*
Duncan, John. (2010) *How Intelligence Happens.* New Haven, CT: Yale University Press.
Dutton, Kevin. (2010) *Split-Second Persuasion: The Ancient Art and New Science of Changing Minds.* New York, NY: Houghton Mifflin Harcourt.
Eades, Michael R. (2013, December) "Absolute Risk versus Relative Risk: Why You Need to Know the Difference." www.proteinpower.com/drmike/statins/absolute-risk-versus-relative-risk-need-know-difference
Eagleman, David. (2011) *Incognito: The Secret Lives of the Brain.* New York, NY: Pantheon Books.
Ekman, Paul. (2003) *Emotions Revealed: Recognizing Faces and Feelings to Improve Communication and Emotional Life* (2nd ed.). New York, NY: Owl Books.
Fatsis, Stefan. (2008) *A Few Seconds of Panic: A Sportswriter Plays in the NFL.* New York, NY: Penguin Press.

Fields, Douglas R. (2004, April) "The Other Half of the Brain." *Scientific American.*
Flynn, John. (2013, March) "Why Our IQ Levels Are Higher Than Our Grandparents'." TED Talk. www.ted.com/talks/james_flynn_why_our_IQ_levels_are_higher_than_our_grandparents
Foer, Joshua. (2007, November) "Remember This." *National Geographic Magazine.*
Foer, Joshua. (2011) *Moonwalking with Einstein.* New York, NY: Penguin Press.
Fragopanagos, Nikos and Taylor, John G. (2005, July) "Emotion Recognition in Human-Computer Interaction." *Neural Networks.*
Fries, Pascal, Womelsdorf, Thilo, Oostenveid, Robert, and Desimone, Robert. (2008, May) "The Effects of Visual Stimulation and Selective Visual Attention on Rhythmic Neuronal Synchronization in Macaque Area V4." *Journal of Neuroscience.*
Gao, Yu, Raine, Adrian, Venables, Peter H., Dawson, Michael E., and Mednick, Sarnoff A. (2010, January) "Association of Poor Childhood Fear Conditioning and Adult Crime." *American Journal of Psychiatry.*
Gavey, Nicola. (2005) *Just Sex? The Cultural Scaffolding of Rape.* New York, NY: Routledge.
Geary, James. (2011) *I Is an Other: The Secret Life of Metaphor and How It Shapes the Way We See the World.* New York, NY: Harper Collins.
Gierach, John. (1995) *Dances with Trout.* New York, NY: Simon and Schuster.
Gigerenzer, Gerd, Gaissmaier, Wolfgang, Kurz-Milcke, Elke, Schwartz, Lisa, and Woloshin, Steven. (2007, November) "Helping Doctors and Patients Make Sense of Health Statistics." *Psychological Science in the Public Interest.*
Gigerenzer, Gerd, Gaissmaier, Wolfgang, Kurz-Milcke, Elke, Schwartz, Lisa, and Woloshin, Steven. (2009, April/May/June) "Knowing Your Chances." *Scientific American Mind.*
Gilbert, Daniel. (2007) *Stumbling on Happiness.* New York, NY: Vintage Books.
Gladwell, Malcolm. (2009, July 27) "Cocksure." *New Yorker.*
Goldacre, Ben. (2007, February 18) "What's Wrong with Dr. Gillian McKeith PhD?" *Guardian.*
Gould, Stephen Jay. (1996) *Full House: The Spread of Excellence from Plato to Darwin.* New York, NY: Harmony Books.
Grady, D. L., Harxhi, A., Smith, M., Flodman, P., Spence, M. A., Swanson, J. M., and Moyzis, R. K. (2005, July) "Sequence Variants of the DRD4 Gene in Autism: Further Evidence That Rare DRD4 7R Haplotypes Are ADHD Specific." *American Journal of Medical Genetics Part B: Neuropsychiatric Genetics.*
Grandin, Temple. (1976) *Thinking in Pictures: My Life with Autism.* New York, NY: Vintage Books.
Greenberg, Leslie S. (2002) *Emotion-Focused Therapy: Coaching Clients to Work through Their Feelings.* Washington, DC: American Psychological Association.
Griffiths, Thomas, and Tenenbaum, Joseph. (2005, December) "Structure and Strength in Causal Induction." *Cognitive Psychology.*
Hall, James. (2005) *Tools of Thinking: Understanding the World through Experience and Reason.* Chantilly, VA: The Teaching Company.
Hanh, Thich Nhat. (2002) *No Death, No Fear.* New York, NY: Riverhead Books.
Harford, Tim. (2011a) *Adapt: Why Success Always Starts with Failure.* New York, NY: Farrar, Stress and Giroux.
Harford, Tim. (2011b) "Trial, Error and the God Complex." TED Talk, www.ted.com/talks/tim_harford
Harford, Tim. (2013) *The Underground Economist Strikes Back.* New York, NY: Penguin Riverhead.
Havens, Ronald A. (2005) *The Wisdom of Milton H. Erickson: The Complete Volume.* Bethel, CT: Crown Publishing.

Hawking, Stephen. (1988) *A Brief History of Time*. Westminster, MD: Bantam Books.
Hawking, Stephen, and Leonard Mlodinow. (2010, October) "The Elusive Theory of Everything." *Scientific American*.
Haynes, John-Dylan and Rees, Geraint. (2006, July) "Decoding Mental States from Brain Activity in Humans. *Nature Reviews Neuroscience*.
Heard, Heidi L., and Linehan, Marsha M. (1994, March) "Dialectical Behavior Therapy: An Integrative Approach to the Treatment of Borderline Personality Disorder." *Journal of Psychotherapy Integration*.
Heilman, Kenneth M., Blonder, Lee X., Bowers, Dawn, and Valenstein, Edward. (2012) "Emotional Disorders Associated with Neurological Diseases." In *Clinical Neuropsychology*. (5th ed.) New York, NY: Oxford University Press.
Heisenberg, Werner. (1979) *Philosophical Problems of Quantum Physics*. Woodbridge, CT: Oxbow Press.
Held, Barbara S. (1995) *Back to Reality: A Critique of Postmodern Theory in Psychotherapy*. New York, NY: W. W. Norton.
Herbert, Wray. (2010a, March/April) "Extraordinary Perception." *Scientific American*.
Herbert, Wray. (2010b) *On Second Thought: Outsmarting Your Mind's Hard-Wired Habits*. New York, NY: Crown.
Hey, Tony, Tansley, Stuart, and Tolle, Kristen (Eds.). (2009) *The Fourth Paradigm: Data-Intensive Scientific Discovery*. Redmond, WA: Microsoft Research.
Hooker, Evelyn. (1957) "The Adjustment of the Male Overt Homosexual." *Journal of Projective Techniques*.
Huxley, Aldous. (1954) *The Doors of Perception*. New York, NY: Harper and Row.
Ioannidis, John P. A. (2005, August) "Why Most Published Research Findings Are False." *PloS Medicine*.
Jackendoff, Raymond. (1987) *Consciousness and the Computational Mind*. Cambridge, MA: MIT Press.
Jarvik, Jeffrey G. et al. (2003, June) "Rapid Magnetic Resonance Imaging vs Radiographs for Patients with Low Back Pain: A Randomized Controlled Trial." *Journal of the American Medical Association*.
Jaynes, Julian. (2000) *The Origin of Consciousness in the Breakdown of the Bicameral Mind*. New York, NY: Houghton Mifflin Harcourt.
Jensen, Maureen C. et al. (1994, July 14) "Magnetic Resonance Imaging of the Lumbar Spine in People without Back Pain." *New England Journal of Medicine*.
Josipovic, Zoran. (2013, August) "Neural Correlates of Nondual Awareness in Meditation." *Annals of the New York Academy of Sciences*.
Kahneman, Daniel. (2011a, October 19) "Don't Blink! The Hazards of Confidence." *New York Times*.
Kahneman, Daniel. (2011b) *Thinking, Fast and Slow*. New York, NY: Farrar, Strauss and Giroux.
Kahneman, Daniel. (2013, March/April) "What Really Matters." *Psychotherapy Networker*.
Kahneman, Daniel, and Tversky, Amos. (1973, July) "On the Psychology of Prediction." *Psychological Review*.
Kahneman, Daniel, and Tversky, Amos. (1979, March) "Prospect Theory: An Analysis of Design Under Risk." *Econometrica*.
Kandel, Eric. (2006) *In Search of Memory: The Emergence of a New Science of Mind*. New York, NY: W. W. Norton.
Kasser, Jeffrey. (2001) *Philosophy of Science*. Chantilly, VA: The Teaching Company.
Kelso, J. A. Scott. (1995) *Dynamic Patterns*. Cambridge, MA: MIT Press.

Kester, George W. (2010, Spring) "What Happened to the Super Bowl Stock Market Predictor?" *Journal of Investing*.

Kirkpatrick, David. (2009, December 20) "The Conservative-Christian Big Thinker." *New York Times Magazine*.

Kirsch, Irving. (2010) *The Emperor's New Drugs: Exploding the Anti-Depressant Myth*. New York, NY: Basic Books.

Kirsh, David, and Maglio, Paul. (1994, October) "On Distinguishing Epistemic from Pragmatic Action." *Cognitive Science*.

Kluger Jeffrey (Ed.) (2011) *Your Brain: A User's Guide*. New York, NY: Time Books.

Koch, Christof. (2004) *The Quest for Consciousness: A Neurobiological Approach*. Englewood, CO: Roberts and Company.

Kramer, Peter. (2011, July 9) "In Defense of Anti-Depressants." *New York Times*.

Kravitz, Len. (2007, October) "The 25 Most Significant Health Benefits of Physical Activity." *Fitness Journal*.

La Cerra, Peggy, and Bingham, Roger. (2002) *The Origin of Minds: Evolution, Uniqueness, and the New Science of the Self*. New York, NY: Harmony Books.

Lakoff, George, and Johnson, Mark. (2003) *Metaphors We Live By*. Chicago, IL: University of Chicago Press.

Lane, Richard D., and Nadel, Lynn (Eds). (2000) *Cognitive Neuroscience of Emotion*. New York, NY: Oxford University Press.

Leung, Angela K., et al. (2012, May) "Embodied Metaphors and Creative Acts." *Psychological Sciences*.

Lewis, Michael. (2003) *Moneyball: The Art of Winning an Unfair Game*. New York, NY: W. W. Norton.

Libet, Benjamin. (1982, September) "Readiness Potential Preceding Unrestricted 'Spontaneous' versus Pre-planned Voluntary Acts." *Clinical Neurophysiology*.

Lilienfeld, Scott, Lynn, Steven Jay, Ruscio, John, and Byerstein, Barry. (2010) *Fifty Great Myths of Popular Psychology: Shattering Widespread Misconceptions about Human Behavior*. Malden, MA: Wiley-Blackwell.

Louv, Richard. (2005) *Last Child in the Woods: Saving Our Children from Nature-Deficit Disorder*. Chapel Hill, NC: Algonquin Books.

Luria, A. R. (1987) *The Mind of a Mnemonist: A Little Book about a Vast Memory*, Jerome S Bruner (Trans.). Cambridge, MA: Harvard University Press.

Madanes, Cloe. (2014, March/April) "Soft Shock Therapy." *Psychotherapy Networker*.

Mauboussin, Michael. (2009) *Think Twice: Harnessing the Power of Counterintuition*. Boston, MA: Harvard Business School Press.

McCulloch, Warren S., and Pitts, Walter. (1943) "A Logical Calculus of the Ideas Immanent in Nervous Activity." *Bulletin of Mathematical Biophysics*.

McGonigal, Kelly. (2013, June) "How to Make Stress Your Friend." TED Talk. www.ted.com/talks/kelly_mcgonigal_how_to_make_stress_your_friend

McGrayne, Sharon Bertsch. (2011) *The Theory That Would Not Die*. New Haven, CT: Yale University Press.

McGurk, Harry, and MacDonald, John. (1976, December 23) "Hearing Lips and Seeing Voices." *Nature*.

Meana, Marta. (2012) *Sexual Dysfunction in Women*. Cambridge, MA: Hogrefe.

Meehl, Paul. (1954) *Clinical versus Statistical Prediction*. Minneapolis, MN: University of Minnesota Press.

Merullo, Roland. (2008) *Breakfast with Buddha*. Chapel Hill, NC: Algonquin Books.

Miller, Peter. (2012, January) "A Thing or Two about Twins." *National Geographic Magazine*.

Mishra, Pankaj. (2004) *An End to Suffering.* New York, NY: Farrar, Straus and Giroux.
Moore, Thomas. (1992) *Care of the Soul: A Guide for Cultivating Depth and Sacredness in Everyday Life.* New York, NY: Harper Collins.
Norcross, John C. (Ed.). (1986) *Handbook of Eclectic Psychotherapy.* New York, NY: Brunner/Mazel.
Norden, Jeanette. (2007) *Understanding the Brain.* Chantilly, VA: The Teaching Company.
Novella, Steven. (2012) *Your Deceptive Mind: A Scientific Guide to Critical Thinking Skills.* Chantilly, VA: The Teaching Company.
Ogden, Pat, Minton, Kekuni, and Pain, Clare. (2006) *Trauma and the Body: A Sensorimotor Approach to Psychotherapy.* New York, NY: W. W. Norton.
Oxnam, Robert. (2005) *A Fractured Mind.* New York, NY: Hyperion Books.
Paese, Paul W., and Sniezek, Janet A. (1991, February) "Influences on the Appropriateness of Confidence in Judgment: Practice, Effort, Information and Decision-Making." *Organizational Behavior and Human Decision Processes.*
Park, Alice. (2010, October 14) "Forget Pain Pills, Fall in Love Instead." *Time.*
Pascual Olivier et al. (2005, October) "Astrocytic Purinergic Signaling Coordinates Synaptic Networks." *Science.*
Patterson, Scott. (2010) *The Quants.* New York, NY: Crown Business.
Paulos, John Allen. (2009, December 10) "Mammogram Math." *New York Times Magazine.*
Pert, Candace B. (1998) *Molecules of Emotion: The Science Behind Mind-Body Medicine.* New York, NY: Simon and Schuster.
Peters, Ole. (2011, October) "Optimal Leverage from Non-ergodicity." *Quantitative Finance.*
Piff, Paul. (2013, October) "Does Money Make You Mean?" TED Talk. www.ted.com/talks/paul_piff_does_money_make_you_mean
Pinker, Steven. (1994) *The Language Instinct.* New York, NY: Harper Perennial Modern Classics.
Pinker, Steven. (1997) *How the Mind Works.* New York, NY: W. W. Norton.
Pinker, Steven. (2007) "The Stuff of Thought: Language as a Window into Human Nature." Altadena, CA: The Skeptics Society, DVD 178.
Pinker, Steven. (2011) *The Better Angels of Our Nature.* New York, NY: Viking.
Pols, Edward. (1992) *Radical Realism: Direct Knowing in Science and Philosophy.* Ithaca, NY: Cornell University Press.
Popper, Karl. (1963) *Conjectures and Refutations: The Growth of Scientific Knowledge.* New York, NY: Routledge and Kegan Paul.
Poundstone, William. (2010) *Priceless.* New York, NY: Hill and Wang.
Principe, Gabrielle, Bruck, Maggie, Ceci, Stephen, and Greenhoot, Andrea. (2013) *Children's Memory: Psychology and the Law.* Hoboken, NJ: John Wiley and Sons.
Quiroga, Rodrigo Quian, Fried, Itzhak, and Koch, Christof. (2013, February) "Brain Cells for Grandmother." *Scientific American Mind.*
Rakel, David P. et al. (2009) "Practitioner Empathy and the Duration of the Common Cold." *Family Medicine.*
Ramachandran, Vilayanur S. (2005) *A Brief Tour of Human Consciousness: From Imposter Poodles to Purple Numbers.* New York, NY: Pi Press.
Ramachandran, Vilayanur S. (2009) "The Neurons that Shaped Civilization." TED Talk. www.ted.com/talks/vs_ramachandran_the_neurons_that_shape_civilization
Ramachandran, Vilayanur S., Blakeslee, Sandra, and Sacks, Oliver. (1999) *Phantoms in the Brain: Probing the Mysteries of the Human Mind.* New York, NY: William Morrow.
Ramscar, Michael, Hendrix, Peter, Shaoul, Cyrus, Milin, Peter, and Baayen, Harald. (2014, January) "The Myth of Cognitive Decline: Non-Linear Dynamics of Lifelong Learning." *Topics in Cognitive Science.*

Reingold, Eyal M., and Sheridan, Heather. (2011, August) "Eye Movements and Visual Expertise in Chess and Medicine." In *The Oxford Handbook of Eye Movements*, Simon P. Liversedge, Iain Gilchrist, and Stefan Everling (Eds.). Northamptonshire, UK: Oxford University Press.

Resick, Patricia, Monson, Candice, and Chard, Kathleen. (2008) *Cognitive Processing Therapy: Veteran/Military Version*. Washington, DC: Department of Veterans Affairs.

Robinson, Daniel. (1989) *Aristotle's Psychology*. New York, NY: Columbia University Press.

Rogers, Annie G. (1996) *A Shining Affliction: A Story of Harm and Healing in Psychotherapy*. New York, NY: Penguin Books.

Ross, Michael. (1989, April) "Relation of Implicit Theories to the Construction of Personal Histories." *Psychological Review*.

Rothschild, Babette. (2006) *The Body Remembers: The Psychophysiology of Trauma and Trauma Treatment*. New York, NY: W. W. Norton.

Rounder, Jeffrey N. (2013, April) *Bayesian Inference in Psychology*. pcl.missouri.edu/jeff/sites/pcl.missouri.edu.jeff/files/t_3.pdf

Rubin, Eugene. (2014, February 5) "Physicians Who Take Their Own Lives." *Psychology Today*.

Satir, Virginia. (1983) *Conjoint Family Therapy*. Palo Alto, CA: Science and Behavior Books.

Sax, Leonard. (2007) *Boys Adrift: The Five Factors Driving the Growing Epidemic of Unmotivated Boys and Underachieving Young Men*. New York, NY: Basic Books.

Schacter, Daniel L. (2001) *The Seven Sins of Memory: How the Mind Forgets and Remembers*. New York, NY: Houghton Mifflin.

Schaller, Susan. (2012) *A Man Without Words*. Oakland, CA: University of California Press.

Schedlowski, Manfred, and Pacheco-Lopez, Gustavo. (2010) "The Learned Immune Response: Pavlov and Beyond." *Brain, Behavior and Immunity*.

Scheiber, Marc H., and Hibbard, Lester S. (1993, July) "How Somatotropic Is the Motor Cortex Hand Area?" *Science*.

Schoonover, Carl. (2010) *Portraits of the Mind: Visualizing the Brain from Antiquity to the 21st Century*. New York, NY: Abrams.

Schwartz, Casey. (2011, February 11) "Why Some People Choose Anxiety." *Newsweek*.

Schwartz, Jeffrey M., and Begley, Sharon. (2002) *The Mind and the Body*. New York, NY: Harper Collins.

Schwartz, Richard. (1997) *Internal Family Systems*. New York, NY: Guilford Press.

Schwarzkopf, D. Samuel, and Rees, Geraint (2013, March 25) "Subjective Size Perceptions Depends on Central Visual Cortical Magnification in Human V1." www.plosone.org/article/info%3Adoi%2F10.1371%2Fjournal.pone.0060550

Sejnowski, Terry, and Tobi Delbruck. (2012, October) "The Language of the Brain." *Scientific American*.

Senghas, Ann. (1995) "The Development of Nicaraguan Sign Language via the Language Acquisition Process." In D. MacLaughlin & S. McEwen (Eds.), *Proceedings of the Boston University Conference on Language Development*, 19, 543–552. Boston: Cascadilla Press.

Shenk, Joshua Wolf. (2009, June) "What Makes Us Happy?" *Atlantic Monthly*.

Sherry, David F., and Schacter, Daniel I. (1987) "The Evolution of Multiple Memory Systems." *Psychological Review*.

Shubin, Neil. (2008) *Your Inner Fish*. New York, NY: Random House.

Simon, Dan. (2012) *In Doubt: The Psychology of the Criminal Justice Process*. Cambridge, MA: Harvard University Press.

Simon, Herbert. (2002) "What Is an Explanation of Behavior?" In David G. Myers (Ed.), *Intuition: Its Powers and Perils*. New Haven, CT: Yale University Press.

Skeptic's Dictionary. "Zener ESP Cards." www.skepdic.com/zener.html

Skinner, B. F. (1948) " 'Superstition' in Pigeons." *Journal of Experimental Psychology.*
Smith, Kerri. (2013, October 23) "Mind-Reading Technology Speeds Ahead." *Scientific American.*
Song, Hyunjin, and Schwarz, Norbert. (2008, October) "If It's Hard to Read, It's Hard to Do: Processing Fluency Affects Effort Prediction and Motivation." *Psychological Science.*
Sousa, David A. (2012) *Brainwork: The Neuroscience Behind How We Lead Others.* Bloomington, IN: Triple Nickel Press.
Spruston, Nelson. (2008, March) "Pyramidal Neurons: Dendritic Structure and Synaptic Integration." *Nature Reviews Neuroscience.*
Stanovich, Keith. (2009) *What Intelligence Tests Miss: The Psychology of Rational Thinking.* New Haven, CT: Yale University Press.
Sterling, Theodore D. (1959) "Publication Decision and the Possible Effects of Inference Drawn from Tests of Significance—or Vice Versa." *Journal of the American Statistical Association.*
Steyvers, Mark, Griffiths, Thomas, and Dennis, Simon. (2006, July) "Probabilistic Inference in Human Semantic Memory." *Trends in Cognitive Sciences.*
Tammet, Daniel. (2006) *Born on a Blue Day.* New York, NY: Free Press.
Tetlock, Philip. (2006) *Expert Political Judgment.* Princeton, NJ: Princeton University Press.
Thayer, Richard. (1985) "Mental Accounting and Consumer Choice." *Marketing Science,* 4 (3), 199–214.
Thayer, Richard H. (1999, September) "Mental Accounting Matters." *Journal of Behavioral Decision Making.*
Tippett, Krista. (2010) *Einstein's God: Conversations about Science and the Human Spirit.* New York, NY: Penguin Books.
Tong, David. (2012, November 13) "The Unquantum Quantum." *Scientific American.*
Turner, Erick H., Matthews, Annette M., Linardatos, Eftihia, Tell, Robert A., and Rosenthal, Robert. (2008, January 17) "Selective Publication of Antidepressant Trials and Its Influence on Apparent Efficacy." *New England Journal of Medicine.*
Tversky, Amos, and Kahneman, Daniel. (1974) "Judgment under Uncertainty: Heuristics and Biases." *Science.*
University of California–San Diego. (2013, April 22) "Gone, but Not Forgotten: Scientists Recall EP, Perhaps the World's Second-Most Famous Amnesiac." *ScienceDaily.* www.sciencedaily.com/releases/2013/04/130422154947.htm
Vaish, Amrisha, Grossmann, Tobias, and Woodward, Amanda. (2008, May) "Not All Emotions Are Created Equal: The Negativity Bias in Social-Emotional Development." *Psychological Bulletin.*
Vaillant, George. (2012) *Triumph of Experience: The Men of the Harvard Grant Study.* Cambridge, MA: Belknap Press.
Van Petten, Cyma, and Kutas, Marta. (1987) "Ambiguous Words in Content: An Event-Related Potential Analysis of the Time Course of Meaning Activation." *Journal of Memory and Language.*
Varela, Francisco, Thompson, Evan, and Rosch, Eleanor. (1991) *The Embodied Mind: Cognitive Science and Human Experience.* Cambridge, MA: MIT Press.
von Baeyer, Hans Christian. (2013, June) "Quantum Weirdness? It's All in Your Mind." *Scientific American.*
Vyshedskiy, Andrey. (2008) *On the Origin of the Human Mind.* Mobile Reference.
Wager, Tor D., Phan, Luan K., Liberzon, Israel, and Taylor, Stephan F. (2003) "Valence, Gender and Lateralization of Functional Brain Anatomy in Emotion: A Meta-Analysis of Findings from Neuroimaging." *Neuroimage.*

Wang, X. T., and Dvorak, Robert D. (2010, February) "Sweet Science: Fluctuating Blood Glucose Levels Affect Future Discounting. *Psychological Science*.

Weed, Lawrence, MD. (1972, March) "Medical Records that Guide and Teach." *New England Journal of Medicine*.

Weed, Lawrence, MD, and Weed, Lincoln. (2011) *Medicine in Denial*. CreateSpace Independent Publishing Platform.

Wegner, Daniel. (2002) *The Illusion of Conscious Will*. Cambridge, MA: MIT Press.

Weil, Andrew. (2011) *Spontaneous Happiness*. New York, NY: Little, Brown and Company.

Westly, Erica. (2010) "Abuse and Attachment." *Scientific American Mind*.

"Who is Volunteering for Today's Military?" www.defense.gov/news/Dec2005/d20051213 mythfact.pdf

Whybrow, Peter. (2005) *American Mania: When More Is Not Enough*. New York, NY: W. W. Norton.

Willcox, Gloria. (2001) *Feelings: Converting Negatives to Positives*. Morris Publishing.

Wilson, Timothy D., Lisle, Douglas L. J., Schooler, Jonathan W., Hodges, Sara D., Klaaren, Kristen J., and LaFleur, Suzanne J. (1993, June) "Introspection about Reasons Can Reduce Post-Choice Satisfaction." *Personality and Social Psychology Bulletin*.

Wittgenstein, Ludwig. (1921) *Tractatus Logico-Philosophicus*. New York, NY: Routledge Classics, 2001.

Wittgenstein, Ludwig. (2009) *Philosophical Investigations* (4th ed.), P.M.S. Hacker and J. Schulte (Eds.). Wiley-Blackwell.

Wolfe, Jeremy, and Robertson, Lynn (Eds.). (2012) *From Perception to Consciousness: Searching with Anne Treisman*. Oxford Series in Visual Cognition.

Wolman, David. (2012, March 14) "The Split Brain: A Tale of Two Halves." *Nature News*.

Yuste, Rafael, and Church, George. (2014, March) "The New Century of the Brain." *Scientific American*.

Zunshine, Lisa. (2006) *Why We Read Fiction: Theory of Mind and the Novel*. Columbus, OH: The Ohio State University Press.

INDEX

Note: Page numbers in *italics* indicate illustrations.

absolute risk 199–200
abstraction 16, 33, 170, 175
access: to consciousness 143; to information/access consciousness 143–5
action, bias toward 131–2
action potential 56
addictions and abstinence 194–5
adenosine 61
ADHD (attention deficit hyperactivity disorder) 17
adrenarche 62
affective states, definition of 29–30
agency and discerned patterns 15
aggression, belief in direct expression of 194
aging and memory 111
agnosia 162
agreement, method of 35–6
Amirault day care case 107–8
amygdala 49, 79, 88–9, 110
analog: consciousness as mental state as 142; perception as 3, 7, 205
analogy 7, 15–16, 181
analytical statements 34
anatomy, early beliefs about 42–3
anchoring effect 126, 193, 196
anesthetics 145–6
antidepressant drugs 59–60, 187–9, 203
antisocial behavior 79

anxiety: alcohol abuse and 195; categories of disorders of 72; depiction of 77; mind-body connection in 8; obsessive-compulsive disorder and 110; panic attacks and 241–2; valence of 73
anxious-ambivalent attachment 82
anxious-avoidant attachment 82
Apgar scale 218
apoptosis 55
argument from authority 176
argument from final consequences 176
artificial intelligence 133–4
ascending reticular activating system 145
aspects 207
association: of ideas 99; as tool in processing sensory stimuli 13–14
association areas 48–9, *50*
association pathways 48
astrocytes 61
attachment theory 82–4
attention 118, 144
attention deficit hyperactivity disorder (ADHD) 17
auditory pareidolia 15
autism spectrum disorders 26, 27
auto-associators 98–9, *99*
autonomic nervous system 63
availability heuristic 193, 205
axon 47
axon hillock 56

back pain and technology 183–5
Bayes, Thomas 36–7, 233–4
Bayesian probability theory 114–15, 226
Bayesian statistics 192, 202
behavior: as area of study 11; emotions and 79–86
behavioral economics 179, 180–1
behavioral objectives, manuals of 237
behavioral psychology 9
behaviorism 93, 222
bias: processing of memories and 108–9; toward selves 39; *see also* cognitive biases
bifurcated self 168
binary concepts 84
binding problem 162
biochemistry of emotions 74–7
biogenic amines 59
biology, classification system within 170
body: interaction with brain and environment 133–40; sense of self and 154
Boolean logic 114
borderline personality disorder 87
boundaries 206
boys and nature deficit disorder 129
brain: comparison of computer to 92, 97, 97–8; development of 54–5; environment of scarcity and 180; glia cells in 60–3; information processing as activity of 93–4; interaction with body and environment 133–40, 139–40; networks of 169; organization of 43–9, *45*, *49*, *50*, 51; plasticity of 56, 57; resources required for 115; sex of 163–4; thinking and 116–20; trauma and 63–5; understanding of 51–3; *see also* neurons
brain/body connection 65–7
Brain Research through Advancing Innovative Neurotechnologies (BRAIN) Initiative 53, 140
brainstem 45, 47, 154–5
breast cancer screening 191–4
Broca's area 46
Brodmann's areas 48, *50*

Capras delusion 77
caricature heuristic 128
catecholamines 59
categories, creation of 14
caudal area of brain 45
causality in language 207
causal structure 36

causation: concepts of 151; correlation and 176, 191; hypothesis of 230, 236–7; overview of 94; theory of 228–9
cause-and-effect analysis 35–8, 83–4
CBT (cognitive-behavioral therapy) 188, 189–90, 222
cell body 47, *47*
cell doctrine of memory 102
cell phones, radiation exposure from 57–8
central nervous system 21, 44–5
cerebellum 47, *49*
cerebral cortex 46
cerebral hemispheres 45
change bias 108
"chemical imbalance" theory of depression 187–8
chemical theory of synaptic transmission 102
childhood abuse: brain, trauma, and 63; drawings by survivor of *158–9*; memories of 107; survival and 51
childhood psychiatric disorders 17
chimps, communication of 45–6
Chomsky, Noam 5–6, 170–1
Clark, Andy 133, 134, 135–6, 137–8, 139, 169, 240
classical conditioning 9
cognition: as area of study 11; definition of 29; emotion and 72, 77; evolutionary model of 214; improving 215–20; maximizing 215–20; model of 133–4; *see also* thinking
cognitive-behavioral psychology: definition of emotion 70; embodied cognition and 136; on emotion and thought 30; foundation of 80; overview of 10
cognitive-behavioral therapy (CBT) 188, 189–90, 222
cognitive biases: in breast cancer screening recommendations 192–4; in psychotherapy 223–4, 240; survival and 123–6; *see also specific biases*
cognitive dissonance 16
cognitive emotions 153
cognitive errors and flood of information 176–7
cognitive processing therapy (CPT) 64–5
cognitive scaffolding 123, 136
cognitive therapy 222, 238
color discrimination 7
combat trauma 64–5, 113
commissural pathways 48
compatibilism 152–3

computational model of thought 93–101, 175
computed tomography (CT) scan 52–3
computer, comparison of brain to 92, 97, 97–8
computer technology 213
concept cells 105
cones 21
confidence and persuasion 197
confirmation bias 14, 131, 132, 156, 184–5, 204, 224, 236–7
conflicts, internal psychological 195
connectionism 99
conscience, development of 79–80
consciousness: neurobiology of 145–9; in neurological model of thinking 118; overview of 141–5
conscious will 149–54
consistency and conscious will 152
consistency bias 108
conspiracy theory 15, 204
consumer choice and emotion 76
consumerism and persuasion 196–8
content problems and dysrationalia 39–40
contiguity 99
continuous reciprocal causation 137–8
control groups 184
conversion disorder 160
cootie heuristic 128–9
cornea 21, *22*
corpus callosum 46
correlation 176, 191, 202
correspondence bias 161
cortisol 181
critical thinking 220
cytoarchitecture 48
cytokines 66

Damasio, Antonio 30, 71, 144, 154–5
dance and movement therapies 5
data 133
data collection 231–3
data mining 176
day science 106
death, awareness of 130–1, 166–8
decisions, making: consumerism, persuasion, and 196–8; memory and 239; overview of 120–2; survival and 122–31
decline effect 203–4
decoy heuristic 126–7
deduction 15, 34
default heuristic 131

definitions 4–5
Dehaene, Stanislas 3, 143, 146–8
dendrites 47
deoxyribonucleic acid (DNA) 54–5, 201
depression: conceptualizations of 217; cytokines and 66; depression 66; medication for 59–60, 187–9, 203; neurotransmitters and 59; pharmacology and 185–91; rumination and 110
design heuristic 127
determinism 152–3
deterministic models 40–1, 92, 224–5
development of brain 54–5
Diagnostic and Statistical Manual (DSM) 71, 72, 155, 185
diagnostic categories 231
dialectic 15
dichotomous thinking 152–4
diencephalon 47
diet and cognitive functioning 67
difference, method of 36
diffusion tensor imaging 53
digital, interpretation of external world as 3, 7, 205
dissociative identity disorder 156–8, *158–9*
distributed internal representations of experiences 13, 137
DNA (deoxyribonucleic acid) 54–5, 201
DNA methylation 84
doctrine of four causes 36
dopamine 59
dorsal area of brain 45
drugs, psychotropic 185–91, 222–3
dualism 7, 30
dysrationalia 38–40, 199–200

ear and hearing *24*, 24–6
eclecticism 232
economy: as emergent system 218; investing and 177–83
efficient cause 36
egocentric bias 109, 111
Einstein's razor x
Einstellung Effect 215
electroencephalogram (EEG) 52
eliminativism 12
embodied, active cognition 136–9, 169
embodied action 134
embodiment 86, 88
emergence, concept of 216–18
emotion: access consciousness and 144; as area of study 11; behavior and 79–86; biochemistry of 74–7; cognitive 153;

components and functions of 72; consumer choice and 76; decision making and 121–2; definition of 70–1; dichotomy with thinking 68–70; language and 77–9; memory and 75, 112–13; models of 72–3, 76; neurological explanations of 71; prediction and 181–2; psychotherapy and 86–7; stress and 87–9; as subjective experience 68; thought and 29–30; valence of 73; value system and 71–2
emotional transformation 87, 88
empathy 197–8
empirical will 151
empiricism 45–6, 70
enaction 137
endorphin 75
enkephalin 75
environment: adaptation to threats in 122–3; interaction with brain and body 133–40; nurture and 84; of scarcity 180
epigenetics 84
episodic memory 100, 103
epistemology 70
ergodic system 181, 224
estradiol 163
evidence-based treatment and mammography 191–4
evolution 10–11
exclusivity and conscious will 152
exercise, aerobic 60
experience, emotional coloring of 144
expertise, development of 218–19
explicit memory 103
extrinsic network 169
eye and vision 21, *22*, 23, *23*, 134
eyewitness testimony 102

fallibility of memory: bias in processing 108–9; emotion and 112–13; errors of commission and 105–8; errors of omission and 105; gist, distilling 110–11; injury, insult, and 115; mnemonic techniques for 111–12; model of 114; persistence and 109–10
false memories 106–8
false positives with mammography 192
family therapy 234–5, 237, 241–3
fast thinking 128, 204, 215–16, 230, 239, 244
fate, awareness of 166–8
feeling 72; *see also* emotion
"Feeling Wheel, The" 76
fiction, reading 162

fight-or-flight response 72
final cause 36
financial crisis 177–8
fissures in brain 46
flashbacks 63
flying, fear of 29
Flynn Effect 93
*f*MRI (functional MRI) 53, 146–7
focusing illusion 216
foraging heuristic 128
foramen magnum 44–5
forebrain 47
formal cause 36
fourth paradigm 175–6
fraud in research 204
free will 150–4
frequency theory 36–7
frontal lobe 48, *49*, 51
functional impairment 20
functional MRI (*f*MRI) 53, 146–7
fundamental error of attribution 161, 240
future, concepts of 207
future bias 127

gambling, investing compared to 178, 181–3
gamma waves 147
gender and sex 162–6
genes and memory 104
gesture and language 45–6
gist, distilling 110–11
glial cells 43–4, 55, 60–3
Grandin, Temple 27
gray matter 47–8
grim reaper heuristic 130
gyri 46

habituation 101
"hard wired" 123
Harford, Tim 11, 176, 219
health care: addictions and abstinence 194–5; back pain and technology 183–5; delivery of 183; depression and pharmacology 185–91; mammography and evidence-based treatment 191–4; specialization in 236–7; statistics and 198–201
hearing *24*, 24–6
Herbert, Wray 122–8, 130, 207
hermaphrodism 163
heuristics 123–31
higher order thinking 132–3
hindbrain 47
hindsight bias 108–9, 111, 207

hippocampus 46
holistic system of visual identification 171
homunculus 137
hormones and cognitive functioning 66
Human Brain Project 53, 140
Human Connectome Project 53, 140
humans, distinguishing characteristics of 170–1
hypnosis 29, 139, 198
hypothalamus 47
hypothesis of causation and resolution 230
Hz 147

id 195
ideas, association of 99
idiographic nature of research 225
illusions: of control 178; perceptual 23; of validity 205, 224
immortality tale 167
implicit memory 103, 137
incongruity, neurology of 198
induction 15, 34
inflammation and depression 66
information: cognitive errors due to flood of 176–7; definition of 133, 176; processing of 93–4, 121, 122; sharing of, among brain areas 148
input, sensory 26–32
"inside" view 182
instinct, language of 6
intelligence 92–101, 134
internal milieu 154
interneurons 104
interpretation: differences in 3; language as digitizing 227; as process 31; in psychotherapy 210–13; of sensory input 27–32, 70
intrinsic network 169
intuitive physics 124–5, 206–9
intuitive psychology 93
intuitive theories 100–1
investing and economy 177–83
ionic hypothesis of memory 102
ions 57
IQ tests 93
irrational thinking 240

James, William 70, 88, 142
judicial/justice system 102, 130

Kahneman, Daniel 178–9, 196, 205, 216, 219, 230, 239, 244
knowledge, definition of 133
knowledge hierarchy 133, 174–6

knowledge representation 94–5, *95*
Koch, Cristof 145–6

La Cerra, Peggy 172–3
language: brain as empowered by 138; characteristics of 5–6, 7; complexity of 6; connection between gesture and 45–6; as digitizing interpretations 227; emotions and 77–9; as expression of thinking 5; mental synthesis and 170–1; as metaphorical 2; neuronal network model and 100; physics in 206–8; private 4; as process 7–8; psychotherapy and 5; public 138, 139; reading and 3; sound waves and 4
lateral area of brain 45
lateral prefrontal cortex 51
law, definition of 38
learning 101, 103–4
legacy, immortality through 168
lens 21, *22*
lexical priming 6
ligands 74
limbic association cortex 49, *50*
limbic system 48, 75, 164
location 206, 208
logic, as binary 213
logical positivism 33, 34–5, 210
long-axon neurons 54
long-term memory 102, 104–5

magical thinking and fishing 151
magnetic resonance imaging (MRI) 53
magnetoencephalography 53
maladaptive emotion 86
mammography and evidence-based treatment 191–4
MAO (monoamine oxidase) inhibitors 59
marriage, as emergent system 217–18
Material cause 36
McGurk effect 27
meaning: ability to make 214, 219; creation of 3, 44; as observer dependent 85; psychotherapy as quest for 190–1
meaning bias 204, 223–4
medial area of brain 45
medial temporal lobes 49
mediating circuits 104
medical issues *see* health care
medulla oblongata 47
memory: aging and 111; competitions 133; creating 101–5; decision making and 239; emotion and 75; fallibility of 105–15; fluid nature of 102; for

information read 115; in neurological model of thinking 118–19; as tool in processing sensory stimuli 12–13
memory binding 106
memory conjunction 106
mental accounting 120–1
mentalese 5, 96
mental representations 94–6, *95*, 144
mental synthesis 148–9, 151, 170–1
mesencephalon 47
metacognition 29, 220; *see also* thinking about thinking
metaphors 2–3, 238, 240–1
metencephalon 47
midbrain 47
middle childhood 62
Mill, John Stuart 35–6
mimicry heuristic 125
mind/body connection 65–7
mirror neurons 85, 161–2, 168–9
misattribution 106
modulating circuits 104
momentum heuristic (propensity effect) 124, 182, 207
monoamine oxidase (MAO) inhibitors 59
mood 72
moral decision making 129–30
Morgan Stanley 177
mortality rate 201
motivation and change 173
motor cortex 137
MRI (magnetic resonance imaging) 53
mu waves 161, 168–9
myelencephalon 47
myelin sheath *47*, 48, 55, 61–2

narrative therapy 229
naturalist heuristic 129
natural selection 10–11
nature and nurture 84
negative emotional valence 77–8
negativity bias 73
neural correlates of consciousness 146
neural model *98*
neural networks 98–100, 172–3
neural oscillation 147
neural plate 54
neural tube 54
neurobiology of consciousness 145–9
neurological model of thinking *116*, 116–20, *117*
neuronal ensembles *116*, *117*, 148
neurons: connecting diverse 55–60; description of 43–4; intelligence and 96–8, *98*; mirror 85, 161–2, 168–9; parts of *47*, 47–8; receptors on 74; short- and long-axon 54
neuropeptides 66
neuroscience, as area of study 11
neurotransmitters 58–9, 61, 64, 187
night science 106
nomothetic method 225
non-dual awareness 169
non-ergodic system 225
non-science, defining line between science and 33–4
norepinephrine 59
no-self, concept of 168
nostalgia 130
nuclei 48
null hypothesis 202
numerical heuristics 125–7
nurture and nature 84

objective data 235–6
obscenity 77–8
observer effect 4
obsessions 214
obsessive-compulsive disorder 110
Occam's razor ix
occipital lobe 48, 49, *49*
off-label purposes, prescriptions for 188–9
oligodendrocytes 61–2
omission bias 193
ontology 69
operationalization of terms 32
opiate receptors 74–5
opsin 21
optic disc 21
optic nerve 21, *22*
orbitofrontal lobe 51
organs of Corti 25
oscillation 147
"outside" view 182
overconfidence, psychology of 178
oxytocin 75, 88, 165

pain, perception of 73–4
panic attacks 241–2
parallel architecture 92
parallelism 175
pareidolia 14–15
parietal lobe 48, 49, *49*, 51
parieto-occipital-temporal association cortex 49, *50*
path dependence 11–12, 215, 224
patient/problem categories, specification of 228

pattern discernment 3–4, 14–15, 218, 240
peptides 75
perception: active nature of 137; as analog 3; as area of study 11; overview of 16–21; personal interpretation of 190; of reality 91, 134–5, 205–14
periaqueductal gray area 75
personality 155–8, 160–1
personalization 128, 240
person-permanence thinking 167
persuasion and consumerism 196–8
pharmacology 185–91, 222–3
phenomenal consciousness 143
phenomenal will 151
philosophy, task of 213
phobias 69
phonemes 15
phrenology 43
Pinker, Steven: on aspects of consciousness 143–5; on auto-associators 98–9; on conceptions of mind 91–2; on emotion and swearing 77–8, 79; on improving content of thinking 215; on information 176; on intelligence 93–4, 99–101; on judges 81; on language 5, 6, 7, 206–7; on mental representation 96; on pedestrian poetry 2; on rates of violence and murder 131
pinna 24, *24*
placebo effect 187
plasticity of brain 56, 57
point of view 186
polarization of neurons 56
political life and persuasion 197–8
polypeptides 75
pons 47
Ponzo illusion 23
positive emotional valence 78
positron-emission tomography (PET) 53
posterior parietal cortex 51
post modern therapy 229
posttraumatic stress disorder (PTSD) 31–2, 110
Prader-Willi syndrome 80
pragmatism 232
prediction 181–2, 205, 218
Preferred States Inventory 76
prefrontal association cortex 49, *50*
prefrontal cortex 48, 120–1
prepositional database 94–5, *95*
present, concepts of 207
presynaptic axon terminal 57, *58*
primary emotion 86
primary rational awareness 91

priority and conscious will 152
private language 4
probabilistic framework 92
probability theory 36–7
problem causation, theory of 228–9; *see also* causation
problem conceptualization model: overview of 229–30, 230–6; problem resolution 230, 236–7; therapeutic process 238–44
Problem-Oriented Medical Record 233, 235
problem resolution, theory of 228, 229
procedural memory 103
processing, faulty, and dysrationalia 38–9
propensity effect (momentum heuristic) 124, 182, 207
propranolol 113
proprioceptive 16
prospect theory 178–9, *180*, 194, 196
prostate cancer 198–9, 201
proteins and memory 104
psychoanalysis 9, 195, 222
psychology: classical, intuitive 9–16, 135–6; definition of 10; intuitive 93; of overconfidence 178; study of 68; *see also* cognitive-behavioral psychology
psychosurgery 52
psychotherapeutic intervention 230
psychotherapy: benefits of 88; causation and resolution in 236–7; confident thinking and 182; emotions and 78, 86–7; interpretation in 210–13; language and 5; memory and 106, 112–13; overview of 7; problem conceptualization in 230–6; public language and 138; purpose of 9; science and 221–5; science-based model of 226–30; sensorimotor 56–7; suggestibility and 106–8; therapeutic process in 238–44; visual capacity used in 214–15
psychotic disorders 17–18
P3 waves 147
PTSD (posttraumatic stress disorder) 31–2, 110
publication bias 203, 243
pupil 21, *22*
puzzle solving 78, 136

Qbism 226–7
qualia 145
qualitative analysis 177
quants/quantitative analysis 177
quantum entanglement 213

quantum theory 208–10, 226
qubits 213

radiation exposure from cell phones 57–8
rationalism 46, 70
rationalization 16, 120
rational thinking 30–1, 38–41
Readiness Potential 150
reading, adaptation of brain to challenge of 3
realism 207–8
reality, perceptions of 91, 134–5, 205–14
reason, as tool in processing sensory stimuli 15–16
recall 102
receptor specificity 74
recognition 102
recursion 100, 175
reductio ad absurdum 191
reductive materialism 190–1
reflection on emotion 87
regression to mean 203–4
reification 33, 158
relative risk 199–200
relativism 210
relativity, theory of 209
reliability, inter-rater 71
replicability of research 203
research: control groups in 184; on depression 187–8; fraud in 204; as idiographic 225; on psychotherapy 223; publication bias and 243; replicability of 203
resemblance 99
resolution *see* problem resolution
restraint bias 194
resurrection theme 167–8
reticular formation 48
retina 21, *22*
retinal ganglion cells 21
Retrieving Effectively from Memory model 114
risk aversion 179, 196–7
rods 21
rostral area of brain 45

scale 206
Schacter, Daniel 105–6, 107, 108, 109, 110
schizophrenia 6
science: in language 206–8; limitations in abilities to interpret findings from 205–15; psychotherapy and 221–5; rationality and 38–41; role of computing in 175–6; *see also* scientific method; scientific thinking

Scientific American Mind magazine ix
scientific method 7, 9, 35
scientific skepticism 220
scientific thinking 32–8, 184
sculpting 241
secondary emotion 86
secondary rational awareness 91
secure attachment 82
selective serotonin re-uptake inhibitors (SSRIs) 59–60, 187–9
self: awareness of fate and 166–8; concepts of 239; consciousness and 141–9; conscious will and 149–54; definition of 144–5; gender, sex, and 162–6; as human 170–1; sense of 154–8, 160–2; transformation of 171–3
self-awareness, consciousness compared to 142
self-bias 39, 130
self-interest and persuasion 197
self-knowledge 143
selflessness 168–9
self-organizing without central cause 133–9
self-regulation 180
semantic memory 100, 103
semantic network 94–5, *95*
sensation, rich field of 144
senses: hearing 24, *24*–6; integration of input from 26–7; interpretation of input from 27–32, 70; perception and 16–21; vision 21, *22*, *23*, *23*
sensitization 101
sensorimotor psychotherapy 56–7
sensory processing disorders 18–19
sensory stimulation, processing 12–16; *see also* senses
sentience 145
serial architecture 92
serotonin 59, 187
sex and gender 162–6
sexual dimorphism 163–4
shape 206
short-axon neurons 54
short-term memory 102
simplicity and persuasion 197
Simpson's paradox 201
smiling 85–6
soccer and penalty kicks 131
social casework ix
somatic disorders and emotion 87–9
somatic heuristics 123–4
somatic interventions 241
somatosensory system 16, 57
space 206

special pleading 177
speech analysis of emotion 84–5
spinal canal 54
SSRIs (selective serotonin re-uptake inhibitors) 59–60, 187–9
Stanovich, Keith 38–40
statistics, processing 198–205
stereotype bias 109
stereotyping 100–1
stirmergic algorithms 150
Strange Situation experiment 82
stress: behavioral economics and 180–1; emotions and 87–9; neurotransmitters and 64
stress inoculation 80–1
string theory 210
subjective data 235–6
substance 206, 208
suggestibility 106–8
sulci 46
superego 195
superposition 213
supervenience 216
survival: adaptation and 179, 214; argument from authority and 176; childhood abuse and 51; memory systems for 100; role of thought in 122–32; visual identification systems and 171
swearing 77–8
synapse 58, 96
synchronicity of brain areas 148–9
synthetic statements 34–5

tabula rasa 122
technology: back pain and 183–5; computer 213; information and 174–6
telencephalon 46
temperament 84
temporal lobe 48, 49, *49*
terror management 167
thalamus 47
theory, disproval of 184
theory of mind 78
therapeutic process 238–44
thinking: dichotomy with feeling 68–70; higher order 132–3; limitations of 205–14, 212; making decisions 120–2; neurological model of *116*, 116–20, *117*; overview of 90–2; physical underpinnings of experience of 8; as subjective experience 68; visually 28; *see also* cognition
thinking about thinking, as essence of psychotherapy ix, 9; *see also* metacognition
time, concepts of 207, 208–9
transcranial magnetic stimulation 190
transformation of self 171–3
trauma and brain 63–5
tricyclic antidepressants 59
trophic factors 55

universe, expansion of 209–10
utility theory 179, *180*

validity 33
value heuristics 125–6
values and decision making 122
ventral area of brain 45
ventricular system 54
supervenience 216
vestibular 16
vision: mental synthesis and 171; Ponzo illusion *23*; processing of visual stimuli 134; role of eye in 21, *22*, 23
visual analysis system 171
visual art 5
visualization 214–15
visual pareidolia 14
visual processing of emotion 84–5
void heuristic 131
Vyshedskiy, Andrey 116–17, 148–9, 151, 170, 171

water and cognitive functioning 67
Wegner, Daniel 150, 151, 152, 153
white matter 47
willpower 144–5
winner effect 180–1
working memory 103, 122
world, experience of 3, 7, 205
writing 3–4
WYSIATI 219

X-rays 52